Therapeutic Endoscopy and Radiology of the Gut

Therapeutic Endoscopy and Radiology of the Gut

Edited by

JOHN R. BENNETT
M.D., F.R.C.P.
Consultant Physician,
Hull Royal Infirmary

LONDON
Chapman and Hall

First published 1981
by Chapman and Hall Ltd
11 New Fetter Lane, London EC4P 4EE

Phototypeset by Preface Ltd., Salisbury
and printed in Great Britain at the
University Press, Cambridge

ISBN 0 412 22070 9

British Library Cataloguing in Publication Data

Therapeutic endoscopy and radiology of the gut.
1. Endoscope and endoscopy
2. Alimentary canal – Examination
3. Fiber optics
4. Alimentary canal
5.Radiology, Medical
I. Bennett, John R
616.3′3′0754 RC804.E6

ISBN 0–412–22070–9

Contents

Contributors

M. Atkinson, Consultant Physician, University Hospital, Queens Medical Centre, Nottingham, U.K.

J. R. Bennett, Consultant Physician, Gastro-Intestinal Unit, Hull Royal Infirmary, Hull, U.K.

M. K. Bilbao, Professor of Radiology, Department of Diagnostic Radiology, University of Oregon Health Sciences Centre, Portland, Oregon, U.S.A.

H. J. Burhenne, Professor and Head, Department of Diagnostic Radiology, University of British Columbia, Vancouver, Canada.

A. Clark, Consultant Surgeon, Brighton General Hospital, Brighton, U.K.

P. B. Cotton, Consultant Physician, Department of Medicine, Middlesex Hospital, London, U.K.

C. T. Dotter, Professor and Chairman, Department of Diagnostic Radiology, University of Oregon Health Sciences Centre, School of Medicine, Portland, Oregon, U.S.A.

W. L. Gear, Consultant Surgeon, Gloucestershire Royal Hospital, Gloucester, U.K.

D. A. Gilbert, Assistant Professor of Medicine and Assistant Director, University Hospital, Endoscopy Service, University of Washington, Seattle, Washington, U.S.A.

J. Hellemans, Head of the Section of Geriatrics and Consultant in the Section of Gastroenterology, Department of Medicine, University Hospitals, St. Rafaël, Leuven, Belgium.

F. S. Keller, Assistant Professor in the Department of Diagnostic Radiology, University of Oregon Health Sciences Centre, School of Medicine, Portland, Oregon, U.S.A.

A. Lunderquist, Docent in Diagnostic Radiology, Head of Section for Gastrointestinal Radiology and Angiography, Department of Radiology, University Hospital, Lund, Sweden.

R. L. Protell, Assistant Professor of Medicine, University of Washington, Seattle, Washington, U.S.A.

B. J. Prout, Consultant Physician, Royal Cornwall Hospital (Treliske), Truro, Cornwall, U.K.

J. Rosch, Department of Diagnostic Radiology, University of Oregon Health Sciences Centre, School of Medicine, Portland, Oregon, U.S.A.

P. R. Salmon, Consultant Physician, University College Hospital, Rayne Institute, University Street, London, U.K.

K. F. R. Schiller, Consultant Physician, St. Peter's Hospital, Chertsey, Surrey, U.K.

E. Seifert, Professor, 1st Department of Internal Medicine, Städt. Krankenhaus Kemperhof, Koblenz, West Germany.

F. E. Silverstein, Professor of Medicine, University of Washington, Seattle, Washington, U.S.A.

R. Teague, Consultant Physician, Torbay Hospital, Torbay, U.K.

G. Vantrappen, Professor of Medicine, Division of Gastroenterology, Department of Medicine, Akademisch Ziekenhuis, Leuven, Belgium.

C. B. Williams, Consultant Surgeon, St. Mark's Hospital, London, U.K.

K. G. D. Williams, Consultant Surgeon, Farnborough Hospital, Farnborough Common, Orpington, Kent, U.K.

Foreword

It is a singular pleasure to write a foreword to this book. John Bennett is one of the gastroenterologists who have seized on the great opportunities offered by modern fibreoptic endoscopes to improve the treatment of patients. He was himself one of the pioneers to make use of such instruments to treat benign oesophageal strictures by passing a guide-wire through the stricture before employing a Puestow–Eder dilator for the actual dilatation, a method of treatment that has now become universally accepted as the safest and least troublesome. It is therefore not surprising that he has been able to assemble a team of experts in endoscopy and radiology to give us a conspectus of the various ways in which endoscopists and radiologists, either alone or in combination, can carry out a range of therapeutic manoeuvres that were impossible only a few years ago.

When fibreoptic endoscopes with facilities for obtaining biopsy specimens under direct vision were introduced in the late 1960s, their diagnostic potential was rapidly realized, but their use as therapeutic tools was slower to be appreciated and development on this side is still in progress. Some of the therapeutic applications are now completely established. Perhaps the most striking example is colonoscopic polypectomy, here excellently reviewed by Christopher Williams, who has great experience with the technique. Another well-established method, which I have already mentioned, is the use of a fibreoptic endoscope to facilitate dilatation of benign oesophageal strictures and there can be no doubt that this method is a great advance on its forerunners, as will be obvious from the information in Michael Gear's chapter. The method of inserting a prosthetic tube in malignant stricture of the oesophagus, devised by Michael Atkinson, is already widely used. The chapter by Klaus Schiller on the removal of foreign bodies gives a vivid picture of the ingenuity and dexterity that have been exercised in this field.

At the other end of the scale, the applications of lasers for such purposes as the control of upper gastrointestinal haemorrhage is still at a research stage, although the future possibilities look promising, as will be evident from Paul Salmon's chapter.

I am particularly pleased that John Bennett has included several radiologists in his team of contributors. Radiology has always been of great importance as a diagnostic method in gastroenterology and it is essential that physicians and surgeons should work in co-operation with their radiologist colleagues if the best results are to be obtained. It is encouraging that radiologists, like endoscopists, are not confining themselves simply to diagnosis but are developing their own methods of therapy. Quite apart from this, there are several therapeutic methods which need to be carried out with the endoscopist and the radiologist working together.

I feel sure that this book will prove to be an inspiration to many endoscopists and radiologists who have not yet ventured to embark on therapeutic techniques. It gives me great satisfaction to congratulate the Editor on his choice of subjects and contributors, and to express my hope that the book will prove to be the great success that it deserves to be.

S. C. Truelove

Preface

Operative surgery was unfairly castigated by Lord Cohen of Birkenhead as 'that accessory branch of therapeutics', and even its most ardent exponent would hardly deny that it is a means to an end; the desired end being usually the improvement or removal of a pathological condition. If that end can be achieved other than by open operation, then it is right that such means should be explored. This book records and discusses the results of two recent avenues of such exploration.

Access to the alimentary tract is now easily possible both by illuminated, flexible, fibreoptic endoscopes (inserted orally or *per anum*), and by needles and catheters under radiological control. These techniques began as purely diagnostic manoeuvres, and the therapeutic potential of fibreoptic endoscopy, in particular, was called into question (notably in a notorious letter in which a surgeon described the fibreoptic endoscope as an 'expensive piece of illuminated spaghetti'). The ingenuity and imagination of endoscopists and radiologists, supported by the constructional skills of manufacturing companies, have now made many therapeutic procedures possible without the need for surgical operation. These exploits at first seemed like legerdemain, but their practical value and feasibility are now well established.

With an ageing population we increasingly meet patients ill-fitted to withstand the stresses imposed even by modern anaesthesia and surgery; moreover, costs of medical care continue to rise. Procedures carried out by endoscopy or under radiological control have lower morbidity and mortality, and involve a shorter hospital stay, two great advantages over the operative techniques they displace. It seems certain that their application will increase.

In this book, experts in the various techniques describe them so that other endoscopists and radiologists may safely undertake them; they also record the outcome of these procedures so that they may be judged against the alternatives by referring doctors. We have thus combined an instruction manual with a scientific exposition of results, in the belief that anyone with patients' welfare at heart will more readily place at their disposal the best that can be provided in 1981. Although many of the techniques are in regular and common use they are still being developed, while others (particularly approaches to gastro-intestinal haemorrhage) are insufficiently assessed to justify wholesale adoption; these stand as pointers to the future. Many will have been refined even in the short time this book has been in preparation, and there are techniques not mentioned in the book which have been at least the subject of experimental work – endoscopic vagotomy, for example (T. V. Taylor, personal communication). Above all we show how medicine has again taken modern technology and harnessed it for patients' welfare.

John R. Bennett

1 Some aspects of fibreoptic instruments

JOHN R. BENNETT

That so many operative and therapeutic techniques can be performed with fibreoptic endoscopes only a dozen years after they came into common use is attributable as much to the instrument designers' skills as it is to the ingenuity of the operators. Most of the techniques described in this book can be carried out with the standard endoscopes likely to be found in any endoscopic unit, and differences between instruments from the various manufacturers are small in detail, though not unimportant. Some instruments have been specifically designed for operative procedures, notably those with two channels, but although they simplify some manoeuvres, they are not widely used and chiefly have a place in highly specialized centres. No procedure described in this book necessitates a special endoscope.

The purpose of this chapter is to mention a few of the endoscope characteristics which are important for operative work. Most of the information will be familiar to practised endoscopists, and the discussion chiefly serves to evaluate particular characteristics of available instruments to guide those with less experience of operative endoscopic procedures. Manipulative tools are dealt with in individual chapters.

1.1 OESOPHAGOGASTRODUODENOSCOPES

By definition these are forward (end) or fore-oblique viewing instruments so that the oesophagus can be well seen. A forward view is obviously essential for any operative work in the oesophagus.

1.1.1 **Direction of view**

Most are forward viewing. A fore-oblique view (30° up, giving a field of view 90° diagonal, 60° vertical and horizontal) is given by the Olympus GIF K2, and is recommended for varices injection (See Chapter 4) though a forward-viewing endoscope can be used. Fujinon make the FG/QBF forward-viewing instrument with a 105° field of view, while the Machida PFS B instruments also have a moving optical system.

1.1.2 **Tip angulation**

As operative techniques are likely to involve awkward manoeuvring, the extent of tip deflection is important. The main forward viewing 'standard' instruments (ACMI TX8, Olympus GIF D3) offer 180° in one direction, the Olympus flexing to only 100° laterally, while the ACMI TX8 flexes to 180° in all four directions. The Fujinon FG/QBF has 210° flexion in one plane, 90° in the other.

1.1.3 **Forceps raisers**

In operative work it is convenient to be able to flex an instrument passed down the channel independently of movements of the endoscope tip. This facility is found in 'standard' oesophagogastroduodenoscopes only in the Olympus GIF K2 and GIF D3; they are included in the special operating instruments Olympus TGF 2D also.

1.1.4 **Endoscope calibre**

The 'standard' endoscopes are between 12.4 and 12.8 mm in diameter. When there is narrowing of the gut lumen, or in the elderly or children, it can be useful to have a narrower instrument. For a few years there have been 'paediatric' endoscopes – particularly the Olympus GIF P2 (8.8 mm diameter) and ACMI TX7 (9.5 mm diameter) with narrower biopsy channels. A recent Olympus instrument, the GIF Q, is only 11 mm in diameter, as is the Fujinon FG/QBF, both having 2.8 mm biopsy channels.

1.1.5 **Biopsy channel**

The bore of the biopsy channel is especially important for operative work as this determines the size of instrument which can be introduced (except in special circumstances when tools are taped to the outside of the endscope). The channel sizes of 'standard' instruments are 3.0 mm (ACMI), 2.9 mm (Olympus) and 2.6 mm (Machida). The GIF Q and FG/QBF, despite their small calibre, have channels of 2.8 mm, and the Olympus GIF P2 is 2.1 mm. The Olympus TFG ID instrument has a single, large channel 5.0 mm in diameter, the endoscope calibre being 14.4 mm.

1.2 SPECIAL OPERATING UPPER GI ENDOSCOPES

Endoscopes with two channels, allowing two manipulating tools to be operated simultaneously (e.g. a snare and a forceps) have advantages in their range of procedures, but may have a larger calibre and less flexibility. The ACMI TX82 has channels of 3.6 mm and 2.6 mm diameter with the same 12.5 mm shaft calibre as the TX8 as well as 180° tip flexibility in four directions. The Olympus TGF 2D has bigger channels – 3.7 mm and 2.8 mm (the smaller channel has a forceps raiser), but a bigger shaft size – 14.4 mm, and tip flexibility of 180° and 80° vertically, 100° laterally.

The Olympus TFG 1D has only a single channel but it is particularly wide (5.0 mm).

1.2.2 **Specialized endoscopes**

Endoscopes have been adapted for a single therapeutic purpose. Notable examples are a balloon mounted on a gastroscope used for pneumatic dilatation in achalasia (see Chapter 6), and a forward viewing endoscope made by Way with two channels, a slot in the distal flange, and a proximal balloon designed for the controlled sclerosant injection of oesophageal varices (see Chapter 4).

1.3 SIDE-VIEWING UPPER GI ENDOSCOPES

A side-viewing endoscope is essential for work in the duodenum – particularly papillotomy and other biliary manipulations – but it has potential advantages in the stomach also. An end-viewing instrument may be so close to the stomach wall, particularly the lesser curvature, that any operative procedure becomes difficult or impossible because of the tangential approach. A side-viewing endoscope allows a face-on view with the operating tool projecting straight at the target area. The Olympus GFB2 has a 2.8 mm channel and 70° angle of view, and Olympus also have the TGF 2S with two channels, both with forceps raisers. Lateral flexion of its tip is only 50° however. Machida offer the FGS-BL with forceps raisers.

The other side-viewing instruments are designed as duodenoscopes. These are the Olympus JFB3 (shaft diameter 10.5 mm, channel 2.1 mm), the Fujinon FD/QB (shaft 10.5 mm, channel 2.2 mm), ACMI TX6 (shaft 10.0 mm, channel 2.0 mm) and the Machida FDS11 (shaft 10.6 mm, channel 2.0 mm). All of these seem satisfactory for ampullary cannulation and related procedures.

1.4 COLONOSCOPES

1.4.1 **Length**

Colonoscopes vary in length from 1855 mm down to 1115 mm, and there are also 'flexible sigmoidoscopes' of about 650 mm length. While total colonoscopy may frequently be possible with the shorter colonoscopes this cannot always be achieved. The question of how complete a colonoscopy should be is discussed in Chapter 17.

1.4.2 **Channel diameters**

In the single channel instruments the channel bore in the Olympus instruments is 2.8 mm, ACM 2.8 mm, Fujinon 2.8 mm and Machida 2.6 mm. All have 13 mm shafts. The single channel instruments have the best flexibility characteristics for ease of introduction.

1.4.3 **Double-channel colonoscopes**

For polypectomy, the only common colonoscopic operative procedure, it is sometimes useful to have two channels in order to manipulate two snares, or a snare and a forceps, particularly in difficult circumstances – for example, when there is haemorrhage (see Chapter 17). The double-channel endoscopes are thicker and less easily introduced because of their reduced flexibility. The shaft is 16.3 mm (Olympus) or 16.0 mm (ACM), but the biopsy channels are generous – 3.3 mm and 4.0 mm (ACM), 3.8 mm and 2.9 mm (Olympus).

1.5 'THE BEST SET'

The more instruments available to an operator, the greater will be his versatility. However, economics dictate that the range of endoscopes in any unit has to be limited. Most of the procedures described in this book can safely be performed with a reasonable expectation of success in an endoscopy unit equipped with three instruments – a 'standard' forward-viewing gastroduodenoscope, a side-viewing duodenoscope and a long, single-channel colonoscope. Which extra endoscopes are obtained will be dictated by the work-load. Specialists in colon work may wish to have a double-channel colonoscope. Anyone doing much oesophageal work requires a 'paediatric' gastroduodenoscope. A side-viewing gastroscope will be a boon to anyone doing several hundred gastroscopies a year for biopsies of gastric ulcers alone, quite apart from more complex operation procedures.

Each year further technical advances are made by the instrument manufacturers, and by the time this book appears there may be new products on the market. All instrument manufacturers have agents who are willing to give current information and who will usually allow endoscopists an opportunity to try and compare instruments from their range.

2 Benign oesophageal strictures

M. W. L. GEAR

Benign strictures of the oesophagus are usually due to reflux oesophagitis, but may follow the ingestion of corrosives. Rare causes are inflammation adjacent to an area of ectopic gastric mucosa, an oesophageal web associated with severe iron deficiency anaemia, or the ingestion of corrosive tablets such as 'Clinitest' or potassium chloride.

2.1 DIAGNOSIS

2.1.1 **History**

The presenting history is usually dysphagia, relentless and progressive in malignant strictures, whereas in benign stricture the severity of symptoms may vary. Associated or preceding symptoms may be present: posture-related substernal pain or reflux in patients with oesophagitis and hiatus hernia; pronounced weight loss and anorexia in patients with malignant disease.

2.1.2 **Radiology**

The barium swallow and meal is the first investigation in assessing the cause of dysphagia. The site, extent and surface outline of the stricture may be clearly seen in most cases. However, the accuracy in differentiating benign and malignant strictures is not adequate to allow decisions on treatment to be made. In a personal series of 135 strictures, radiology was uncertain or incorrect in 28% of all strictures and in 41% of malignant strictures, when compared with the final diagnosis (Eastman, Gear and Nicol, 1978). A tissue diagnosis must be made at endoscopy (see Section 2.1.3 below).

Radiology may also be misleading in assessing the size of lumen in oesophageal stricture, and again, direct measurement at endoscopy is required.

Radiology can give useful information about the adequacy or

otherwise of the anti-reflux mechanism of the cardia (when films are taken with the patient in the head-down position) thus supplementing evidence obtained from the history. Barium should also be allowed to enter the stomach and duodenum and further films taken, as conditions such as carcinoma of the gastric fundus, or pyloric or duodenal stenosis may affect the management of an oesophageal stricture. This is an important requirement in investigation as it may not be possible to pass even a small diameter endoscope through a tight stricture and abnormalities distal to the stricture will not be seen.

A chest radiograph should be obtained at the same time as the barium examination. Patients with gastro-oesophageal reflux may have sustained nocturnal inhalation of gastric contents producing basal changes in the lungs. In patients with malignant strictures, evidence of primary or secondary tumour in lungs or mediastinum may be seen.

2.1.3 **Endoscopy**

All patients with an oesophageal stricture must have an endoscopic examination. This should be performed with a flexible fibreoptic instrument. There is no doubt that this is substantially safer than the old-fashioned rigid oesophagoscope which is still widely used. Williamson (1975) reports six cases of perforation in 270 examinations carried out with a rigid instrument, whereas the British Society of Digestive Endoscopy (Schiller *et al.*, 1972) reported only 11 oesophageal perforations in 24 000 examinations with modern fibrescopes.

(a) *Technique*

Any end-viewing fibrescope is suitable provided that it has an adequate diameter side-channel for taking tissue specimens (Fig. 2.1). Most diagnostic endoscopy examinations may be carried out with local anaesthesia and intravenous sedation. The patient is examined in the left lateral position. The instrument is gently introduced past the cricopharyngeal sphincter and advanced down the oesophagus to the stricture. The distance from the incisor teeth is noted, using the centimetre marks on the shaft of the fibrescope. True strictures can be distinguished from spasm (e.g. achalasia) by feeling the resistance to onward movement of the endoscope while maintaining the lumen centrally in the field of view. The nature of the stricture is judged visually, benign lesions usually being smooth walled with or without the inflammatory changes of oesophagitis, while malignant strictures usually reveal nodular tissue protruding into the lumen. Ulceration may be present in both types of stricture. Visual examination alone is not a reliable guide and must be combined with a diagnosis from tissue specimens to reach maximum accuracy (see below). Photographs are

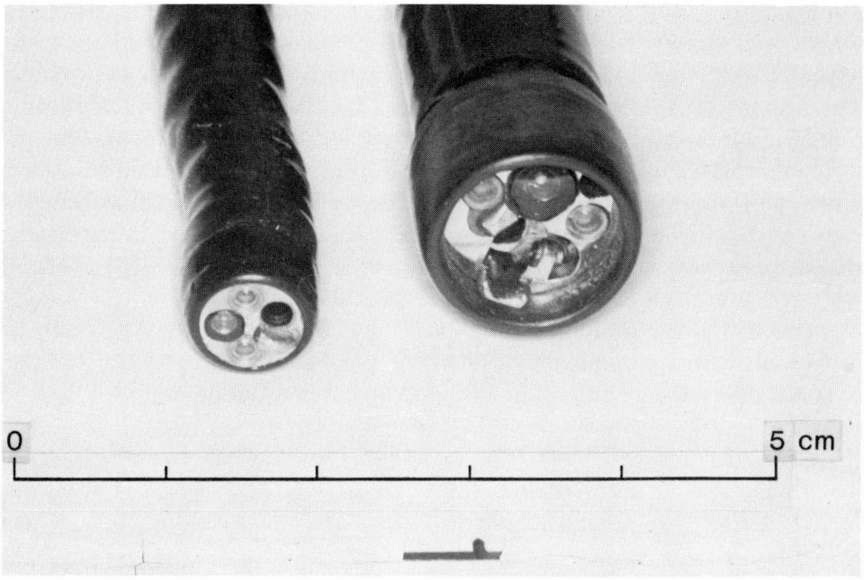

Fig. 2.1 Distal ends of the large and small fibrescopes (Olympus GIF D3 and GIF P2).

useful for record purposes and for comparison with pictures taken after appropriate treatment.

The size of the lumen is difficult to judge endoscopically without an objective standard. A simple measuring device such as that illustrated in Fig. 2.2 should be used. The cytology brush is then passed down the

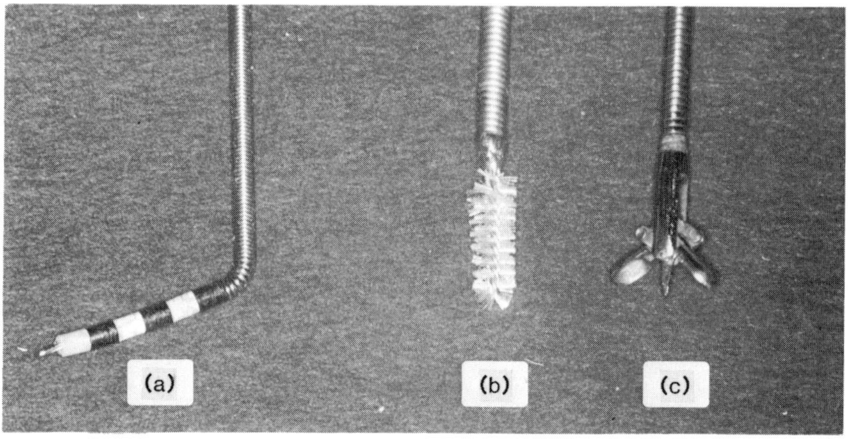

Fig. 2.2 (*a*) Measuring device (2 mm graduations); (*b*) cytology brush; (*c*) biopsy forceps, opened to show central spike.

side-channel and guided onto the face and into the lumen of the stricture, where it is drawn backwards and forwards vigorously several times to abrade the surface and thus obtain cells from as wide an area as possible. The brush is withdrawn, slides are made, and later suitably stained using standard cytological techniques.

The biopsy forceps with a central spike (Fig. 2.2) is then used to obtain a series of specimens from different sites on the face and, if technically possible, from the lumen of the stricture. The specimens are immediately shaken out in formalin–saline mixture and then microscope slides prepared using standard histological techniques.

If the size of the lumen permits, the endoscope (which may be changed for an instrument of smaller calibre) is passed through the stricture to obtain a complete examination of the stomach and duodenum.

(b) *Results*

The diagnostic accuracy of the methods described above is studied in the report of Eastman, Gear and Nicol (1978). The main findings are set out in Tables 2.1 and 2.2.

The study consisted of 135 endoscopic examinations in 115 patients. In 75 examinations (69 patients) the final diagnosis was of a malignant stricture and in 60 examinations (46 patients) the final diagnosis was of a benign stricture. The endoscopic diagnosis was correct in 90% of examinations, uncertain in 3% (four cases) and incorrect in 7% (10 cases). The 10 incorrect endoscopic diagnoses consisted of three false positive and seven false negative diagnoses. Four of the seven false negative diagnoses (i.e. tumour tissue was *not* obtained) were made in patients who were examined following treatment for a malignant stricture. This had involved a resection in three cases and radiotherapy in one case. If these four cases are excluded, the accuracy of diagnosis increases to 92%.

Table 2.1 Comparison of endoscopic diagnosis and its component parts with final diagnosis for all strictures.

Report	*Correct* %	*Uncertain* %	*Incorrect* %
Endoscopic appearance (n = 135)	82	9	9
Cytological report (n = 100)	81	6	13
Histological report (n = 121)	73	12	15
Endoscopic diagnosis (n = 135)	90	3 (4 cases)	7 (10 cases)

35 cytology specimens and 14 histology specimens were either not taken or were inadequate for assessment.

Table 2.2 The contribution of tissue specimens in achieving a correct diagnosis of malignancy at endoscopy.

	No. of cases	%
Malignant tissue present on both histological and cytological examination	32	49
Malignant tissue present on histological examination alone	17	26
Malignant tissue present on cytological examination alone	11	17
Diagnosis endoscopic appearance alone	5	8
Total	65	100

It should be emphasized that tissue biopsy without cytology will result in a higher percentage of incorrect diagnoses. Other authors who have supported the use of cytology in addition to tissue biopsy are: Prolla *et al.* (1971); Bedine and Cocco (1972); Boddington (1974); Hishon *et al.* (1976) and Mortensen and Mackenzie (1979).

2.2 MANAGEMENT

2.2.1 **General medical management**

The symptoms resulting from reflux oesophagitis (with or without associated stricture), 'heartburn', central substernal chest pain, pain on swallowing hot liquids and varying degrees of dysphagia may all be substantially or even completely alleviated by intensive medical management. The patient should be advised on simple measures to reduce gastro-oesophageal reflux:

Weight reduction.
Raising the head of the bed and sleeping propped up.
Avoidance of bending and stooping.
Abandoning tight clothes around the abdomen.
No smoking.

Symptomatic relief (and perhaps some improvement in the degree of inflammation) may be obtained with alkalis taken regularly and frequently. Combinations of alkali with alginate compounds (Gaviscon) or with polymethyl-siloxane (Polycrol, Asilone) may be effective in some patients. Despite disappointing controlled trial results, metoclopramide (Maxolon) 10 mg before meals and at night is sometimes helpful.

Cimetidine (Tagamet) has been shown in clinical trials to relieve the symptoms of oesophagitis (Behar *et al.*, 1978; Wesdorp *et al.*, 1978 and

Lepsien *et al.*, 1979). However, Powell-Jackson, Barkley and Northfield (1978) and Behar *et al.* (1978) commented on the failure of cimetidine to improve the endoscopic and histological changes. Further studies are required.

Medical measures, directed primarily against reflux oesophagitis, may produce considerable improvement in dysphagia, which may in part be due to oesophageal spasm or oedema. The endoscopic findings should suggest those strictures which are suitable for simple medical treatment on an out-patient basis. Severe symptoms may justify an intensive course of treatment as an in-patient.

Failed medical treatment – the persistence of symptoms despite the measures outlined – is a clear indication for endoscopic dilatation, surgery or both (see Section 2.3.2 below). Dysphagia may be the predominant symptom at presentation, reflux symptoms having waned as the stricture became tighter. In patients with dysphagia, endoscopic dilatation should be considered initially along with other non-surgical measures. A decision for surgery can be made later when improved swallowing has been achieved. Most strictures due to reflux will recur unless the reflux is abolished by surgery. However, many patients with strictures are elderly, and repeated dilatation may have to be accepted as the safest form of management.

2.2.2 **Endoscopic dilatation**

(a) *History*

Prior to the development of modern endoscopic methods, dilatation of oesophageal strictures was a difficult and hazardous procedure usually carried out under general anaesthesia. There was a substantial perforation and mortality rate (four perforations with one death in 100 patients: Raptis and Milne, 1972; three deaths in 38 patients, a mortality rate of 7.9%: Williamson, 1975).

A further problem using the rigid oesophagoscope and bougienage was that tight, tortuous strictures were often impassable. Thus direct surgery to the stricture was required, with greatly increased risks to the patient; 50% of patients treated by Raptis and Milne (1972), 52% treated by Logan (1965) and 63% of those reported by Williamson (1975) were treated surgically. The problems of the risk of perforation and failure to dilate oesophageal strictures are largely overcome by the use of wire-guided dilators at fibreoptic endoscopy.

(b) *Indications*

Any patient with a stricture which will not admit the larger size of endoscope (i.e. with a lumen smaller than 12 mm) should be considered

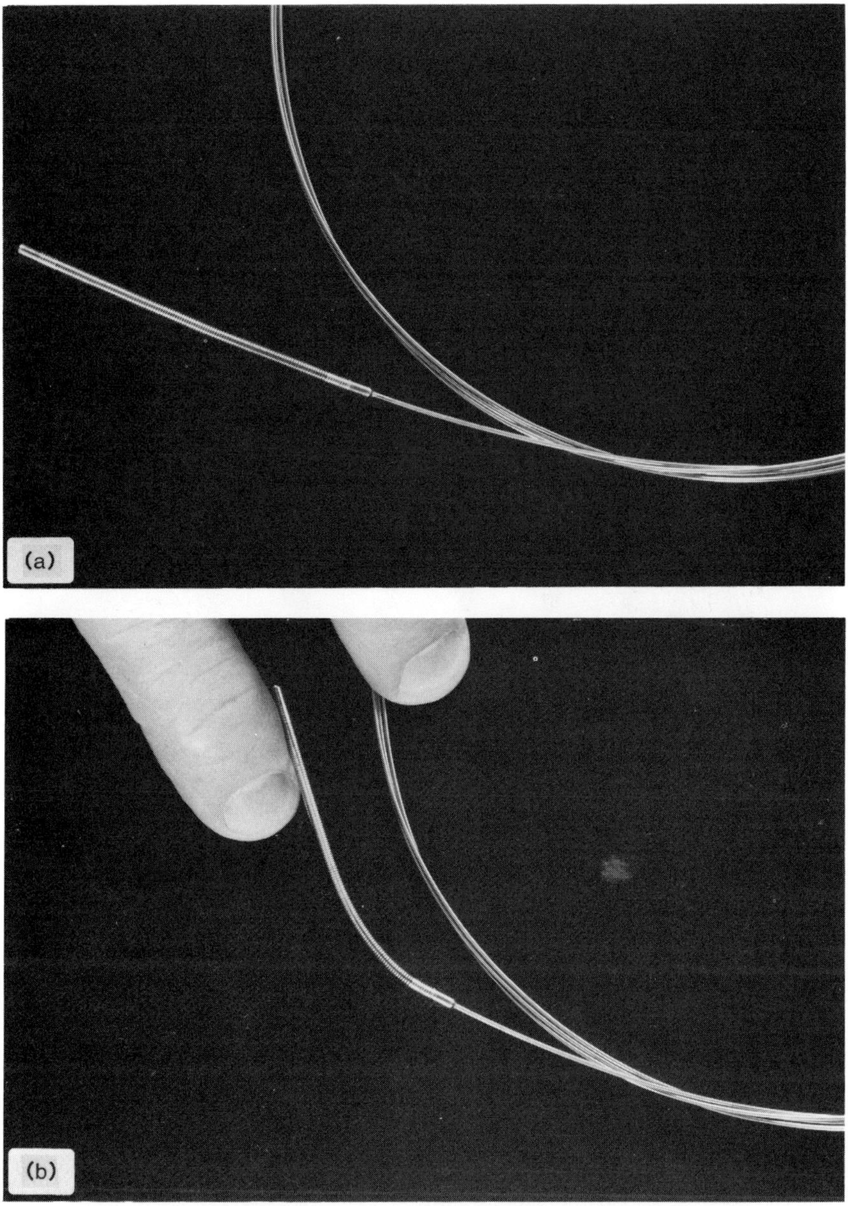

Fig. 2.3 (*a*) and (*b*) Guide-wire, showing flexible spring tip.

for endoscopic dilatation. The only contraindications are patients with a recent myocardial infarct or severe respiratory insufficiency. However, even these patients may require dilatation if the stricture tightens progressively.

(c) *Technique*

(i) *Instruments.* An end-viewing endoscope, with a side-channel large enough to allow the passage of the guide-wire (2 mm) (Fig. 2.3) is suitable. It is an advantage to have a small diameter (9 mm) end-viewing

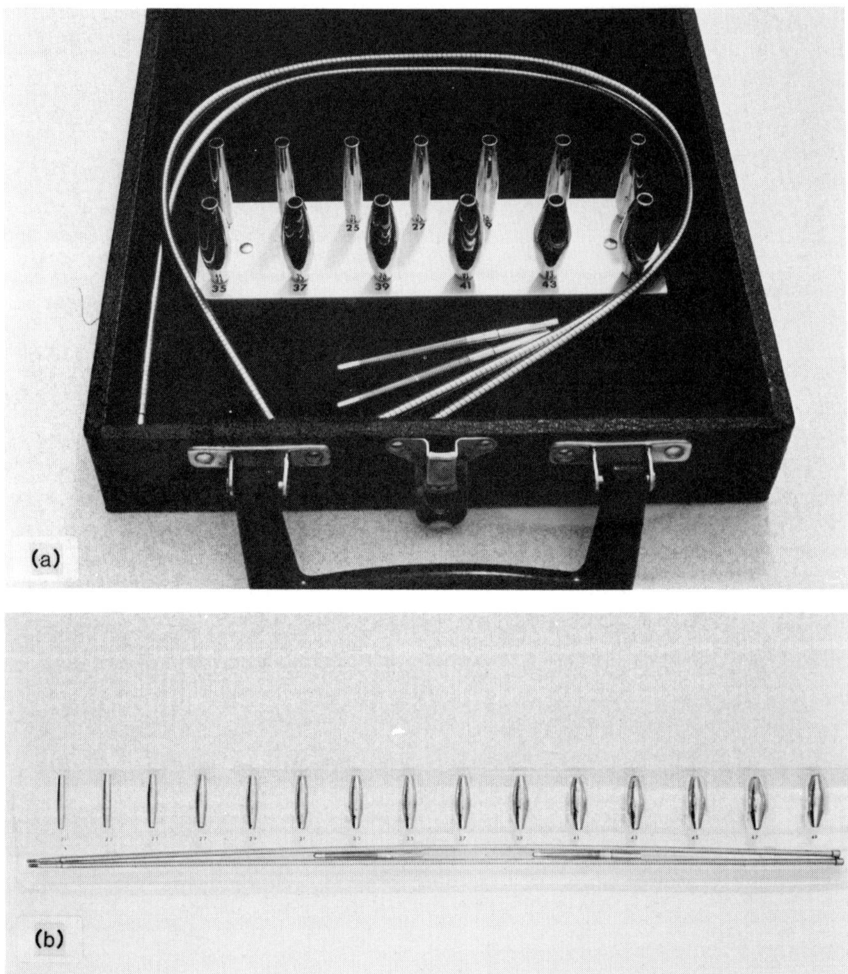

Fig. 2.4 (*a*) Set of Eder–Puestow dilators in box; (*b*) dilators ready for use in Gloucester dispenser. Note two extra large sizes (sizes: French gauge).

instrument available. The guide-wire occasionally becomes impacted, either within a tortuous stricture or, having passed through the stricture, in the hiatus hernia. It is then often possible to guide the small diameter endoscope through the angles in the stricture and hiatus hernia and on into the stomach. The guide-wire is then easily placed across the stricture.

The Eder–Puestow dilators (Fig. 2.4) were described initially for use before the developments in fibreoptics (Puestow, 1955), but Lilly and McCaffery (1971) reported the advantages of placing the guide-wire under direct vision at endoscopy. The set consists of a guide-wire with a flexible spring tip and graduated olive-shaped dilators from 7 mm to 15 mm (Fig. 2.5) It has been found to be an advantage to have two larger dilators made, 15.7 mm and 16.25 mm, as suggested by Dowling (1976). A new type of plastic dilator with gradually increasing diameter has been designed by Celestin (1979) (Fig. 2.6). This new dilator is used over the same guide-wire, but no results have been reported.

If the stricture is of small diameter, or tortuous, then it is wise to perform the first dilatation under a general anaesthetic, again on a day-care basis.

(ii) *Dilatation*. The patient normally lies in the left lateral position for dilatation as for diagnostic endoscopy. This lessens the risk of inhalation of regurgitated gastric contents. (Under a general anaesthetic a cuffed endotracheal tube is used; dilatation may then be carried out safely with the patient supine.) The flexibility of both guide-wire and the staff of the assembled dilator allows dilatation without extending the patient's neck; even patients with a severe kyphosis may undergo this procedure.

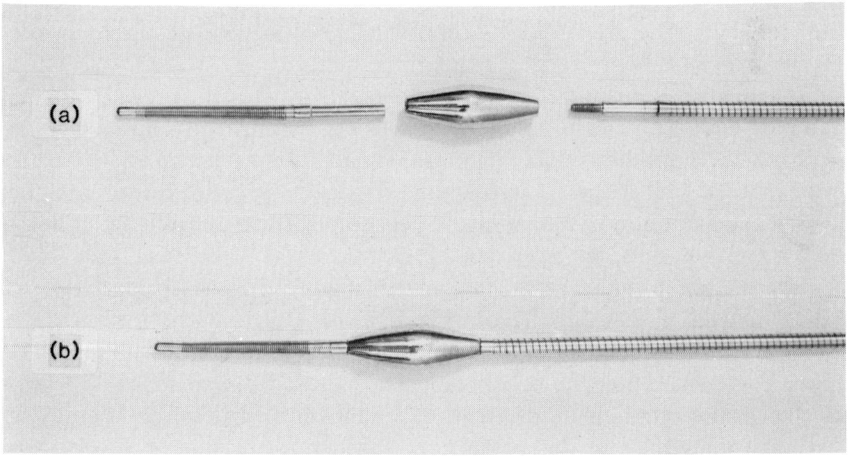

Fig. 2.5 Single dilator (*a*) component parts; (*b*) assembled.

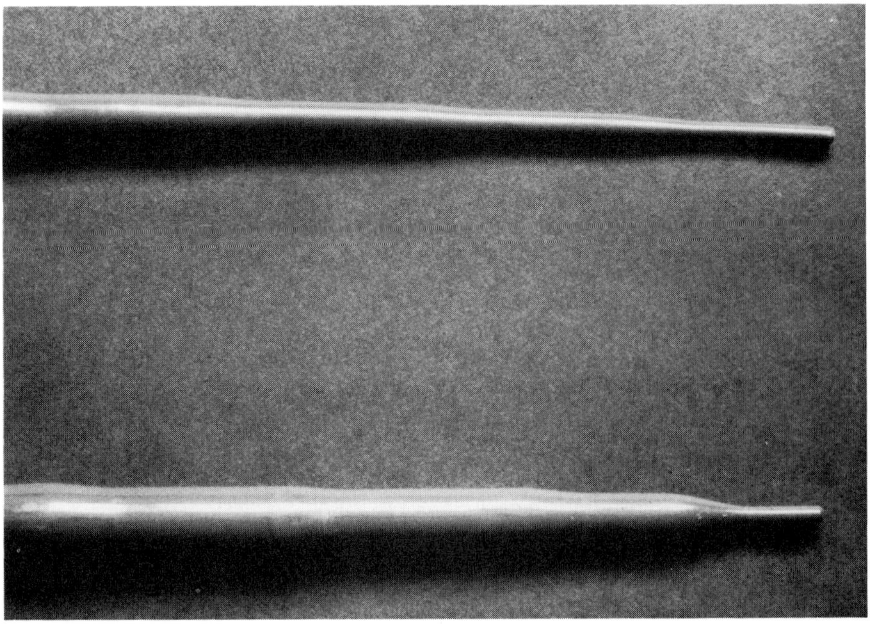

Fig 2.6 Prototype plastic 'stepped' dilator, designed by Mr. R. Celestin.

Once the stricture has been measured, the guide-wire is advanced through the stricture under direct vision. In most cases the wire passes on to curl up in the stomach; but if there is any tendency for the guide-wire to impact, the small diameter endoscope may be used as described above. It is also helpful, when dilating difficult strictures, to be able to see the direction taken by the guide-wire tip using X-ray image intensification (Fig. 2.7*a*, *b*, *c*). This may allow the guide-wire to be directed successfully through tortuous strictures too narrow to allow the passage of the small diameter endoscope. The endoscope is then withdrawn, taking care not to displace the guide-wire. If there is any doubt as to whether the guide-wire is still in place across the stricture, a second guide-wire may be laid alongside the first as a check on the position, following the line of the oesophagus outside the patient.

The graduated dilators are then threaded over the guide-wire and gently pushed across the stricture. It is important that the guide-wire is not allowed to form an acute angle as the 'feel' of the resistance of the stricture is lost. Thus the dilator and staff must be kept moving relative to the guide-wire throughout the dilatation manoeuvre. It may be necessary to withdraw the guide-wire slightly as the dilator is advanced. An extra length of guide-wire is then re-introduced as the dilator is withdrawn. If the stricture is soft and dilates easily, the next dilator used can be two sizes bigger than the previous one, while a tight stricture will require the use of each dilator up the scale of sizes. The majority of strictures may be dilated fully on the first occasion, but the degree of resistance encountered should determine the point at which it is unwise to dilate further. The procedure may be repeated at two-week intervals for a tight stricture until dilatation to full size is achieved.

(iii) *After-care*. The usual precautions must be taken for patients who have had intravenous sedation with diazepam. Patients should be observed closely by trained nursing staff for at least two hours after dilatation. They must be accompanied home and advised not to drive, not to go out alone, not to use machinery or take business decisions for the next 24 hours. The greatest risk is that of perforation. Any complaint

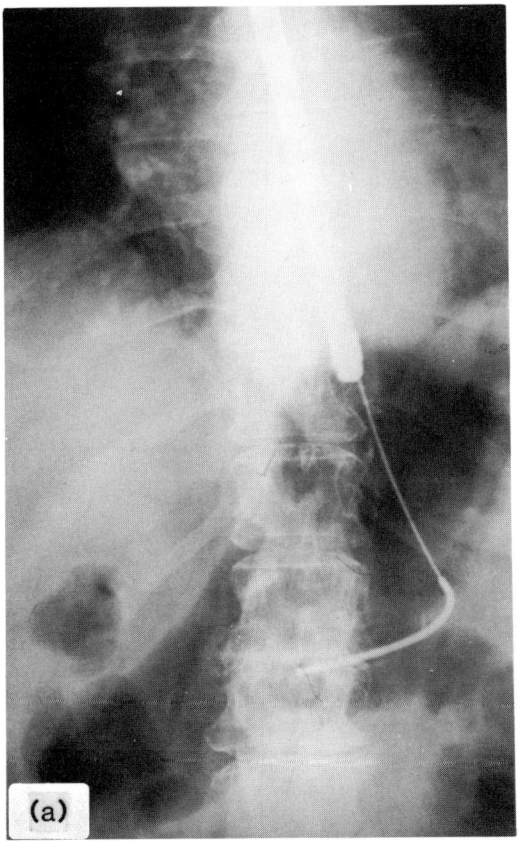

Fig. 2.7 (*a*) X-ray picture showing small fibrescope in the stomach, having negotiated a stricture, with guide-wire passed through side channel.

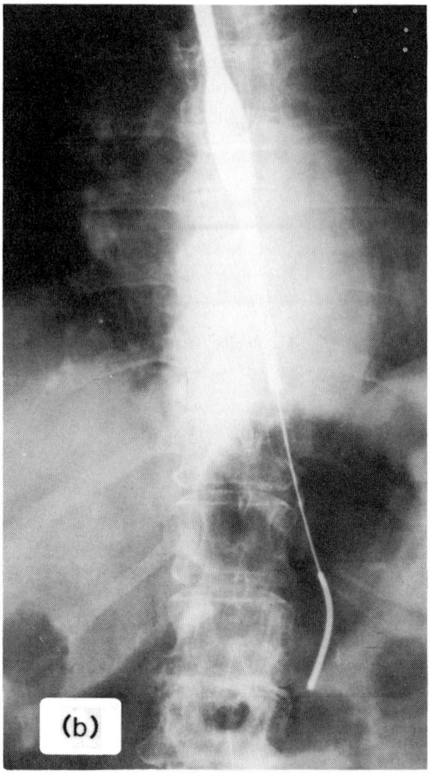

Fig. 2.7 (b) Dilator, about to negotiate a stricture, sliding down over guide-wire.

of cervical, thoracic or abdominal pain should result in immediate admission of the patient for observation. Patients who are allowed home should be warned of the need to consult a doctor if pain develops. There is evidence that the majority of endoscopic perforations will recover on conservative management provided that treatment is instituted early (Wesdorp *et al.*, 1980).

2.3 RESULTS OF ENDOSCOPIC DILATATION

Since the early reports (Price, Stanciu and Bennett, 1974; Royston, Dowling and Gear, 1976) an extensive experience of endoscopic wire-guided dilatation has been accumulated. There is now no doubt that the technique has revolutionized the management of benign oesophageal stricture. The benefits that have accrued are:

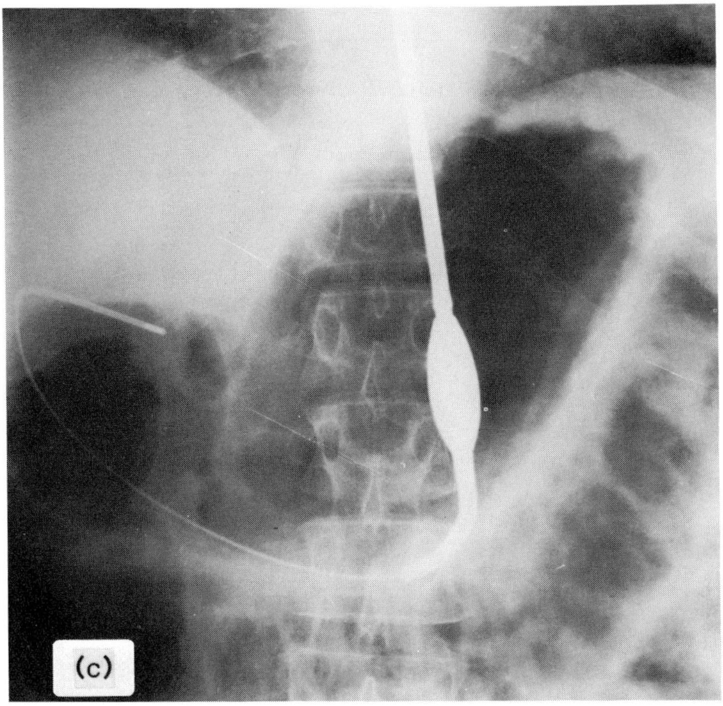

Fig. 2.7 (*c*) Dilator through stricture into stomach.

A safer technique with fewer complications.
Dilatation under local anaesthetic and intravenous sedation, avoiding general anaesthesia.
Out-patient management in most cases.
Dilatation may be repeated at short intervals if necessary.
Hazardous transthoracic surgery and resection can be avoided, as few strictures are impassable.
If surgery is indicated, anti-reflux operations may be carried out through the abdomen in the knowledge that subsequent dilatation of the stricture (if necessary) is simple and safe.

2.3.1 **Detailed results**

The series described by Ethell, Dowling and Gear (1979) is summarized below: 414 dilatations were carried out on 165 patients presenting consecutively in two district general hospitals in Northampton and Gloucester. The age range was from 22 to 95 years with an average of 68.2 years (Table 2.3).

Table 2.3 Age distribution of 165 patients undergoing oesophageal dilatation.

	Age group							
	20–29	*30–39*	*40–49*	*50–59*	*60–69*	*70–79*	*80–89*	*90–99*
No. of patients	2	2	6	22	49	57	25	2

(a) *Anaesthesia*
363 dilatations (87.6%) were performed using intravenous sedation with diazepam (Valium), often supplemented by pentazocine (Fortral) or pethidine and 51 (12.4%) were performed under general anaesthesia.

(b) *Aetiology of the stricture*
The majority were due to reflux oesophagitis. Other causes were: persistent stricture after hiatus hernia repair; transient dysphagia due to a tight repair; corrosive stricture; postradiotherapy stricture and anastomotic stricture after previous resection and anastomosis for malignancy. Some cases with malignant strictures were dilated before the diagnosis was made with certainty (Table 2.4).

(c) *Frequency of dilatation*
The frequency and number of dilatations required to maintain adequate swallowing varied greatly (Table 2.5). Many strictures are confined to the mucosa of the oesophagus, dilate with ease to full size and do not require further dilatation. Over half the patients in the series were in this category. The fibrosis in other strictures is transmural and may extend into the mediastinal tissues around the oesophagus. Such strictures require gradual dilatation in stages to reach full size and often narrow down again within a few weeks. If surgery for reflux is contraindicated because of age or cardio-respiratory disease, dilatation may be required over long periods. Twelve patients in the series required dilatation on more than five occasions, the interval between dilatations averaging two to three months.

Table 2.4 Aetiology of strictures.

Reflux oesophagitis	104
Oesophageal carcinoma	38
Following repair of hiatus hernia	7
Following oesophageal resection	9
Corrosive	2
Carcinoma of bronchus	2
Others	3

Table 2.5 Number of dilatations/patient.

	No. of dilatations												
	1	*2*	*3*	*4*	*5*	*6*	*7*	*8*	*9*	*10*	*11*	*14*	*15*
No. of patients	79	25	30	12	7	3	1	2	1	1	2	1	1

(d) *Failure to dilate*

It was not possible to pass the guide-wire through the stricture in five patients. All were subsequently found to have a malignant stricture. All benign strictures in the series reported above were successfully dilated.

(e) *Complications*

There were only two complications (1.2%) with one death (0.6%). An elderly man developed pneumonia (probably due to inhalation) with recovery and a 76-year old woman died following conservative treatment for perforation.

2.3.2 **Indications for surgery**

The use of wire-guided endoscopic dilatation has reduced the need for surgery. During the study reported above (Ethell, Dowling and Gear, 1979) no patient was referred for thoracic surgery for benign stricture.

When dysphagia has been relieved by endoscopic dilatation the patient's symptoms should be reviewed. Persistent reflux with nocturnal pain and pain on swallowing is often severe enough (despite medical measures) to warrant surgery. Rapid return of dysphagia, with a requirement for frequent dilatations, is a clear indication for surgery. In most cases, once reflux has been controlled, no further dilatations are required.

The age and general infirmity of many patients with benign oesophageal stricture may preclude surgery. Continuing reflux symptoms and the need for repeated dilatation may have to be accepted. The only alternative is intubation of the stricture (see Chapter 3).

2.3.3 **Surgical techniques**

(a) *Intubation at operation*

Bristol *et al.* (1979) reported the use of the Celestin tube introduced at operation in 33 patients. However, five patients (15%), all over 70 years of age, died and a number of other complications were recorded.

(b) *Endoscopic intubation*

Endoscopic techniques of insertion (see Chapter 3 on malignant strictures) should be safer. However, it might be expected that reflux of gastric contents through the tube would occur, producing inflammation (and stricture) at a higher level in the oesophagus. In the Gloucester endoscopy department Celestin tubes have been used for benign strictures on four occasions since the development of the endoscopic method of insertion. Two of these patients have developed strictures proximal to the tube within a few months of insertion (Fig. 2.8).

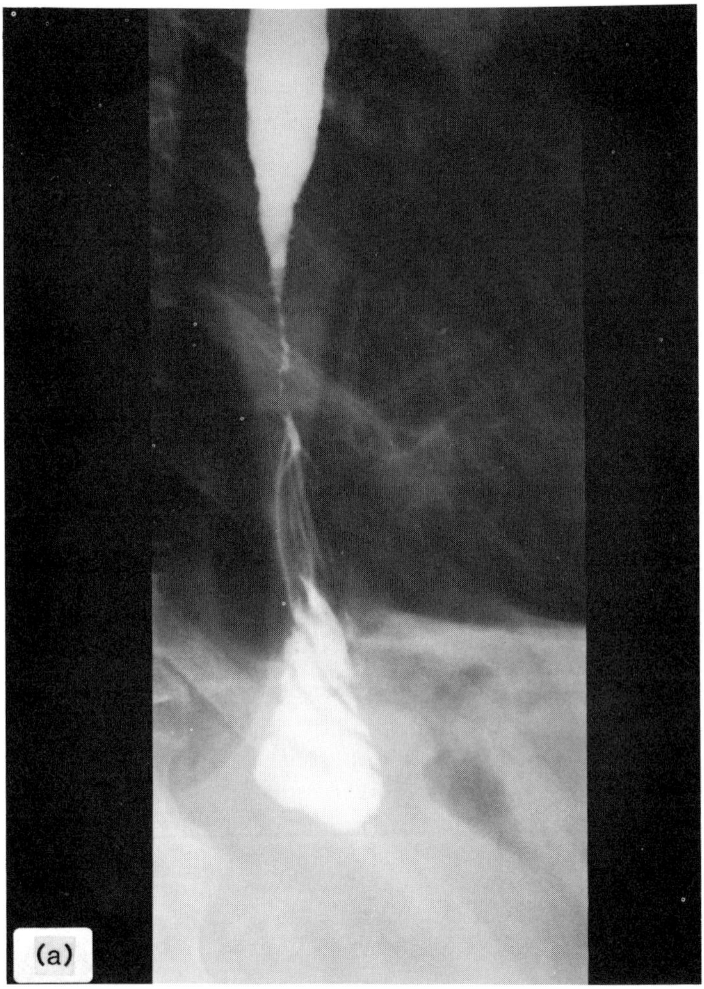

Fig. 2.8 (*a*) Barium swallow appearances of a severe stricture due to bile reflux proximal to an oesophago-jejunostomy anastomosis after total gastrectomy.

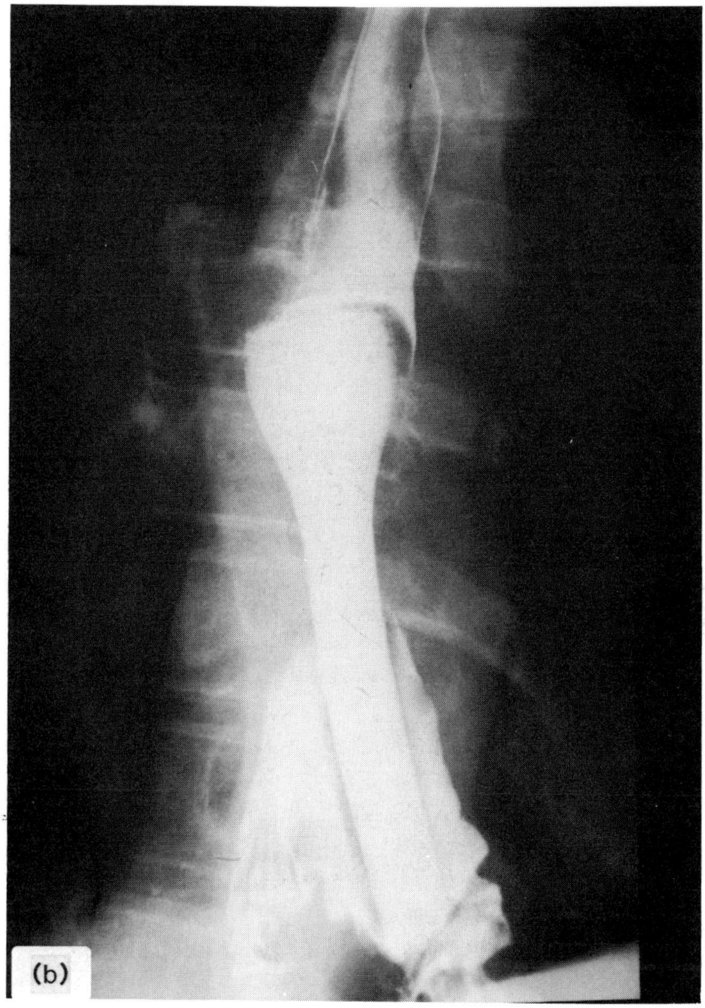

Fig. 2.8 (*b*) After progressive dilatation over many months, a Celestin tube was introduced endoscopically in an attempt to avoid the need for further dilatation.

(c) *Control of reflux*

An extensive surgical literature on the control of gastro-oesophageal reflux has built up since Allison (1951) drew attention to the pathology of the condition (Fig. 2.9). Approach to the oesophageal hiatus has been advocated from above and below the diaphragm and a variety of techniques have been used to restore competence to the cardia. In this brief summary two techniques only will be mentioned.

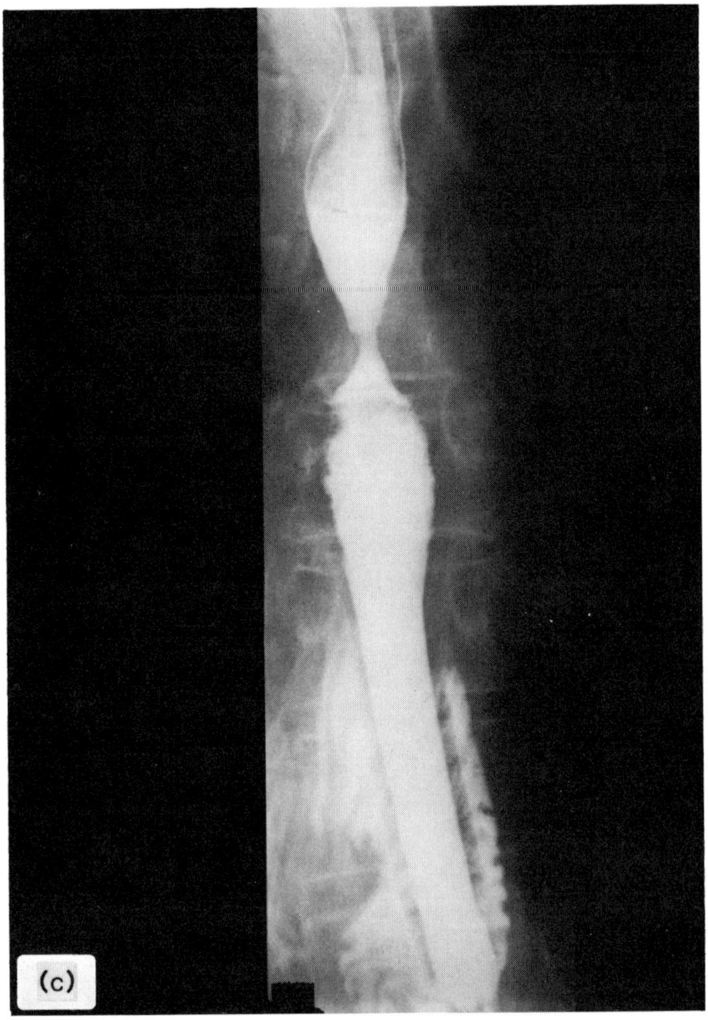

Fig. 2.8 (*c*) Bile reflux through the Celestin tube produced another stricture proximally. The new stricture was dilated, the tube removed and a bile-diverting Roux-en-'Y' anastomosis performed. The stricture then remained patent.

Fig. 2.9 Typical severe irregular stricture due to gastro-oesophageal reflux. (*a*) Before dilatation; (*b*) after two dilatations and a Nissen fundo-plication operation. No further stricturing over the three years of follow-up.

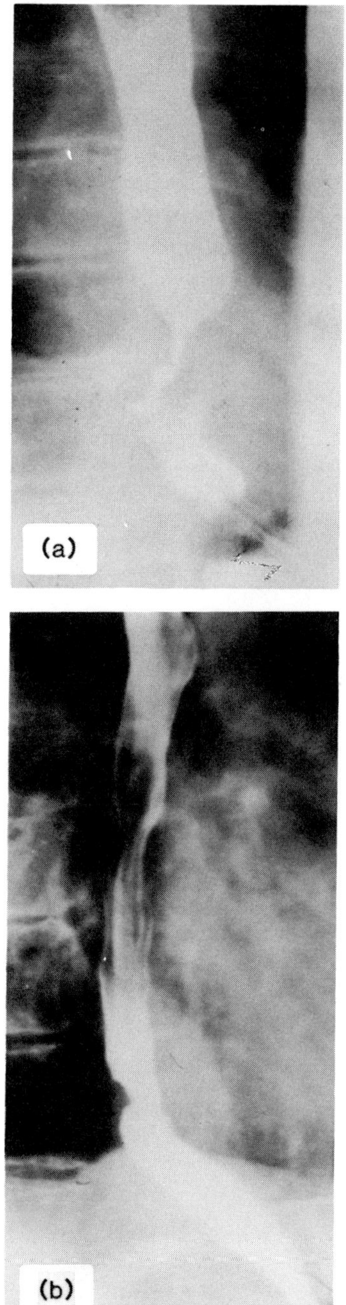
(a)
(b)

Nissen (1964) described a method of 'fundo-plication' combined with repair of the hiatus which has become the most widely used abdominal operation for the control of reflux. This method is effective but may be difficult to apply in patients with severe stricture, with perioesophagitis producing shortening and fixation of the oesophagus in the mediastinum. In this especially difficult situation an alternative approach to the problem has been subjected to a controlled clinical trial (Spencer *et al.*, 1980). Patients with severe inflammation and stricture due to reflux were randomly allocated to the standard Nissen or to an antrectomy with bile-diverting anastomosis as described by Royston, Dowling and Spencer (1975). The theoretical and practical advantages of the technique of antrectomy with bile diversion result from the reduction of the quantity of acid and bile in the stomach. There is, therefore, no need to perform a procedure to control reflux. Dramatic resolution of inflammation and reversal of the stricturing process may result.

EQUIPMENT

Eder–Puestau dilators are supplied by KeyMed Ltd., KeyMed House, Southend-on-Sea, Essex, U.K.

REFERENCES

Allison, P. R. (1951). Reflux oesophagitis, sliding hiatal hernia and the anatomy of repair. *Surg. Gynec. Obstet.*, **92**, 419–31.

Bedine, M. S. and Cocco, A. E. (1972). A comparison of washing and brushing cytology and biopsy in the diagnosis of malignant disease of the esophagus, stomach and colon. *Gastrointest. Endosc.*, **19**, 75–76.

Behar, J. *et al.* (1978). Cimetidine in the treatment of symptomatic gastroesophageal reflux: a double-blind controlled trial. *Gastroenterology*, **74**, 441–8.

Boddington, M. M. (1974). The cytologist's view point. In: *Topics in Gastroenterology*, **2**. (eds S. C. Truelove and J. Trowell), Blackwell Scientific, Oxford.

Bristol, J. B. *et al.* (1979). Treatment of benign oesophageal strictures by intubation. *Gut*, **20**, A458.

Celestin, L. R. (1979). Personal communication.

Dowling, B. L. (1976). Personal communication.

Eastman, M. C., Gear, M. W. L. and Nicol, A. (1978). An assessment of the accuracy of modern endoscopic diagnosis of oesophageal stricture. *Br. J. Surg.*, **65**, 182–5.

Ethell, A. T., Dowling, B. L. and Gear, M. W. L. (1979). Wire-guided dilatation of oesophageal stricture. (In preparation)

Hishon, S. *et al.* (1976). Cytology in the diagnosis of oesophageal cancer. *Lancet*, **1**, 296–7.

Lepsien, G. *et al.* (1979). Treatment of reflux oesophagitis with cimetidine. *D. Med. Wsch.* **104**, 901–6.

Lilly, J. O. and McCaffery, T. D. (1971). Esophageal stricture dilatation: a new method adapted to the fibreoptic esophagascope. *Am. J. Dig. Dis.*, **16**, 1137.

Logan, A. (1965). Symposium on Peptic Stricture of the Oesophagus. *Thorax*, **20**, 288.

Mortensen, N. J. M. and Mackenzie, E. (1979). Prospective study of brush cytology in the diagnosis of carcinoma of the oesophagus. *Gut*, **20**, A433.

Nissen, R. (1964). The treatment of hiatal hernia and oesophageal reflux by fundo-plication. In: *Hernia*. (eds L. M. Nyhus and H. N. Harkins), Lippincott, Philadelphia, pp. 488–96.

Powell-Jackson, P., Barkley, H. and Northfield, T. C. (1978). Effect of cimetidine in symptomatic gastro-oesophageal reflux. *Lancet*, **2**, 1068–9.

Price, J. D., Stanciu, C. and Bennett, J. R. (1974). A safer method of dilating oesophageal strictures. *Lancet*, **1**, 1141–2.

Prolla, J. C. *et al.* (1971). Further experience with direct vision brushing cytology of malignant tumours of upper gastrointestinal tract. Histopathologic correlation with biopsy. *Acta Cytol.*, **15**, 375–8.

Puestow, K. L. (1955). Conservative treatment of stenosing diseases of the oesophagus. *Postgrad. Med.*, **18**, 6.

Raptis, S. and Milne, D. M. (1972). A review of the management of 100 cases of benign stricture of the oesophagus. *Thorax*, **27**, 599–603.

Royston, C. M. S., Dowling, B. L. and Gear, M. W. L. (1976). Oesophageal dilatation using the Eder–Puestow dilators. *Am. J. Surg.*, **131**, 697–700.

Royston, C. M. S., Dowling, B. L. and Spencer, J. (1975). Antrectomy with Roux-en-'Y' anastomosis in the treatment of peptic oesophagitis with stricture. *Br. J. Surg.*, **62**, 605–7.

Schiller, K. F. R., Cotton, P. B. and Salmon, P. R. (1972). The hazards of digestive endoscopy: a survey of British experience. *Gut*, **13**, 1027.

Spencer, J. *et al.* (1980). (In preparation)

Wesdorp, E. *et al.* (1978). Oral cimetidine in reflux oesophagitis: a double-blind controlled trial. *Gastroenterology*, **74**, 821–4.

Wesdorp, E. *et al.* (1980). Treatment of iatrogenic esophageal and/or cardia perforations. *Abs. IV Eur. Cong. Gastroint. Endoscopy*, Georg Thieme Verlag, Stuttgart, New York.

Williamson, R. C. N. (1975). Peptic oesophageal stricture. *Br. J. Surg.*, **62**, 448–54.

3 Intubation of oesophagogastric neoplasms

MICHAEL ATKINSON

Neoplasms arising in the oesophagus or at the cardia of the stomach rapidly cause severe dysphagia leading to profound nutritional impairment which contributes significantly to the very poor outlook these growths carry. Under-nutrition is a major cause of death; it reduces resistance to infection, impairs immunological competence and delays wound healing, so diminishing the patient's ability to withstand radical treatment with surgery or radiotherapy. Mortality is further increased by the high incidence of aspiration pneumonia from overflow of oesophageal contents into the respiratory tract. Blockage of the gut lumen by encroaching tumour and by impaction of food in the narrowing often prevent even the passage of liquids, so adding fluid depletion and uraemia to the patient's troubles.

Every patient with swallowing difficulty should be seen and investigated without delay if management is to be effective and complications avoided. Rapidly progressing dysphagia is a very distressing symptom which demands urgent relief if the patient is to be made comfortable, whether or not radical treatment is possible.

3.1 HISTORICAL BACKGROUND

In the last century carcinoma of the oesophagus causing dysphagia was generally treated by gastrostomy which carried a high mortality, mainly from sepsis. This led to a search for other methods of providing nourishment and orogastric tube feeding, a technique used by John Hunter in the 18th century, was applied by Durham (1881) to feed a woman with dysphagia resulting from carcinoma of the larynx. Charles Symonds, then Assistant Surgeon to Guy's Hospital, devised a short gum elastic oesophageal tube with a boxwood funnel (Fig. 3.1) which he inserted through the narrowed area (Symonds, 1885). It could be removed for cleaning by silk threads attached to the funnel brought out through

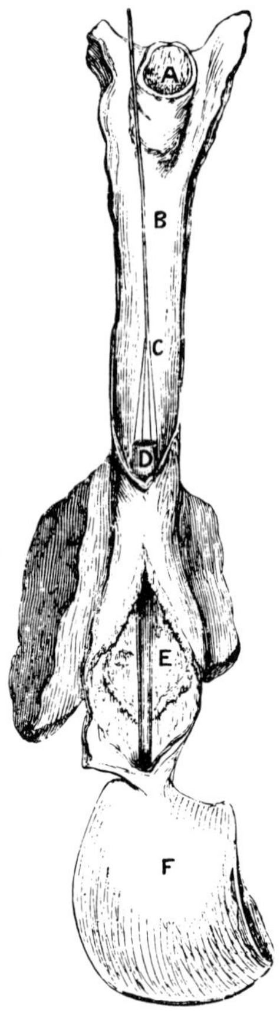

Fig. 3.1 Symond's tube *in situ* showing silk threads (C) attached to funnel (D) and brought out through the mouth.

the mouth and looped over the patient's ear. This device was used in the first recorded instance of successful oral insertion of a prosthetic tube through a malignant oesophageal stricture in order to relieve dysphagia.

Guisez (1914) described a rubber tube of 14 mm bore with a distal end resembling that of a de Pezzer catheter which was stretched on an introducer and passed under direct vision through a rigid oesophagoscope (Fig. 3.2). Guisez's method was developed further by Souttar who at oesophagoscopy inserted a tube made of coiled German silver wire expanded into a funnel at its proximal end (Fig. 3.3). After dilatation by bouginage the tube was mounted on an introducer and passed into the oesophagus over a guidewire. In 1927, Souttar reported 50 intubations by this method with two deaths resulting from the procedure and an average duration of life after intubation of 5.8 months. The limiting

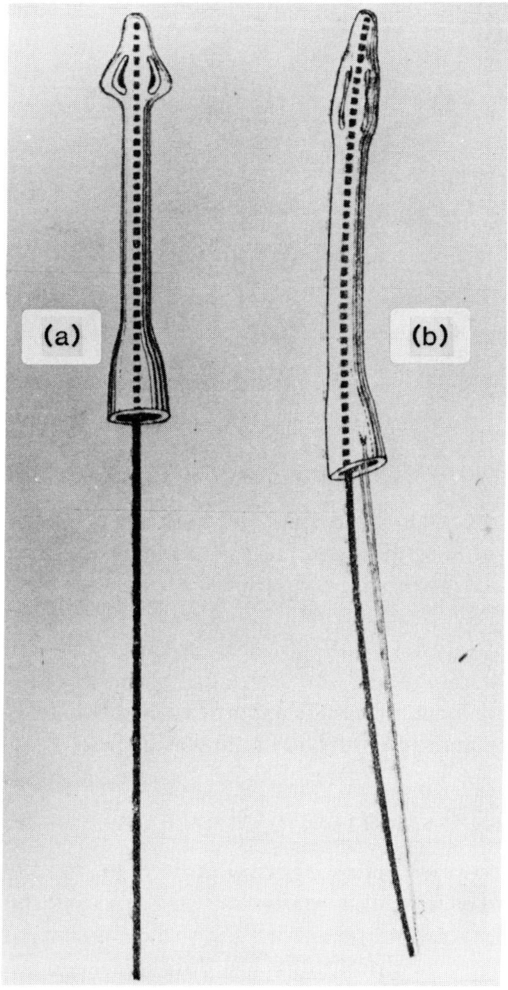

Fig. 3.2 Guisez's tube and its introducer.

factor of Souttar's tube was its narrow bore and its tendency to displace distally, so that he later used a wider funnel made of rubber.

Operative methods of tube insertion became popular during the 1950s mainly because larger tubes could be inserted by this means and because growths at or near the cardia often presented difficulties with the rigid oesophagoscope. The method which came into widespread use for the next 20 years was that of Mousseau *et al.* (1956). They used laparotomy and pull-through of a neoplex tube with its end tapered into a leader which was passed blind through the mouth. When this appeared in the stomach it was pulled down until the tube was in a satisfactory position

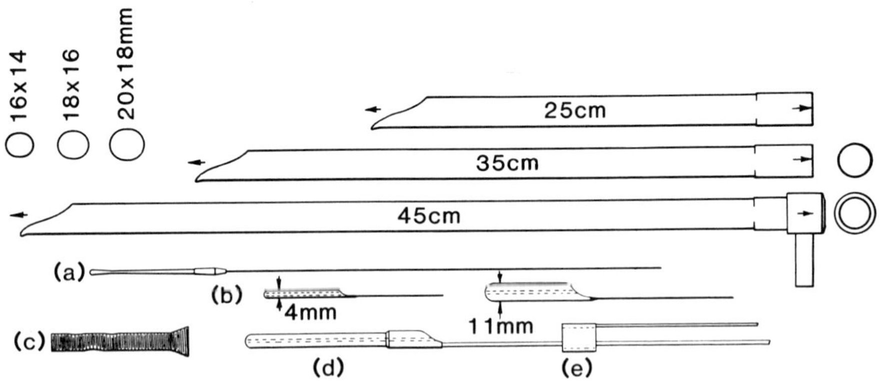

Fig. 3.3. Souttar's tube and accessory instruments for intubation. (a) Flexible bougie; (b) aluminium dilators to pass over shaft of A; (c) flexible wire tube; (d) (e) introducer and releasing ring.

and the end cut off at the required length. Tubes of polyethylene and latex rubber with a nylon spiral incorporated in the wall to prevent kinking were later introduced by this method (Gourevitch, 1959; Celestin, 1959). Until the recent application of fibreoptic endoscopic methods, laparotomy and pull-through remained the standard method of intubation. In a review of the literature, Johnson *et al.* (1976) found excellent improvement in swallowing after Mousseau–Barbin intubation but the average operative mortality rate was 23%.

3.2 ENDOSCOPIC METHODS OF INTUBATION

Rigid and fibreoptic endoscopes continue to be employed in the placement of tubes through malignant strictures of the oesophagus or cardia. Whichever endoscope is used the principal stages in the procedure are the same: firstly as a preliminary endoscopy to establish the diagnosis by biopsy or cytology and to determine the cell type of growth, secondly to dilate the lumen of the malignant stricture and thirdly to insert a prosthetic tube.

3.2.1 **Rigid oesophagoscopic methods**

Weisel *et al.* (1959) passed a funnel ended tube over a filiform bougie inserted through the malignant stricture pushing the tube with a rigid oesophagoscope. O'Connor *et al.* (1963), reviewing the outcome in 342 patients with oesophageal cancer so treated and using polyethylene tubes usually 8–12 cm in length, reported the remarkable figure of only two deaths from the procedure.

Lewis *et al.* (1973) placed a lumen finder through the stricture under direct vision down a rigid oesophagoscope and used this to guide metal olive dilators through the stricture before inserting a latex tube reinforced with a stainless steel coil in its wall (Haering tube) along the lumen finder pushed from behind by a metal olive engaged in the funnel of the tube. They found intubation of growths at the oesophagogastric junction to be difficult because of a high perforation rate, a greater difficulty in positioning the tube satisfactorily and the subsequent occurrence of symptomatic reflux through the tube. Nevertheless, they encountered no deaths from the procedure in 17 patients.

A tube introducer with small lateral projections engaging in holes in the wall of the tube to give a positive grip which could subsequently be released was devised by Schetrumpf (1973). The tube could be tailored to any length and the small side holes were considered to help in preventing displacement since they were invaded by growth of the tumour which acted as an anchor.

3.2.2 **Fibreoptic endoscopic methods**

The development of fibreoptic endoscopes has provided the oesophagoscopist with instruments which will negotiate bends in the oesophagus and cardia and at the same time provide a clear view. Consequently the lower oesophagus and cardia are more accessible, particularly in patients with kyphoscoliosis, which is common in the elderly age group in which oesophageal cancer most frequently occurs. The use of the fibreoptic endoscope, if necessary combined with radiological screening, has greatly facilitated the accurate positioning of a guidewire through tight neoplastic strictures. Metal olive dilators of the Eder Puestow type may be slid over the wire to open up the lumen preparatory to intubation.

3.3 RECENT ENDOSCOPIC METHODS FOR THE INSERTION OF OESOPHAGEAL PROSTHETIC TUBES

The several methods in current use are all based on the principle that the tube must be advanced into position over a guide in order to reduce the risk of false passage and perforation. The guide may be a bougie, the oesophagoscope itself or a steel wire.

A filiform bougie was used for this purpose by Weisel *et al.* (1963) and Boyce (1973) used a mercury filled rubber Maloney bougie. Once this is in position the tube is slipped over it and advanced by pushing from behind with a pusher tube engaging in the funnel of the prosthesis. A silk suture tied to the distal end of the Maloney bougie prevents the prosthetic tube being pushed over the end of the bougie and enables it to be withdrawn, if necessary, during its positioning.

With the advent of fibreoptic endoscopes such as the ACMI TX7 (diameter 9.5 mm) or the Olympus GIF P2 (diameter 8.8 mm) it became possible to slide the prosthesis over the instrument itself by means of a pusher tube mounted behind it on the endoscope. The flexibility of the endoscope enables the tube to be passed round bends in the lumen of the oesophagus or cardia. This method has the advantage of simplicity and in the hands of Tytgat *et al.* (1976) has given good results in a large series of patients (den Hartog Jager *et al.*, 1979). Using a tube made of transparent material (Tygon) the growth can be viewed through its wall and this is of help in positioning the tube correctly. To prevent compression or kinking of the tube when in position its wall must have a certain stiffness which means that, for it to pass easily over the endoscope if on a bend, its bore must be appreciably greater than the outer diameter of the instrument and there is some danger that the leading end of the tube might tear soft growths during passage. Retrieval of the tube is difficult using this method but pushing tubes have been devised with a balloon incorporated in the distal end which, when inflated within the funnel of the tube, provides more positive control of its movement and enables it to be withdrawn. Celestin *et al.* (1980) has developed a latex tube system working on the same principle (Fig. 3.4).

In recent years the Eder Puestow method of dilating peptic oesophageal strictures has come into widespread use. The Puestow stainless steel guidewire, passed down the biopsy channel of the endoscope can be positioned through the stricture under direct endoscopic vision which has made dilatation of strictures, particularly those in the lower oesophagus or at the cardia, a much safer procedure (see Chapter 2). The technique has been adapted to guide prosthetic tubes through neoplastic strictures. Initially the tube was mounted on the

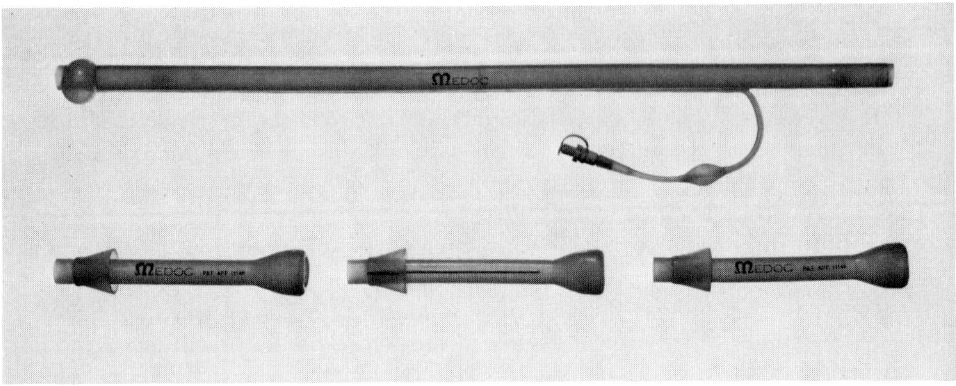

Fig. 3.4. Latex introducer with balloon for passing over the flexible endoscope, together with flanged tube (Celestin).

staff of the Eder Puestow introducer itself using the largest metal olive that would pass through the lumen to provide a smooth leading end (Atkinson and Ferguson, 1977). To prevent displacement of the tube during withdrawal of the Eder Puestow staff and olive, a wide bore rammer engaging with the funnel of the tube was used to hold it in position. This method worked well, but the leading end of the tube still presented a roughened projection and there was no easy means of withdrawing the tube once in position. Gillison *et al.* (1977) employed a Number 28 Foley catheter over the flexible Eder Puestow system, inflating the balloon of the catheter against the inner wall of the tube to provide more positive control and to enable its withdrawal if this became necessary.

3.3.1 **Design of equipment**

In designing a tube and introducer the following requirements should be met.

1. The method must be relatively simple and applicable to patients who are elderly, malnourished, often kyphoscoliotic and who have poor respiratory reserve.
2. Trauma must be reduced to a minimum by providing a flexible assembly with a smoothly tapered leading end.
3. The tube used should not kink when bent, should have a proximal funnel sufficiently large to prevent distal displacement through the growth and yet small enough to pass through the pharynx, cricopharyngeal region and oesophagus without causing trauma. It should preferably have a device on its distal end to prevent proximal displacement.
4. The procedure should be reversible to enable removal of tubes which have undergone displacement, structural deterioration or have been blocked by food material which cannot be removed by the usual methods.

3.4 THE NOTTINGHAM INTRODUCER

This tube introducer is designed to slide over a Puestow guide-wire previously inserted through the neoplastic stricture (Atkinson *et al.*, 1978). The principle used is to grip the tube from within by means of an expanding cup which becomes wedged firmly in the tube lumen. The instrument consists of an inner flexible stainless steel spiral tube upon the distal end of which is mounted the expanding Delrin plastic cup behind a tapered spiral spring leader (Fig. 3.5). Over this is slid a second spiral tube, the end of which is expanded into an olive. This olive enters and expands the Delrin cup when the second tube is slid along the first. A

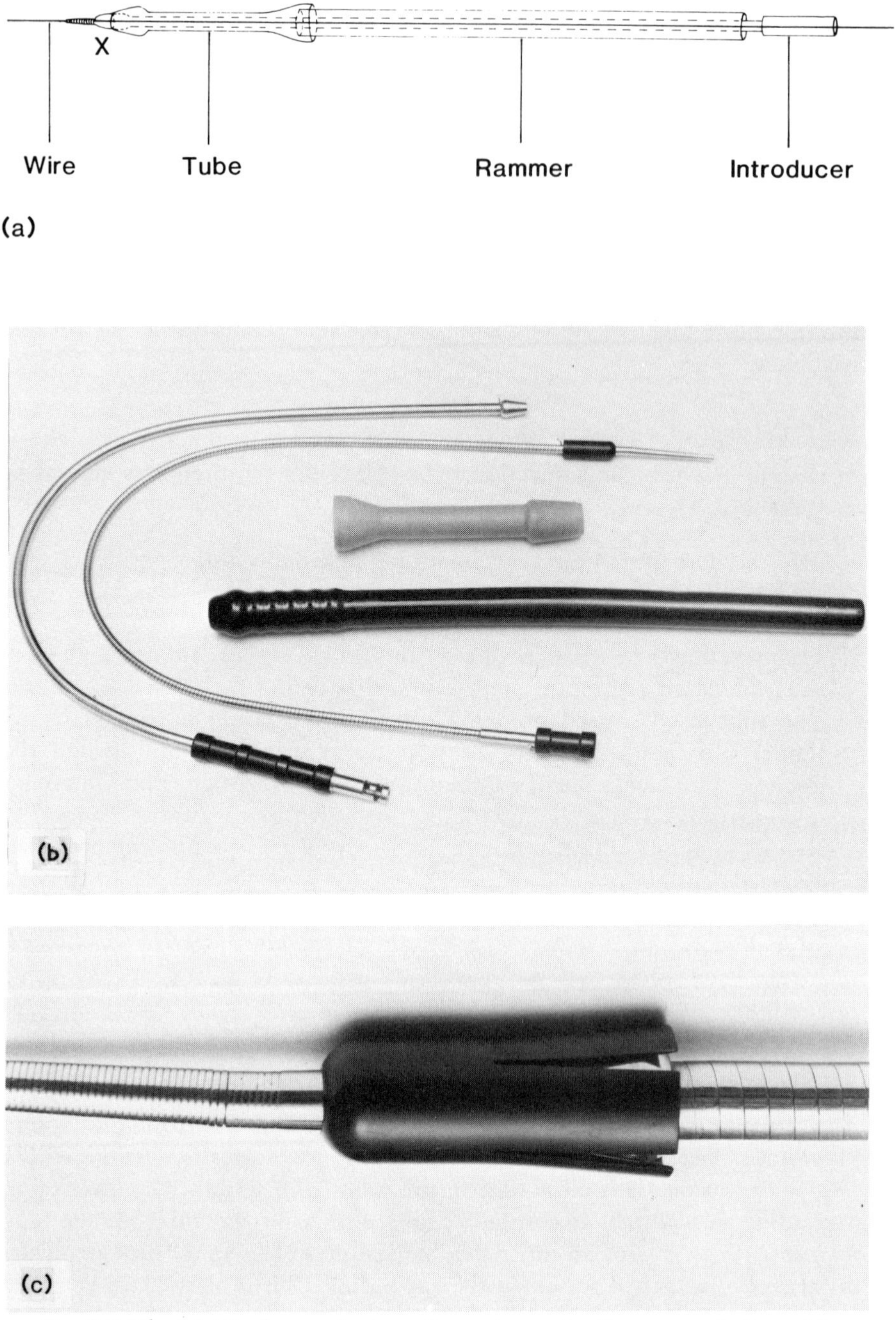

Fig. 3.5 The Nottingham tube introducer shown in diagrammatic form (a), dissembled in (b) together with the tube and rammer and in (c) in close up, with the Delrin cup expanded by the metal olive.

bayonet lock on the proximal end of the introducer enables the cup to be locked in the expanded position, so holding the prosthetic tube firmly until the lock is released. The whole assembly is flexible yet sufficiently rigid to transmit the forces involved in inserting the tube. They are easily dismantled for cleaning and sterilization. (Different sized olives and cups are available for use with tubes of different bores.) A stout plastic rammer is slid over the introducer behind the prosthesis and engages with its funnel. This serves to hold the tube in position while the introducer and guide-wire are withdrawn through it after it has been placed in satisfactory position.

3.4.1 **Procedure for intubation**

Normally the diagnosis would have been confirmed at an earlier endoscopy and the cell type of the growth determined by biopsy and cytological examination. This is important in view of the likelihood that squamous growths may be treated subsequently with radiotherapy. Once the tube is in position the growth is not easily accessible for biopsy. The procedure for intubation is carried out in four stages:

1. Endoscopic insertion of the Puestow guide-wire.
2. Dilatation of the stricture by the Eder Puestow dilators.
3. Endoscopic assessment of the extent of the neoplasm.
4. Insertion of the prosthetic tube.

(a) *Preparation of the patient*

The majority of patients requiring intubation are unable to swallow solid food and in many dysphagia is severe enough to cause fluid depletion necessitating intravenous replacement. Physical and radiological examination of the chest to look for aspiration pneumonia is an important preliminary measure, for if this is present urgent physiotherapy and antibiotics may be needed before intubation is undertaken.

(b) *Anaesthesia*

Intubation may be done under general or local anaesthesia. The size of the funnel of the tube and the introducer assembly causes discomfort during its passage through the pharynx and in the unanaesthetized patients may lead to respiratory obstruction. For these reasons the procedure is best done under general anaesthesia but the anaesthetist must be made aware of the danger of regurgitation of oesophageal contents during induction and have suction to hand. The procedure may be performed using intravenous diazepam, pethidine and topical anaesthesia.

(c) *Placement of the guide-wire*
It is usually possible to insert the Puestow guide-wire without difficulty under endoscopic control. If the guide-wire does not pass easily, X-ray screening using an image intensifier is essential; any retrograde angulation of the flexible leader of the guide-wire indicates impingement on the wall of the stricture or of the gut beyond. By gently withdrawing the wire until its tip has straightened out and by altering slightly the direction of passage of the wire by angling the tip of the endoscope the stricture can usually be negotiated. It is advisable to pass 20 cm of wire beyond the narrowing. The endoscope is then removed, taking care not to withdraw the wire. A narrow endoscope such as the Olympus GIF P2 may be manoeuvred through wider strictures before dilatation but it is still necessary to insert the guide-wire and pass the larger olive dilators.

(d) *Dilatation of the neoplastic stricture*
The stricture is dilated by the Eder Puestow metal olives to a number 45 French gauge (14.3 mm diameter) or if possible to a number 50 (16 mm diameter). Care must be taken by the operator and his assistant not to kink the guide-wire as this causes hold-up of the dilators and if it occurs beyond the pharynx the resistance encountered may be confused with that from the stricture itself. Neoplastic strictures vary considerably in the resistance they offer to dilatation, and those recurring at the site of anastomosis after previous surgical resection, with resulting fibrotic scarring, are often quite tight. Any sudden loss of resistance suggests the neoplasm has split and may be perforated.

(e) *Endoscopic assessment of the length of the stricture*
After dilatation the guide-wire is removed and the endoscope inserted to assess the extent of the neoplasm. Bleeding after dilatation may obscure vision and if so the blood must be washed away. The distance of the upper end of the lesion from the incisor teeth is measured to permit accurate positioning of the tube, and the length of the stricture provides an indication of the length of tube needed. If the growth is in the oesophagus near the cardia, diaphragmatic movement with respiration may cause trauma to the muscosa or tube displacement proximally and it is better to use a longer tube that can be carried through the cardia so that its distal end is in the stomach. At this stage a complete endoscopic search of the stomach, pylorus and duodenum should be made for other lesions. With the endoscope in the pyloric antrum the guide-wire is reinserted and the instrument again withdrawn.

(f) *Insertion of the prosthetic tube*
A tube of suitable length is selected or cut to size and mounted on the Nottingham introducer with the rammer behind engaging in its funnel.

The whole assembly is liberally lubricated and lubricant is smeared on the end of the rammer to prevent it jamming in the funnel. The distance of the proximal end of the growth to the incisors is measured from the root of the funnel and marked on the rammer. The whole assembly is slid along the guide-wire until the mark on the rammer is opposite the incisor teeth. The introducer is then released and it and the guide-wire are withdrawn, the tube being held in position by means of the rammer. The rammer is then disengaged from the funnel by giving it a sharp twist and it is withdrawn, watching the tube on the X-ray screen to make sure it remains in position during the manoeuvre. A thin endoscope is then reinserted to check the position of the tube, and pass through it into the stomach beyond to make sure that the distal end is not occluded by pressure against the wall of the stomach or lower oesophagus.

(g) *Aftercare*

On recovering consciousness the patient is nursed in the sitting position and six hours later a chest radiograph is taken to look for evidence of perforation such as air in the mediastinum or soft tissue of the neck. The position of the tube can be checked on the lateral chest film and if satisfactory the patient is allowed oral fluids and given a soft diet next day. He must be instructed to masticate his food carefully and to wash it down with draughts of fluid. Fizzy drinks such as soda water are useful to wash out any remaining food material from the tube after a meal. If difficulty in swallowing persists, barium studies are needed to check the function and position of the tube. Most patients are able to leave hospital within three to seven days after intubation except for those who go on to receive radiotherapy.

3.5 PROSTHETIC TUBES

The prosthetic tube should be made of non-irritant material which will not undergo denaturation or structural deterioration with time. It should be radio-opaque to enable its position subsequently to be checked radiologically and it should be flexible yet should not kink when bent. The lumen should be at least 1 cm in diameter and the proximal funnel should be sufficiently large to prevent the prosthesis passing beyond the stricture. It should preferably be fitted with a distal shoulder or other device to prevent proximal displacement yet this must not be so large as to preclude its removal by endoscopic means should this become necessary in the future.

3.5.1 **Material**

Metal tubes such as the Souttar tube may cause pressure necrosis of the growth and most tubes are now made of plastic or latex rubber. Tygon polyvinyl tubes may be made to measure from tubing of 10, 12 or 14 mm diameter by cutting to approximate length and moulding the proximal end into a funnel after softening it in hot mineral oil. As it cools the Tygon hardens and any rough projections at the ends may then be filed smooth. The tube should be cut to exceed the tumour length by 4–6 cm. Tygon tubes are durable although they undergo hardening with time and may cause pressure necrosis leading to haemorrhage and ulceration. The method is time-consuming since the tube is constructed during the intubation procedure.

Latex rubber is used in the Haering, Celestin and Medoc tubes, but because of its softness a metal or nylon spiral must be incorporated in the wall to prevent kinking when bent. After several months *in situ* the rubber often undergoes denaturation becoming soft, sticky and friable resulting in disintegration of the tube with release of the nylon or metal spiral (MacKenzie *et al.*, 1976). Any latex tube which has been in position in the oesophagus for six months or more should, therefore, be carefully inspected endoscopically and if necessary replaced. Silicone rubber which is more inert than latex rubber is used in the Atkinson tube.

3.5.2 **Shape**

Tubes inserted by the laparotomy and pull-through method are usually stitched in position in the stomach to prevent displacement. A number of devices have been used to prevent proximal migration of tubes inserted at endoscopy (Fig. 3.6). The amputated funnel of the second Celestin tube has been stitched on to the distal end to form a shoulder (Atkinson *et al.*, 1978) and the Medoc tube employs a thin rubber umbrella-like flange for this purpose. The Medoc may also be introduced by the mandril device with its inflatable balloon designed by Çelestin (Fig. 3.7). A Tygon tube with transverse corrugations and a small distal shoulder is used by Tytgat. The Atkinson tube, made of silicone-rubber over a monofilament nylon spiral, has a wide conical funnel and two distal projections to minimize the risk of proximal displacement (Fig. 3.8).

When the tube lies across the cardia, reflux of gastric contents may cause troublesome symptoms of gastro-oesophageal reflux and oesophagitis. To overcome this difficulty Davidenko *et al.* (1975) constructed a polyvinyl tube with a soft latex rubber tube attached to its distal end which acted as a flutter valve to prevent reflux.

A method of slow dilatation by means of a dumb-bell shaped spring

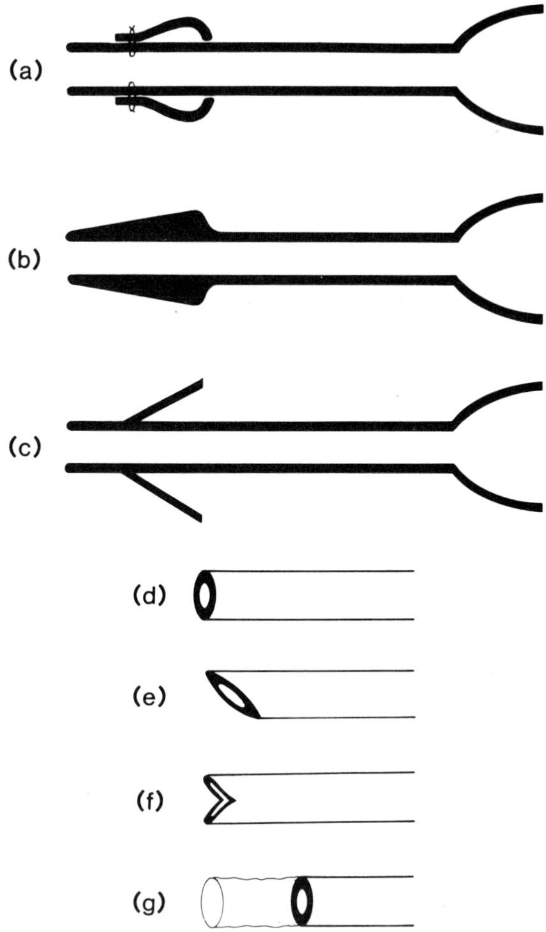

Fig. 3.6 Different types of oesophageal prosthetic tube with retaining devices near their distal ends. (*a*) Celestin tube with the funnel of a second tube sutured on to its distal end to form a shoulder. (*b*) Tube with distal shoulder. (*c*) Tube with distal retaining flange (Medox tube). (*d*), (*e*), (*f*) Different end configurations used to prevent occlusion by contact with the wall of the stomach. (*g*) Anti-reflux flutter valve described by Davidenko.

tube made of stainless steel wire cylindrical braid, which elongates when compressed and returns to its wider diameter and shorter length when released, has been used by Didcott (1973). He found it particularly valuable in strictures high in the oesophagus where there is insufficient space below the cricopharyngeus to accommodate the funnel of a conventional tube.

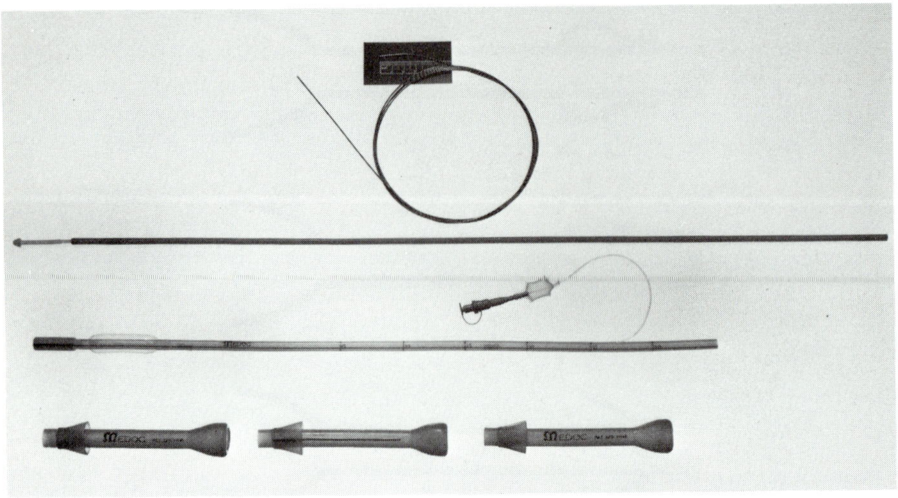

Fig. 3.7 Mandril set for introduction of flanged tubes (Celestin).

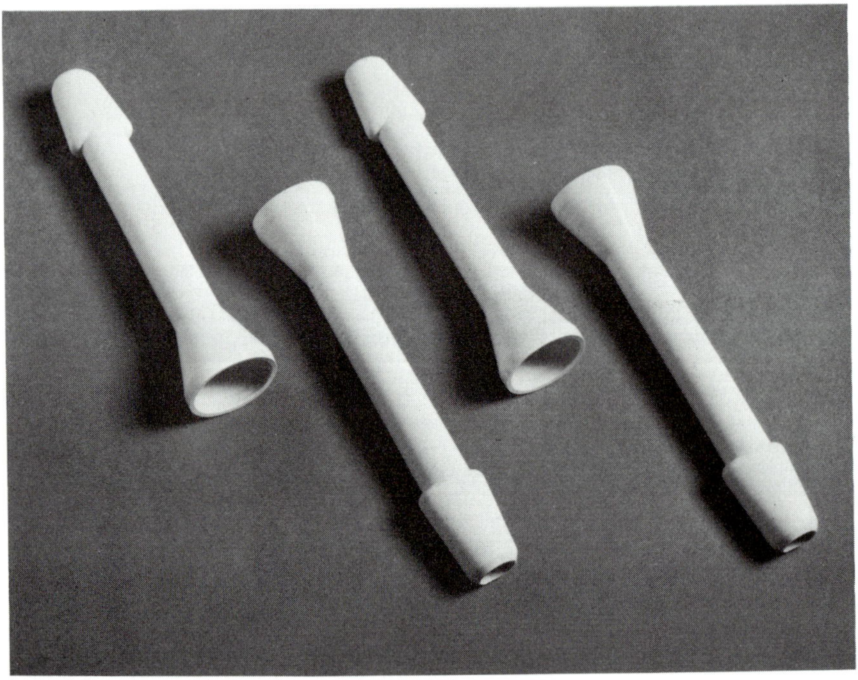

Fig. 3.8 The recently designed Atkinson tube. Note the wide, conical funnel and distal projection to prevent proximal displacement (courtesy of Key-Med Limited).

3.6 ABILITY TO SWALLOW AFTER INTUBATION

The primary object of endoscopic intubation of oesophagogastric neoplasms is to relieve dysphagia and this is the major criterion on which to judge the efficacy of the procedure. Most patients can take an adequate diet after intubation although it is advisable for them to avoid certain foods such as raw apple, hard bread crusts and steak. They learn to take more fluid to wash food down. Careful mastication is essential and if necessary adequate dentures should be provided since bolting meals inevitably causes tube blockage. Few attempts have been made to quantitate swallowing ability after intubation but in a study of 60 patients (Atkinson *et al.*, 1979) more than half could manage a normal diet, omitting only certain hard lumpy foods, and most consumed an adequate if soft diet (Table 3.1). In the great majority improvement in swallowing continued until the patient's death.

3.6.1 **Tracheo-oesophageal fistal**

Breakdown of a neoplasm to cause a tracheo-oesophageal fistula leads to a particularly distressing type of dysphagia with bouts of coughing and choking precipitated by even small sips of liquid. In this group of patients intubation is often strikingly effective in providing symptomatic relief and in alleviating the accompanying respiratory distress (Peura *et al.*, 1978).

3.7 TUBE FUNCTION

3.7.1 **Tube blockage**

This is usually due to inadequate mastication and the delight of being able to swallow again tempting the patient to essay heroic but unwise feats of deglutition. Distension of the upper oesophagus with food causes vomiting which may result in tube displacement.

Table 3.1 Effect of intubation on dysphagia.

Grade of dysphagia	*Before intubation*	*After intubation*
1. Difficulty with certain solids	0 patients	36 patients
2. Soft diet only	4	18
3. Liquids only	25	5
4. Intravenous fluids needed	36	6*
Total	65	65

*All died within a week of intubation.

Tube blockage can usually be cleared by pushing the offending food material through the tube into the stomach with one of the narrower endoscopes of diameter small enough to pass through the tube lumen. If the oesophagus contains much food material this must first be cleared and under these circumstances it is advisable to use general anaesthesia, since the cuffed end of the tracheal tube prevents spillage into the respiratory tract during clearing of the oesophagus by irrigation through a wide bore rubber tube. If the blockage cannot be relieved by these means it is advisable to remove and replace the tube.

3.7.2 Tube displacement

Most prosthetic tubes now used have a large proximal funnel which prevents distal displacement unless the lumen is large. Successful radiotherapy may occasionally shrink the growth and allow the tube to pass through it into the stomach.

Proximal displacement is much more common since tubes inserted by endoscopic means cannot be anchored by sutures. Recurrent bouts of vomiting and blockage of the tube are predisposing factors. To overcome the problem tubes incorporating a shoulder, flange or projections near the distal tip are used. If at a later date it becomes necessary to remove the tube the shoulder can usually be pulled back through the stricture since the presence of the tube for weeks or months serves to dilate the narrowing.

The proximal displacement of a tube necessitates its removal and replacement. This can sometimes be done by grasping the lip of the funnel with grasping forceps, of the type used to remove foreign bodies, passed down the biopsy channel of the endoscope. By this means it may be towed back until the funnel lies in the pharnyx where it can be seen and grasped by Magill's forceps. Care is necessary to avoid damaging the pharynx at this stage. The Nottingham introducer can be used to extract tubes by simply reversing the procedure used for insertion. A guide-wire is passed under endoscopic control down the tube and along this the introducer is advanced until its tip lies in the distal part of the tube. This can usually be assessed by measuring the distance from the incisor teeth along the introducer, but if difficulty is encountered, X-ray screening will confirm whether it is in satisfactory position. The bell is then expanded to grip the tube and the whole assembly is withdrawn gently.

3.7.3 Tube disintegration

Latex tubes left in position in the oesophagus or at the cardia undergo a structural deterioration with time, and whilst the majority of patients do not live long enough for this to reach practical importance, after 6–12 months' disintegration of the latex may release the nylon or metal spiral in the wall which then uncoils. Its end may appear at the anus (MacKenzie *et al.*, 1976). A segment of tube may become completely detached and pass on down the alimentary tract (Atkinson *et al.*, 1979) or if the tube remains *in situ* its wall may collapse causing blockage. It has been suggested that radiotherapy may accelerate structural deterioration in latex tubes but this is yet to be substantiated.

At present the best solution to the problem of deterioration of latex tubes is careful endoscopic surveillance of tubes which have been in position for more than six months and replacement of those in which softening has developed. Once disintegration has occurred, what remains of the tube in the oesophagus should be removed, and if the nylon spiral has become unravelled and its end passed through the pylorus this should be cut and allowed to pass on through the gut. The ultimate solution to this problem must lie in the development of a material more durable than latex which retains its flexibility and elasticity.

3.7.4 **Gastro-oesophageal reflux after intubation**

If the tube is placed across the cardia reflux of irritant gastric contents into the oesophagus usually occurs. This seldom causes more than mild heartburn which can be controlled by antacids and cimetidine, but at times severe oesophagitis can develop and lead to bleeding and ulceration around the upper end of the tube. A tube with a valvular mechanism on the distal end has been described by Davidenko *et al.* (1975) (Fig. 3.6(g)), but in this country gastro-oesophageal reflux is not a sufficiently frequent problem to warrant the use of such a prosthetic tube routinely.

3.8 PERFORATION OF THE GROWTH

3.8.1 **Immediate**

A perforation of the growth may be sustained during the insertion of the tube. If this occurs the procedure should if possible be completed and the patient managed conservatively with intravenous fluids and broad spectrum antibiotics. After a week oral feeding is recommenced and with these measures about 50% of patients make a satisfactory immediate recovery. The perforation rate varies with the skill of the endoscopist, with the debility of the patient and the extent and friability of the growth. If no patients are rejected as being unfit for the procedure a perforation rate of about 10% might be expected (Atkinson *et al.*, 1979).

3.8.2 **Late perforation**

Pressure of the prosthetic tube on the wall of a necrotic friable growth, particularly when this is at the cardia, may cause perforation weeks or months after intubation. Since the process is a more gradual one than when a tear is sustained during intubation, the onset of symptoms of mediastinitis is less dramatic but nevertheless such a perforation is nearly always fatal.

3.9 OUTLOOK AFTER INTUBATION

Intubation of oesophagogastric neoplasms is done primarily as a palliative measure to relieve distressing dysphagia rather than to prolong life. Although the immediate mortality in such an ill group of patients is considerable, about 80% of them are able to return home, swallowing adequately, within a few days of intubation, and both patient and relatives are often grateful that home management is possible during the terminal stages of their illness. The advantages of endoscopic over operative intubation are the lower immediate mortality, the avoidance of wound infection which often follows laparotomy, and the early discharge from hospital which is possible after endoscopic intubation.

Although the average survival is only three months, intubation does at times prolong life for a year or more without other treatment (Fig. 3.9).

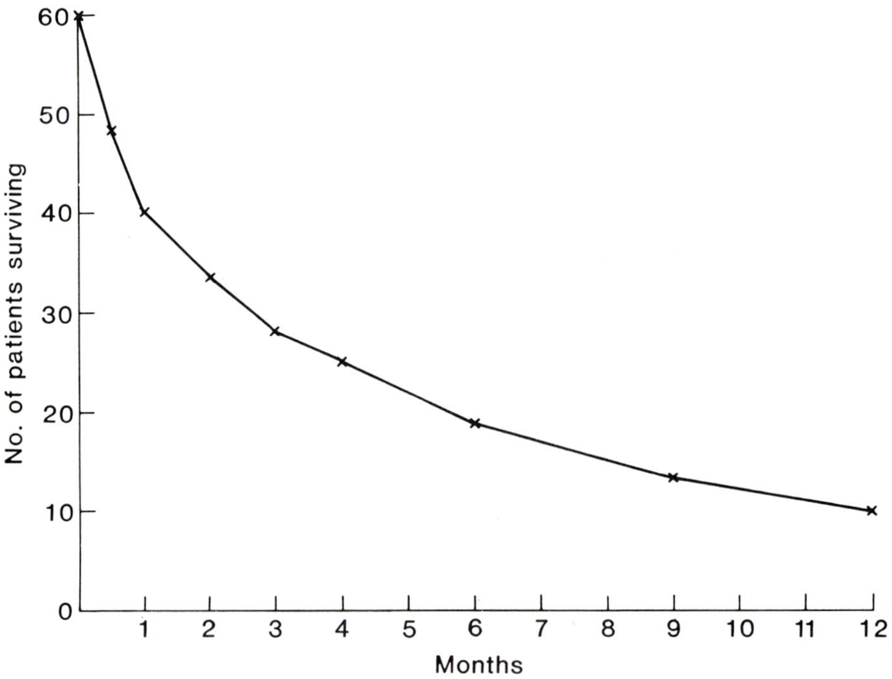

Fig. 3.9 Survival after insertion of a prosthetic tube in 60 patients with inoperable oesophageal or oesophagogastric carcinoma.

In some the nutritional improvement after intubation enables the patient to withstand radical radiotherapy or surgery. Occasionally after successful radiotherapy the tube can be removed without recurrence of dysphagia. Provided the patient is fit enough, radiotherapy should be considered for all squamous carcinomas.

3.10 NASOGASTRIC FEEDING

A prosthetic tube cannot be used when a growth arises ⩽5 cm below the cricoid level because of the intolerable discomfort caused by the presence of the funnel of the tube in the cricopharyngeal region. Growths arising outside the oesophagus and causing severe dysphagia from oesophageal compression are also often unsuitable for the insertion of a prosthetic tube because in the absence of any localized narrowing the tube tends to migrate. In these circumstances it is important to maintain nutrition while radiotherapy is given to shrink the growth with consequent relief of dysphagia. This is particularly important in cancer arising in the upper oesophagus which is commonly more responsive to radiotherapy and carries a better five-year survival after treatment than when it arises lower in the gullet (Pearson, 1977).

Slow nasogastric drip feeding through a soft 1-mm bore polyvinyl chloride tube inserted at endoscopy is useful to maintain nutrition during treatment. The method employed is to pass a stiffening wire down the fine bore PVC tube until its tip lies 2 cm proximal to the tube tip. The biopsy forceps are then passed down the biopsy channel of a narrow diameter endoscope such as the Olympus GIF P2 and the end of the fine bore tube is grasped and withdrawn into the end of the biopsy channel. The endoscope is then passed through the narrowing which, if necessary, has already been dilated, towing the fine bore tube with it until its tip lies in the stomach. The tube is released from the forceps and the stiffening wire keeps it in position whilst the endoscope is withdrawn. The stiffening wire is removed and the end of the tube is brought out through the nose by threading it through the oral end of a Ryle's tube which has been passed through the nose and brought out through the mouth. The Ryle's tube is then removed. Such fine bore nasogastric tubes cause the patient minimal discomfort and through them can be given liquid nourishment by continuous drip (Allison *et al.*, 1979).

REFERENCES

Allison, S. P. *et al.* (1979). Practical aspects of nutritional support. *Res. Clin. Forums*, **1**, 49–57.

Atkinson, M. and Ferguson, R. (1977). Fibreoptic endoscopic palliative intubation of inoperable oesophago-gastric neoplasms. *Br. Med. J.*, **1**, 266–67.

Atkinson, M., Ferguson, R. and Parker, G. C. (1978). Tube introducer and modified Celestin tube for use in palliative intubation of oesophago-gastric neoplasms at fibreoptic endoscopy. *Gut*, **19**, 669–71.

Atkinson, M., Ferguson, R. and Ogilvie, A. L. (1979). The management of malignant dysphagia by intubation at endoscopy. *J. R. Soc. Med.,* **72**, 894–7.

Boyce, H. W. (1973). Non-surgical measures to relieve distress of late oesophageal carcinoma. *Geriatrics,* **28**, 97–102.

Celestin, L. R. (1959). Permanent intubation in inoperable cancer of the oesophagus and cardia. *Ann. R. Coll. Surg.*, **25**, 165–70.

Celestin, L. R. *et al.* (1980). Traitement endoscopique des sténoses oesophagienne par prosthèse Celestin. *Nouv. Presse Med.*, **9**, 2155–57.

Davidenko, N. *et al.* (1975). Intubation des sténoses néoplastiques de l'oesophage – une nouvelle prosthèse avec dispositif anti-reflux. *Nouv. Presse Med.*, **4**, 2396–8.

den Hartog-Jager, F. C. A. *et al.* (1979). Palliative treatment of obstructing esophogastric malignancy by endoscopic positioning of a plastic prosthesis. *Gastroenterology,* **77**, 1008–14.

Didcott, C. C. (1973). Oesophageal strictures. *Ann. R. Coll. Surg.,* **53**, 112–26.

Durham, A. E. (1881). Report of proceedings of clinical society of London. *Lancet,* **ii**, 873.

Gillison, E. W., Khan, J. and Elliott, J. M. (1977). Endoscopic Celestin intubations for inoperable malignant dysphagia – a new use for the Foley catheter. *Gut*, **18**, 941–2.

Gourevitch, A. (1959). Intubation of the cardia for inoperable carcinoma. *Lancet,* **ii**, 258–60.

Guisez, J. (1914). De l'intubation caoutchoutée oesophagienne. *Presse. Med.,* **22**, 85–87.

Johnson, I. R., Balfour, T. W. and Bourke, J. B. (1976). Intubation of malignant gastro-oesophageal strictures. *J. R. Coll. Surg. Edinburgh,* **21**, 225–8.

Lewis, R. J. *et al.* (1973). Per oral esophageal intubation for obstructive carcinoma of the esophagus. *Ann. Thorac. Surg.,* **16**, 148–54.

MacKenzie, I., Whyte, A. S. and Tankel, H. I. (1976). Structural deterioration in Celestin tubes. *Br. J. Surg.,* **63**, 851–2.

Mousseau, M. *et al.* (1956). Place de l'intubation a demeure dans la traitement palliatif du cancer de l'oesophage. *Arch. Malad. Appar. Dig.,* **45**, 208–14.

O'Connor, T. *et al.* (1963). Esophageal prosthesis for palliative intubation. *Arch. Surg.,* **87**, 275–8.

Pearson, J. G. (1977). The present status and future potential of radiotherapy in the management of esophageal cancer. *Cancer,* **39**, 882–90.

Peura, D. A. *et al.* (1978). Esophageal prosthesis in cancer. *Am. J. Dig. Dis.,* **23**, 796–800.

Schetrumpf, J. R. (1973). Permanent intubation in terminal cancer of the oesophagus and cardia – a new tube. *Thorax,* **28**, 533–4.

Souttar, H. S. (1927). Treatment of carcinoma of the oesophagus based on 100 personal cases and 18 post mortem reports. *Br. J. Surg.,* **15**, 76–91.

Symonds, C. J. (1885). A case of malignant stricture of the oesophagus illustrating the use of a new form of oesophageal catheter. *Trans. Clin. Soc.,* **28**, 155–8.

Tytgat, G. N., den Hartog-Jager, F. C. A. and Havercamp, H. J. (1976). Positioning of a plastic prosthesis under fibre-endoscopic control in the palliative treatment of cardio-esophageal cancer. *Endoscopy,* **8**, 180–5.

Weisel, W. *et al.* (1959). Palliative treatment of esophageal carcinoma. *Ann. Surg.,* **149**, 207–16.

4 Oesophageal varices – endoscopic obliteration

K. G. D. WILLIAMS and A. CLARK

In the forty years since the first published account of injection treatment for oesophageal varices (Crafoord and Frenckner, 1939), the choice of treatment after a bleed has included vascular disconnection by splenectomy, decompression by portasystemic anastomosis, and disconnection by oesophageal transection, but recently there has been renewed interest in endoscopic injections. Throughout that time injections have been used as a first treatment after balloon tamponade in a number of centres on the European mainland, notably Vienna (Wodak, 1960) and Bonn (Paquet and Oberhammer, 1978). Several hundred cases are reported from each centre, but there is insufficient information on case selection and liver function, and many patients were later submitted to a portacaval shunt, so that an estimate of the true value of the injection procedure itself is difficult. Similar problems arise in the papers of Macbeth (1955) and Johnston and Rodgers (1973).

Several factors lie behind the present resurgence of interest in the procedure. Portacaval shunting has lost favour in Great Britain following the publication of clinical trials which showed no long-term benefit (Jackson *et al.*, 1971; Resnick *et al.*, 1974; Mikkelsen, 1974; Rueff *et al.*, 1976). Oesophageal transection was reported to have an operative mortality of over 50%, with 24 to 43% of patients surviving over one year (George, 1973; Pugh *et al.*, 1973). Pessimism over the value of this latter procedure may have been exaggerated, as in both series there was a heavy bias towards selecting cases with the worst prognosis. Perhaps the most significant point of the King's College Hospital paper was the appalling mortality (88%) for operations on patients whose liver function grade was C by Childs' method. As these comprise nearly one third of new cases the way was clearly open for a more thorough assessment of non-operative methods of treatment. The problem is increasing, with varices accounting for some 13–24% of new cases in recently collected haematemesis series.

4.1 TECHNIQUES OF INJECTION

4.1.1 **Rigid oesophagoscope**

In the United Kingdom and South Africa the Negus type of rigid oesophagoscope has usually been used, more recently with a slot cut in the side at the tip to allow a varix to intrude for easier injection (Bailey and Dawson, 1975) (Fig. 4.1). Using a rigid needle the operator aims to give an intravenous injection of up 8 ml of ethanolamine oleate before turning to the next varix, the injections being delivered as near to the oesophagogastric junction as possible. The injection procedure is often repeated at intervals of a few weeks until the varices shrink. Variations on this technique are numerous, particularly on the European continent where local anaesthetic is sometimes used and injections given up to three times a week for a short period. Some of the continental endoscopes contain a built-in suction channel which seems to be an advantage over our rigid and fibreoptic techniques because of the time taken to change from suction to injection and back again. Some practitioners inject submucosally beside the varix rather than into it. There is also disagreement about the advisability of concluding the procedure by passing a Sengstaken tube.

4.1.2 **Fibreoptic endoscope**

A flexible needle carrier with retractable needle has been available for some years. It can be used with any of the larger forward-viewing oesophagogastroduodenoscopes. In some centres it is used with the patient under sedation alone, either freehand or with the aid of an inflated gastric balloon which is pulled on to arrest upward blood flow at the time of injection (Kirkham, 1977; Lewis *et al*., 1979).

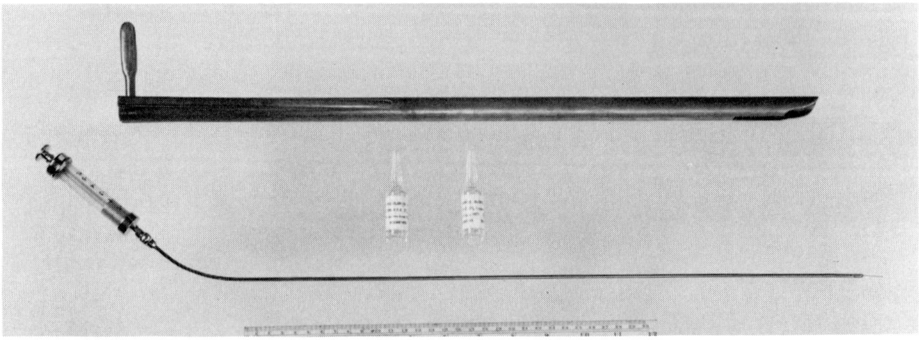

Fig. 4.1 Modified Negus oesophagoscope with rigid Macbeth needle and ethanolamine oleate.

A recent trend has been the use of a balloon inflated above the injection site to dilate the oesophageal lumen and occlude the varices in order to distend them and to prevent sclerosant from leaving the vein (Brunner and Schmidt, 1980; Shapiro and Johanson, 1980; Scott Brooks *et al.*, 1980). Firm evidence that this modification increases the effectiveness or ease of sclerotherapy has not yet accumulated. Our own preference has been to use a general anaesthetic (Ward *et al.*, 1976), together with a flexible outer sheath developed by one of the co-authors (Williams and Dawson, 1979). The sheath is 50 cm long, graduated, and has an internal diameter of 2 cm. A window 3 cm by 0.5 cm is cut 2 cm from the distal end and a mark placed on the same side at the proximal end for orientation (Fig. 4.2). The tube is used in conjunction with an Olympus GIF K gastroscope, and is available from Key-Med. The endoscope is lubricated with a little K-Y jelly and some water, and passed through the sheath. The free tip of the endoscope is passed down the oesophagus and the varices assessed. The outer sheath is then passed down over the endoscope, adjusting the slot to expose the most posterior varix at the oesophagogastric mucosal junction. The tip of the endoscope is flexed to fix it within the outer sheath, and the needle carrier advanced near the varix. The needle is then protruded and the carrier again advanced to pierce the mucosa (Figs. 4.3 and 4.4). Ethanolamine oleate is injected until it runs back out of the tissue or a total of 5 ml has been injected. The needle is then retracted and the carrier withdrawn after dropping the bridge of the endoscope, if that was used in the original aiming procedure. The whole sheath is then rotated to the next varix, thus pressing on the original injection site and allowing the process to be repeated, up to four times at the oesophagogastric junction. Occasionally the swelling produced within the slot is so big that it seems unwise to rotate the sheath. Instead, the endoscope is advanced into the stomach as a guide and the sheath disengaged from the swollen varix by advancing, before rotating to a new position and retracting to the original level. At the end of the series of injections the sheath is again advanced into the

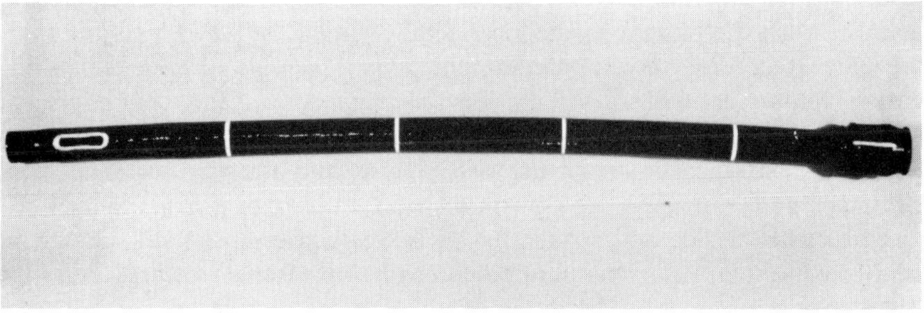

Fig. 4.2 The flexible 50-cm oesophageal varix injection tube.

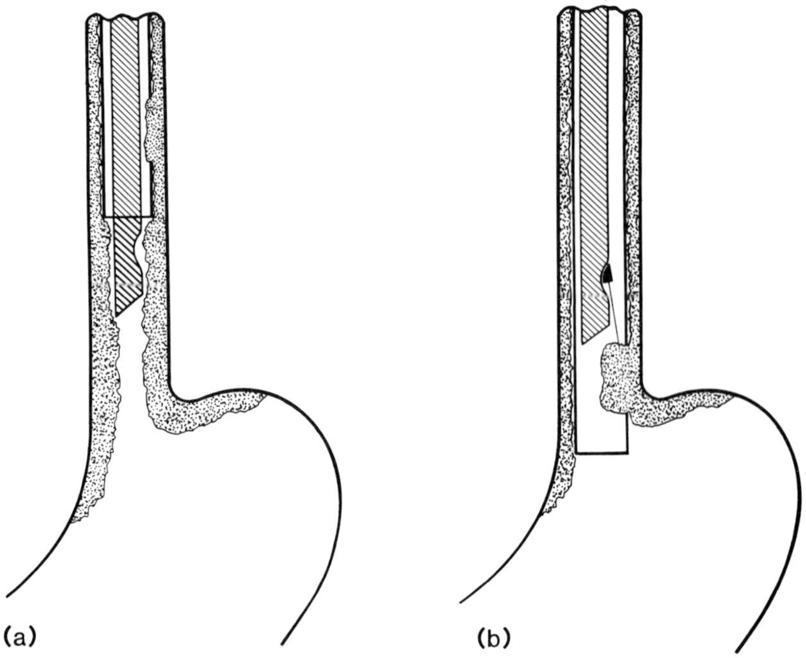

Fig. 4.3 (a) Tube ready to be pushed down gastroscope; (b) varix projecting through window ready for injection.

stomach so as to occlude the injection sites, and possibly the veins running up through the hiatus, for several minutes. The stomach is cleared of all fluid at this time. If there is no bleeding on withdrawing the sheath, major varices are again injected at a level about 5 cm above the original. The continuing appearance of blood or clot within the tube is an indication to return the endoscope and tube through the hiatus for a further period. The Sengstaken–Blakemore tube is hardly ever necessary to control bleeding and has no value in retaining sclerosant in the veins (Barsoum *et al.*, 1978). The endotracheal tube is removed as late as possible with the patient in the left lateral position.

Newer technical developments include the double lumen fibrescope which allows synchronous suction and injection, and a variety of ingeniously constructed proximal balloons on the shaft of the endoscope which distend the lumen of the oesophagus and the varices. The most attractive and expensive is a purpose built fibrescope (Wolf) which has two channels, a slot and a balloon, all in an instrument small enough to be passed under ordinary endoscopic sedation. Initial results with this have been excellent (Brunner and Schmidt, 1980), and further developments are expected.

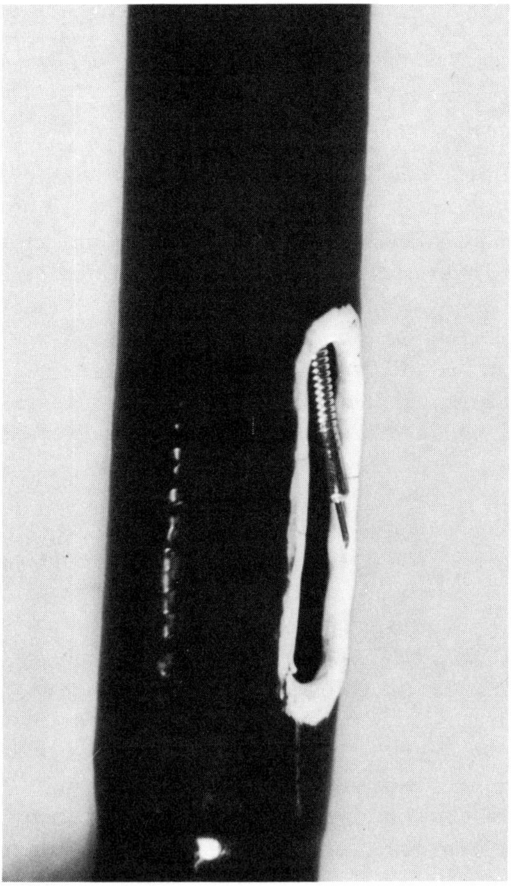

Fig. 4.4 The fine flexible needle projecting into window of tube.

4.1.3 **Site of injection**

It has been suggested that balloons and slots are better since they deliver the injection intravenously while controlling the flow of blood and sclerosant up the varix. Barsoum *et al.* (1978) showed that only a proportion of injections were intravenous. The contrast medium cleared rapidly, regardless of the slot, and well before a controlling Sengstaken tube could be passed. Clark and Wells (1977, unpublished) performed cinevenography in 12 patients, half with the flexible equipment and half with the rigid. In 30 injections only one venogram was produced, and that via the rigid endoscope. Since the same fibreoptic technique produced good results in the King's College Hospital prospective randomized trial (Clark *et al.*, 1980), particular care to introduce the needle into the lumen of the vein seems unnecessary. These considerations are of practical importance because the development of new techniques is clearly affected.

4.1.4 **Complications**

The small number of patients with serious complications prevents comparison of the two types of instrument except in the matter of perforation, which is described below. Other complications are pyrexia (16%), pain (12%), radiographic change at the lung base (9%), oesophageal ulcer (6%), oesophageal stricture (1.5%), and postinjection bleeding (2%). Using the rigid oesophagoscope and performing routine barium examinations after the procedure, Terblanche *et al.* (1979*b*) found three (8%) intramural or small perioesophageal leaks, which were successfully managed conservatively. The other percentages are taken from the King's College Hospital trial.

(a) *Perforation*

Perforation appears so far to be limited to the rigid technique. It is invariably fatal in cirrhosis and has occurred some seven times in the recollection of the King's group in an estimated 180 patients. There were two perforations in Terblanche's first fifteen patients receiving recurrent injections. The cirrhotic died while the other, with an extrahepatic obstruction, survived after major surgery. In retrospective reports, Johnston and Rodgers (1973) describe three perforations in 217 procedures, and Paquet and Oberhammer (1978) 11 in 640 patients. In contrast, patients treated with the flexible injection technique now number over 200 at King's College Hospital, and there have been no perforations.

(b) *Bleeding gastric varices*

These may be revealed at initial endoscopy or later. There are reports of attempted sclerosis by injection, but it is easy to see that this would be particularly difficult if the varix were in the fundus rather than readily accessible below the cardia. The problem has become apparent in a few patients in the King's College Hospital series, some predating the prospective trial. Clearly any method of direct attack on the oesophageal varices is likely to draw the attention of its critics to this problem, as theoretical consequences of obstructing upward flow and increasing the portal pressure. There are no reports of increased portal pressure after these procedures, probably because of the number of pathological connections between portal and systemic veins. More likely, the new increase in survival without oesophageal bleeding allows the gastric varices time to reveal their true potential, and the endoscopist at last has a clear view of them at the time of emergency readmission. The incidence of the problem is not yet known, is probably less than 5%, but may be expected to rise with increasing success in controlling the oesophageal bleeding.

4.1.5 Choice of technique

Rigid endoscopy is used less frequently, even by surgeons, who are turning to the safer fibreoptic technique. Some patients cannot accept the endoscope due to rigidity of the cervical spine, while kyphosis may prevent its passage into the stomach. Injection at the cardia requires some 5 cm of endoscope to be in the stomach. In a large patient the light guides of the endoscope often prevent its rotation, limiting the number of injection sites at the lower level. In contrast, the excellent lighting and optics of a fibreoptic endoscope mean that the gastro-oesophageal mucosal junction can readily be seen and injected confidently. An experienced endoscopist can soon learn the method. The use of the slotted sheath for control and stability has been particularly valuable.

4.2 DISCUSSION

Much confusion has arisen about the uses and usefulness of injection sclerotherapy, for a variety of reasons. Perhaps the most important is the failure of those discussing the procedure to identify clearly the patient population treated, and the type and severity of liver disease. After injection, the application of further different therapeutic measures clouds the results, while the lack of a control group has often deepened the mystery still further. One prospective study in acute haemorrhage (Terblanche *et al.*, 1979*a*), and two prospective randomized controlled studies of recurrent injection (Terblanche *et al.*, 1979; Clark *et al.*, 1980) make the situation clearer.

In extrahepatic portal vein obstruction, the varices respond well to injections, as Crafoord and Frenckner (1939) showed. Since then it has been well shown that patients with this diagnosis fare better than those with cirrhosis (Sherlock, 1964; Grauer and Schwartz, 1979). Nevertheless, most authors continue to include them in their reports. Their presence is misleading in two ways. First they may be unequally distributed between control and treatment groups. Second, they survive to bleed again, so that where an author reports results by the number of bleeding episodes controlled, the number of extrahepatic obstruction cases rises. In the Johnston and Rodgers (1973) report, the 217 procedures included some 30% in extrahepatic obstruction rather than the 5–10% expected normally.

In this discussion we consider the possible application of variceal sclerotherapy in relation to the following possible therapeutic aims.

1. Prevention of initial haemorrhage.
2. Arrest of acute bleeding.
3. Eradication of varices.
4. Prevention of recurrent haemorrhage.
5. Prolongation of life.

4.2.1 **Prevention of initial haemorrhage**

This remains an unlikely prospect. Only a small proportion of patients with varices bleed, and the practical and economic problems of treating every patient make wholesale therapy unlikely. Paquet has carried out a prospective trial in the subgroup with large varices and oesophagitis. The work is unpublished but apparently the injected group had fewer bleeds (6%) than the controls (30%) during the observation period.

4.2.2 **Arrest of acute bleeding**

This is the main claim in many series. In the first part of the King's College Hospital prospective study (Clark *et al.*, 1980) 46 consecutive cirrhotics with proven variceal bleeding were assessed. Forty stopped bleeding with conventional medical management including balloon tamponade. Hence it seems that with *no* treatment other than balloon tamponade and medical support the initial bleed is controlled in some 85% of cases, and this figure is not notably improved by emergency injections in the prospective study from Cape Town (Terblanche *et al.*, 1979*a*). Nevertheless these authors claimed a marked improvement in comparison with a retrospective review in their own unit.

In Belfast (Johnston and Rodgers, 1973), 10 patients were not controlled by injections. It is reasonable to assume that most of these were among the 87 cirrhotics, so making it difficult to be sure of the benefits of early injection. The King's group found emergency rigid endoscopy in the bleeding patient both difficult and dangerous, and were less impressed than some authors with the outcome.

There are no published prospective randomized trials which test the value of emergency injection but Ihre is conducting one in Stockholm where the cases are nearly all alcoholic. At this early stage bleeding control and survival appear much better in the treated group. Again the control group is much worse off than the K.C.H. control patients.

The problem of when to initiate treatment will recede in the face of technical improvements allowing safe injection without anaesthesia in bleeding patients.

4.2.3 **Eradication of varices**

Eradication by repeated injection seems a logical aim, although it cannot readily be achieved in all patients. The clearest account of this approach is from the Karolinska Hospital (Kempe and Koch, 1954). Of the 15 patients who survived splenectomy and the initial few months of injections, six seemed to lose their varices, while nine did not. Terblanche *et al.* (1979*b*) have attacked the varices remorselessly, feeling that any varix is dangerous. The King's College Hospital group have taken the other view, being satisfied with the characteristic white thickened mucosa which appears after a number of injections. Late rebleeding has not been a problem in our series even among those with large persistent varices.

4.2.4 **Prevention of recurrent haemorrhage**

This was clearly achieved in the prospective controlled trials in Cape Town (Terblanche *et al.*, 1979*b*) and London (Clark *et al.*, 1980). The differences in technique, organization and management of the two trials serve only to emphasize the similarity in outcome. Control patients are three to four times more likely to have a further bleed than those given prophylactic injections, and attrition of the control group by deaths from bleeding does not appear to diminish the risk of bleeding among those surviving longer. In the King's College Hospital study, 30% of those at risk rebled each month, while the treated group had only a 10% risk which fell even lower after six months. The mortality for rebleeding remains depressingly high, however it is managed, and emphasizes the need to institute injection therapy as soon as possible after a first bleed, and to repeat it as frequently as possible until variceal shrinkage or mucosal sclerosis appear.

4.2.5 **Prolongation of life**

This ought logically to follow from success in preventing recurrent bleeding, but might be counterbalanced by lethal complications of the injection procedure itself (and the general anaesthesia accompanying it). Again, death might follow from inexorable progression of the liver disease. Five patients died in each group in the Cape Town trial (Terblanche *et al.*, 1979*b*), while among the survivors, only half lived for a year or more, being 30% of the total. Actuarial survival has not been calculated, but there is no apparent benefit for the treated group, perhaps because few in either group died principally from bleeding. This outcome is made particularly likely by the repeated injections given to the control group during their acute bleeding episodes. If the postrandomization

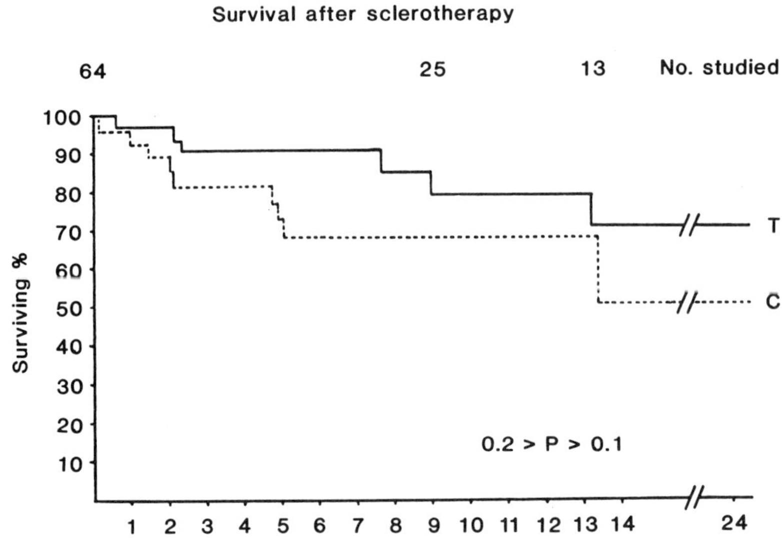

Fig. 4.5 Survival after sclerotherapy. Deaths from haemorrhage were more common in the control group (dotted line) than the treated group (solid line), but the life-table shows no significant differences (log rank sum test).

exclusions are ignored, the controls underwent a total of 19 injection procedures, and the treated group 40.

In the King's College Hospital trial the controls received no injections, and alternative measures for managing rebleeding have proved notably ineffective. Deaths from liver failure alone were equally balanced between the two groups. The overall chance of survival at one year was 81% in the treated group, and 68% in the controls (Fig. 4.5). The early appearance of a significant difference has been counteracted by improved survival in the control group during the second year of the trial. The numbers are now large enough to suggest that survival is not significantly better and that this conclusion will not be overthrown. An important criticism of this study is the lack of intervention in the control group after the first bleed. However, the price of such intervention would have been high. Based on the Childs' grades of our first 16 control patients and the mortality figures from transection in the same unit, the expected mortality would be 44% from operation alone, whereas the number of deaths associated with bleeding was five (32%).

4.3 CONCLUSIONS

Although the evidence for the value of injections in acute haemorrhage has been criticized it seems to have a place in management, particularly in poor risk patients who would almost certainly die from surgery. The value of the procedure in preventing further bleeds seems proved by two separate trials, one of which shows improved survival over a control group who were disadvantaged by having no elective treatment after the first bleed. The survival curve for the treated group compares favourably with the best results in trials of portacaval shunt after haemorrhage, and has been achieved in a group with considerably worse liver function than those submitted to shunt surgery. Hence, sclerotherapy by the fibreoptic technique described ought now to be the reference point for trials of other techniques of long-term management. Developments of technique and assessment of results is proceeding actively in centres throughout the world.

REFERENCES

Bailey, M. E. and Dawson, J. L. (1975). Modified oesophagoscope for injecting oesophageal varices. *Br. Med. J.*, **2**, 540.

Barsoum, M. S., Khattar, N.Y. and Risk-Allah, M. A. (1978). Technical aspects of injection sclerotherapy of acute oesophageal variceal haemorrhage as seen by radiography. *Br. J. Surg.*, **65**, 588–9.

Brunner, G. and Schmidt, F. W. (June, 1980). A modified oesophagoscope for sclerotherapy of bleeding oesophageal varices, *IV Eur. Cong. Gastrointest. Endosc.* (Hamburg). George Thieme Verlag, Stuttgart, New York.

Clark, A. W. *et al.* (1980). Prospective controlled clinical trial of injection sclerotherapy in cirrhotic patients with recent variceal haemorrhage. *Lancet,* **ii**, 552.

Crafoord, C. and Frenckner, P. (1939). New Surgical treatment of varicose veins of the oesophagus. *Acta Otolaryngol.*, **27**, 422.

George, P. (1973). Emergency oesophageal transection in uncontrolled variceal haemorrhage. *Br. J. Surg.*, **60**, 635.

Grauer, S. E. and Schwartz, S. I. (1979). Extrahepatic portal hypertension: a retrospective analysis. *Ann. Surg.*, **189**, 566.

Ihre, T., personal communication.

Jackson, F. C. *et al.* (1971). A clinical investigation of the portacaval shunt: survival of the therapeutic operation. *Ann. Surg.*, **174**, 673.

Johnston, G. W. and Rodgers, H. W. (1973). A review of 15 years' experience. The use of sclerotherapy in the control of acute haemorrhage from oesophageal varices. *Br. J. Surg.*, **60**, 797–800.

Kempe, S.-G. and Koch, H. (1954). Injection of sclerosing solutions in the treatment of oesophageal varices. *Acta Otolaryngolgica,* Suppl., **118**, 120.

Kirkham, J. S. (1977). Personal communication.

Lewis, J., Chung, R. S. and Allison, J. (1979). Sclerotherapy of oesophageal varices. *Arch. Surg.*, **115**, 476.

Macbeth, R. (1955). Treatment of oesophageal varices in portal hypertension by means of sclerosing injections. *Br. Med. J.*, **2**, 877.

Mikkelsen, W. P. (1974). Therapeutic portacaval shunt. *Arch. Surg.*, **108**, 302.

Paquet, K.-J. and Oberhammer, E. (1978). Sclerotherapy of bleeding oesophageal varices by means of endoscopy. *Endoscopy,* **10**, 7–12.

Pugh, R. N. H. *et al.* (1973). Transection of the oesophagus for bleeding oesophageal varices. *Br. J. Surg.*, **60**, 646.

Resnick, R. H. *et al.* (1974). A controlled study of the therapeutic portacaval shunt. *Gastroenterology,* **67**, 843.

Rueff, B. *et al.* (1976). A controlled study of therapeutic portacaval shunt in alcoholic cirrhosis. *Lancet*, **1**, 655.

Scott Brooks, W. *et al.* (1980). Adaptation of the flexible endoscope for endoscopic sclerosis of esophageal varices. *Abstr. IV Eur. Congr. Gastrointest. Endosc.*, Georg Thieme Verlag, Stuttgart, New York.

Shapiro, H. A. and Johanson, C. (1980). Transfibersophogoscopic sclerotherapy for esophageal varices. *Abstr. IV Eur. Congr. Gastrointest. Endosc.*, Georg Thieme Verlag, Stuttgart, New York.

Sherlock, S. (1964). Haematemesis in portal hypertension. *Br. J. Surg.*, **51**, 746.

Terblanche, J. *et al.*, (1979*a*). A prospective evaluation of injection sclerotherapy in the treatment of acute bleeding from oesophageal varices. *Surgery*, **85**, 239.

Terblanche, J. *et al.* (1979*b*). Controlled trial of sclerotherapy in the long-term management of patients after oesophageal variceal bleeding. *Surg. Gynec. Obstet.,* **148**, 323.

Ward, M. E., Davies, T. D. W. and Strunin, L. (1976). Anaesthesia for injection of bleeding oesophageal varices. *Ann. Coll. Surg.,* **58**, 315.

Williams, K. G. D. and Dawson, J. L. (1979). Fibreoptic injection of oesophageal varices. *Br. Med. J.,* **2**, 766.

Wodak, V. E. (1960). Osophagusvarizen-Blutung bei portaler Hypertension; ihre Therapie und Prophylaxe. *Wien. Med. Wschr.,* **27**, 581.

5 Oesophageal varices – obliteration by percutaneous transhepatic injection

ANDERS LUNDERQUIST

The treatment of patients with bleeding oesophageal varices is still an unsolved problem. Many different forms of treatment have been advocated but all seem to have some drawbacks, mainly because progressive disease of the key organ, the liver, cannot be cured.

Standard emergency medical management of these patients (Johnson *et al.*, 1977; Terblanche *et al.*, 1974) includes fresh blood and intravenous pitressin. Patients whose bleeding does not stop during this treatment receive a Sengstaken–Blakemore tube, which in most cases will control the bleeding. However, if bleeding continues, the selection of further treatment is controversial. Emergency portacaval shunt operation carries such a high operative mortality (Orloff *et al.*, 1975) that it is important to try and perform only elective surgery.

On the other hand, it has not been possible to prove that a surgical shunt will increase the length of survival as compared with more conservative methods of treatment (Resnik *et al.*, 1974; Rueff *et al.*, 1976). This has been the stimulus to try other methods such as transoesophageal sclerotherapy (Paquet and Oberhammer, 1978) (see Chapter 4) and percutaneous transhepatic obliteration of the oesophageal varices (Bengmark *et al.*, 1979; Goldman *et al.*, 1976; Lunderquist and Vang, 1974; Lunderquist *et al.*, 1977; Lunderquist *et al.*, 1978; Pereiras *et al.*, 1977; Viamonte *et al.*, 1977) to prevent recurrent variceal bleeding. Both these methods have the advantage of preserved liver perfusion.

This chapter will be concerned with the technique and the evaluation of percutaneous transhepatic obliteration of oesophageal varices in patients with portal hypertension. It should be emphasized that this technique is not established for elective use, but may be valuable in emergencies to arrest active variceal bleeding when other standard techniques have failed.

5.1 TECHNIQUE

Before percutaneous transhepatic catheterization of the portal vein is attempted it is important to show that portal vein thrombosis is not present. This is most easily done by arterial portography, i.e. injection of a large volume of contrast medium into the superior mesenteric artery, usually after the injection of a vasodilator (25 mg priscolin) into the same artery. During the venous return of the contrast medium the portal vein is well demonstrated.

If the portal vein is patent the liver is punctured in the midaxillary line with a long needle sheathed with a radio-opaque polyethylene catheter. The puncture is performed under local anaesthesia usually through the obliterated costophrenic pleura and as straight as possible against the hilum of the liver (Hoevels *et al.*, 1978).

After the needle has been withdrawn the catheter is slowly pulled back, using intermittent aspiration. When blood can be aspirated, a test injection of contrast medium during fluoroscopy will show if the tip of the catheter is in a portal vein branch. If this is the case, a slightly curved guide-wire is manipulated through the portal vein into the splenic vein. The catheter is then pushed over the guide-wire until its tip is in the midportion of the splenic vein. The guide-wire is removed and the portal vein pressure is recorded. Portography is performed by injection of 40 ml of 76% contrast medium at a rate of 8 ml/s using a filming rate of one film/s over 8 s followed by one film every 2 s for 16 s.

Guided by the portographic findings, the veins draining the portal blood to the oesophageal varices are catheterized and obliterated by injection of 0.3–1 ml of isobutyl-2-cyanoacrylate (Bucrylate) (Lunderquist *et al.*, 1978). This monomer has the property of polymerizing immediately on contact with an ionized solution.

In order to prevent its polymerizing within the catheter, a thin coaxial catheter is introduced and the tip advanced 0.5–1 cm beyond the outer catheter. Both catheters are irrigated with 5.5% dextrose solution which, as a non-ionized solution, will prevent the Bucrylate from polymerizing and occluding the catheters when it is finally injected through the inner catheter. After removal of the inner catheter, a test injection of contrast medium will show if the vein has been occluded or whether the procedure has to be repeated. After all veins draining to the oesophageal varices have been occluded, a second portography is performed as a final check. The catheter is then slowly pulled out and a small piece of gelfoam injected into the puncture canal 1–2 cm beneath the surface of the liver to prevent bleeding into the pleura or peritoneal cavity.

A transjugular or transumbilical approach to the portal vein may also be used when gastro-oesophageal varices have to be occluded. Both methods, however, have some drawbacks. Transjugular catheterization is more time-consuming and the manipulation of the catheter more difficult because of the distance to the liver. As for the transumbilical approach, a surgical procedure is necessary to reopen the umbilical vein, and even here the catheter is more difficult to manipulate because the curve of the catheter has to pass from the umbilical vein to the main stem of the portal vein. Another disadvantage of the transumbilical approach is that the radiologist has to have his hands in the radiation field when manipulating the catheter.

5.2 RESULTS

In a first series of 21 patients with portal hypertension (Lunderquist *et al.*, 1977) who had bled or were bleeding from oesophageal varices, obliteration of veins was performed at our institution by injection of thrombin, gelfoam, and etolein. [Etolein (Astra, Sweden) is a sclerosing agent used for injection into varices of the leg.] As a consequence of the occlusion of the outflow tract via the oesophageal varices, portal vein pressure rose by a mean of about five centimetres of water. The philosophy behind this method of treatment was not only to obliterate the bleeding veins but also to increase the perfusion of the liver. When portal pressure rises the blood flow through other portasystemic collaterals (such as inferior mesenteric vein, umbilical vein, and connections to the left renal vein) should theoretically increase (Fig. 5.1).

In 16 cases the procedure was performed electively in patients who previously had bled from oesophageal varices. Five patients were treated when they were actually bleeding, and the bleeding stopped as a consequence of the procedure in four; 12 patients were re-examined by transhepatic portography five days to eight months (median 93 days) after the obliterating procedure. In 10 patients the previously obliterated vein had recanalized and a new obliteration had to be performed. In two patients the previously obliterated left gastric vein was still occluded five and three months later, but in one of the patients the short gastric veins had opened up and drained to the oesophageal varices. No complications occurred that could be referred to the procedure.

The conclusion drawn from these results was that the combination of thrombin, gelfoam, and etolein was not adequate for permanent occlusion of oesophageal varices. In emergency cases, however, the method could be used to arrest haemorrhage when other methods had failed.

Another group with great experience of this technique (Pereiras *et al.*, 1977; Viamonte *et al.*, 1977) did not find the same high degree of recanalization of previously obliterated veins. In a series of 67 patients with successful obliteration of gastro-oesophageal veins 10 patients were re-examined and showed persistent obliteration of the veins.

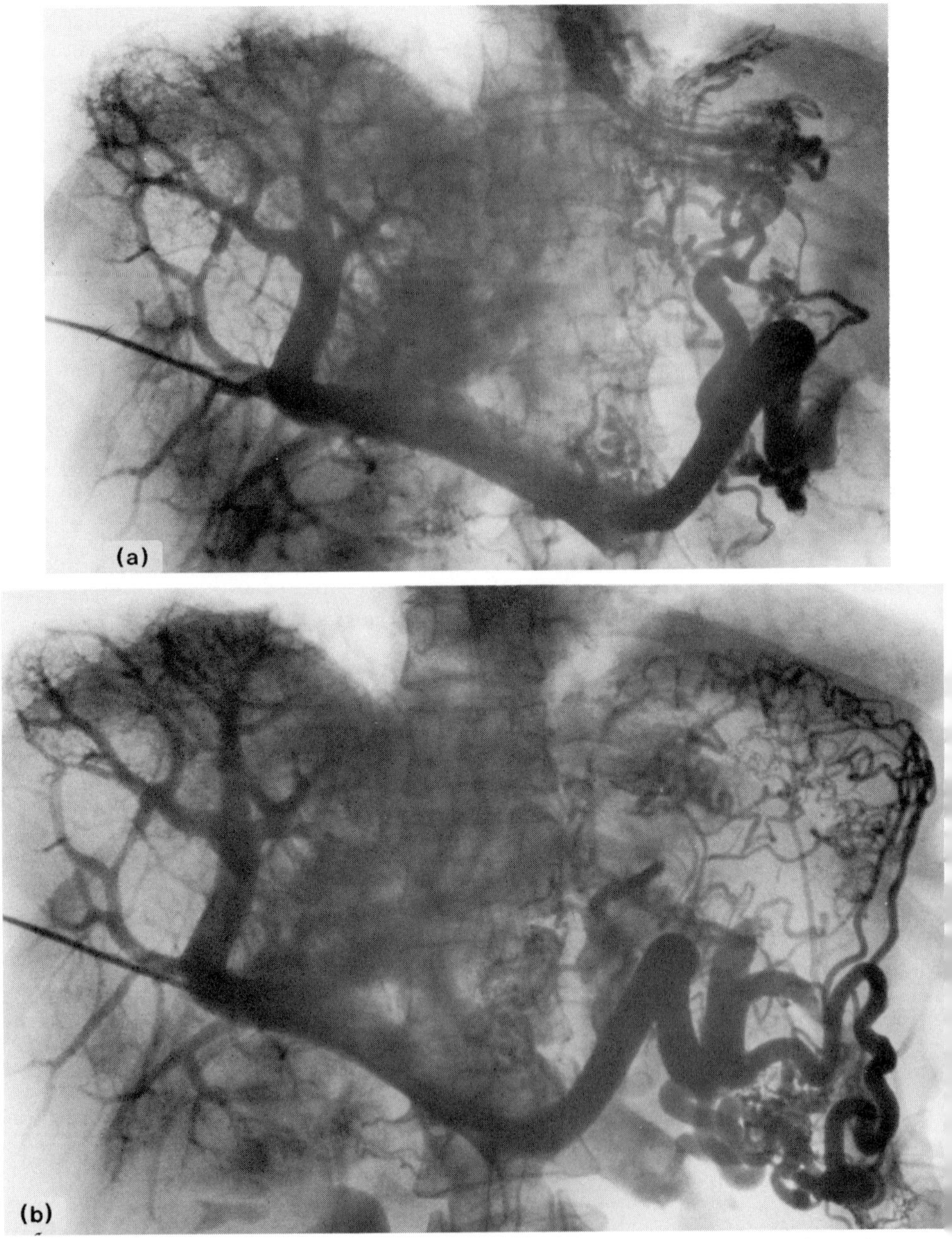

Fig. 5.1 A 34-year-old woman with cirrhosis and bleeding oesophageal varices. Percutaneous transhepatic portography. (*a*) Portal vein pressure 37 cm water. Wide collateral from the splenic vein draining to the oesophageal varices. (*b*) After transcatheter obliteration of the vein feeding the oesophageal varices portal vein pressure rose to 40 cm water. Wide collateral to left renal vein.

To produce permanent occlusion and prevent recanalization, isobutyl-2-cyanoacrylate (Bucrylate) has been tried to occlude the veins draining to the oesophageal varices (Bengmark *et al.*, 1979; Freeny and Kidd, 1979; Goldman *et al.*, 1976; Lunderquist *et al.*, 1978). In a series of 43 patients with portal hypertension we (Bengmark *et al.*, 1979) found frequent rebleeding even after Bucrylate obliteration. Bucrylate obliteration did not totally prevent recanalization but when this occurred the recanalized veins were markedly reduced in size (Fig. 5.2). The main reason for rebleeding was, however, that new collaterals opened up, draining portal venous blood through the oesophageal varices to the azygos and hemiazygos veins. These collaterals usually originated from an extensive network of veins at the upper hilum of the spleen (Fig. 5.3). Other portasystemic collaterals, such as inferior mesenteric vein, paraumbilical vein, and connections to the left renal vein, often dilated but could apparently not drain enough of the portal blood to prevent new veins from draining through the oesophagus.

Fourteen patients were treated on 16 occasions when they were acutely bleeding. One patient was treated three different times for acute bleeding. On 14 occasions the bleeding stopped as a consequence of the treatment, but five of those patients rebled within a week. Mesocaval shunt operation was performed in four and splenectomy in one patient because of rebleeding. Five patients not surgically treated later developed a portal vein thrombosis and died nine days to two years after the embolization procedure.

When varices were obliterated with Bucrylate, some serious complications were recorded. Among 43 patients one died after two days from intra-abdominal bleeding caused by the transhepatic catheterization. Three other patients bled from the site of the puncture but the bleeding stopped after treatment with fresh blood transfusion. One complication that is more difficult to explain is the development of portal vein thrombosis which occurred in six patients, nine days to two years after the embolization procedure. How can a thrombosis develop in the portal vein when other obliterated veins recanalize? It is possible that, when the outflow to the oesophageal varices is blocked, the flow in the portal vein stagnates, predisposing to thrombosis.

It is thus clear that obliteration of gastro-oesophageal varices should not be considered an alternative to surgical or medical treatment in patients who are not actually bleeding. As an *emergency* treatment obliteration of the varices can be performed when other non-surgical methods to stop the bleeding have failed. For this purpose, the technique seems effective. To prevent the development of a portal vein thrombosis the obliterating procedure should be followed by an elective surgical shunt operation as soon as possible.

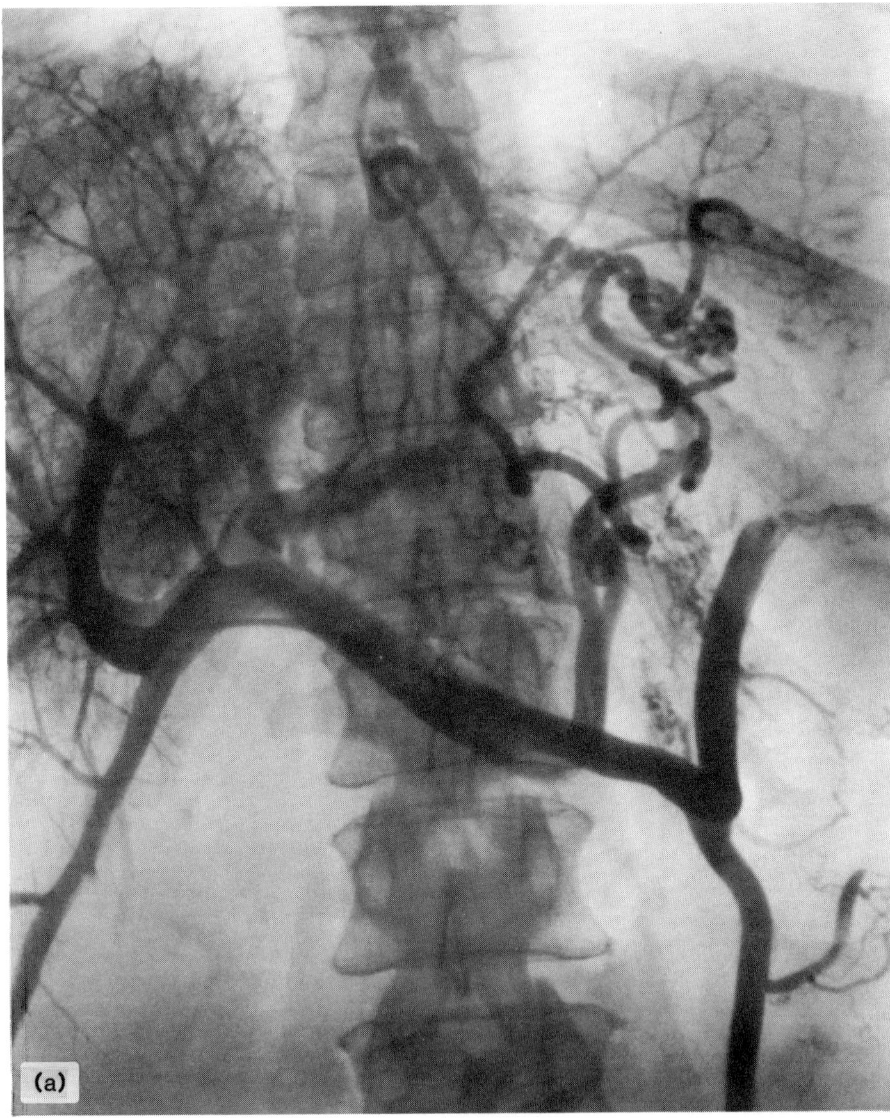

Fig. 5.2 (*a, b, c, d* and *e*) A 57-year-old woman with cirrhosis and bleeding from oesophageal varices. Percutaneous transhepatic portography. (*a*) Portal vein pressure 39 cm water. Wide left gastric vein drain to oesophageal varices. Retrograde flow through wide inferior mesenteric vein.

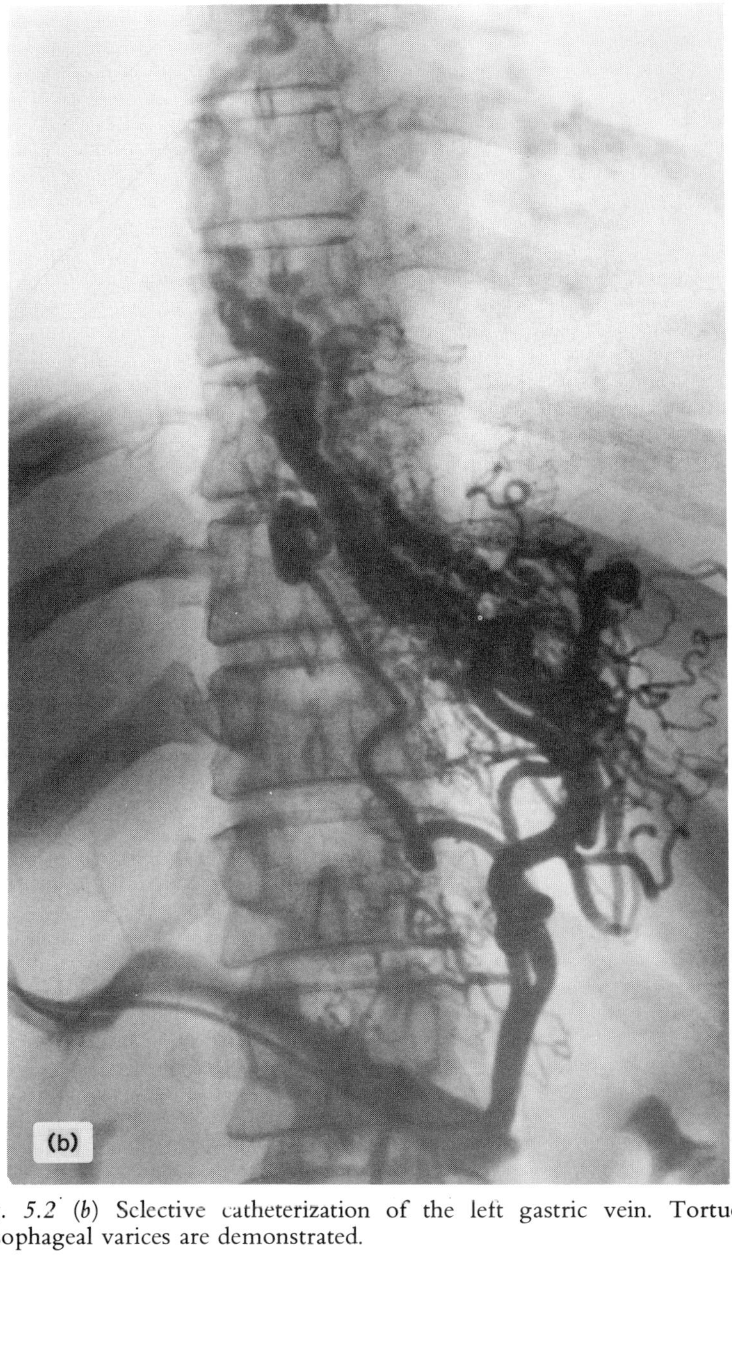

Fig. 5.2 (b) Selective catheterization of the left gastric vein. Tortuous oesophageal varices are demonstrated.

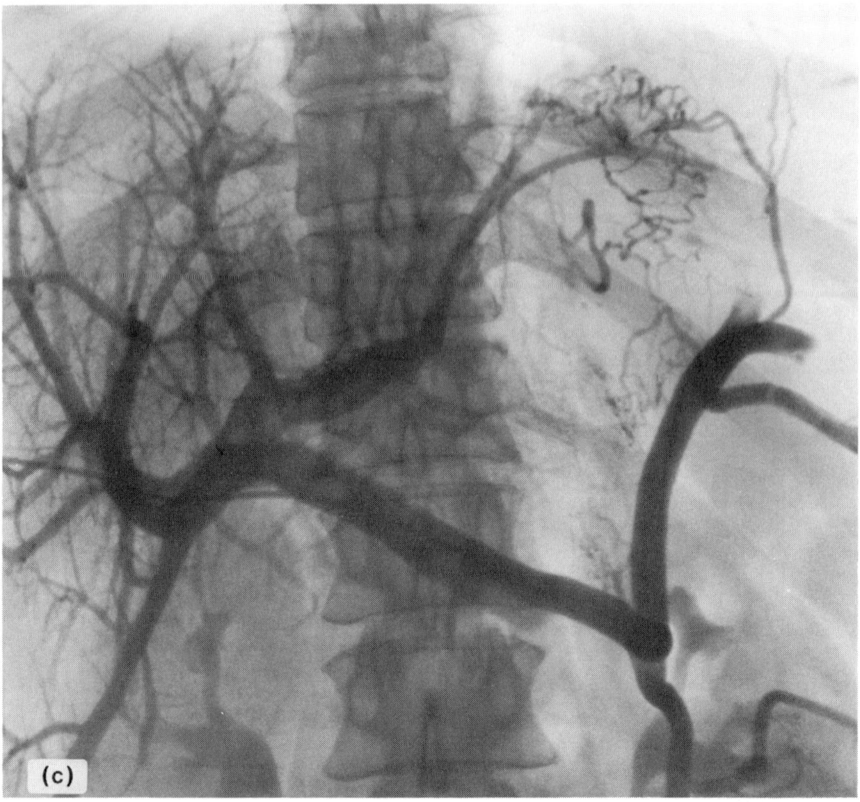

Fig. 5.2 (*c*) Portal vein presure 41 cm water. Left gastric vein obliterated with Bucrylate. No filling of oesophageal varices.

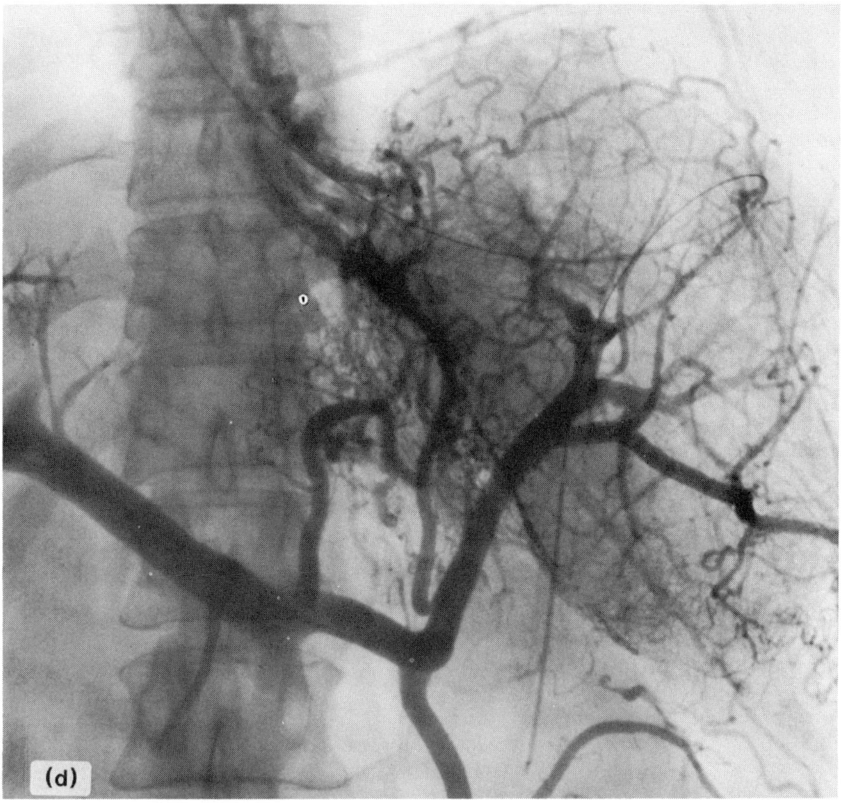

Fig. 5.2 (*d*) Percutaneous transhepatic portography one year after obliteration of left gastric vein. Recurrent bleeding from varices. Portal vein pressure 40 cm water. Left gastric vein (recanalized) and another vein from the splenic vein are feeding oesophageal varices.

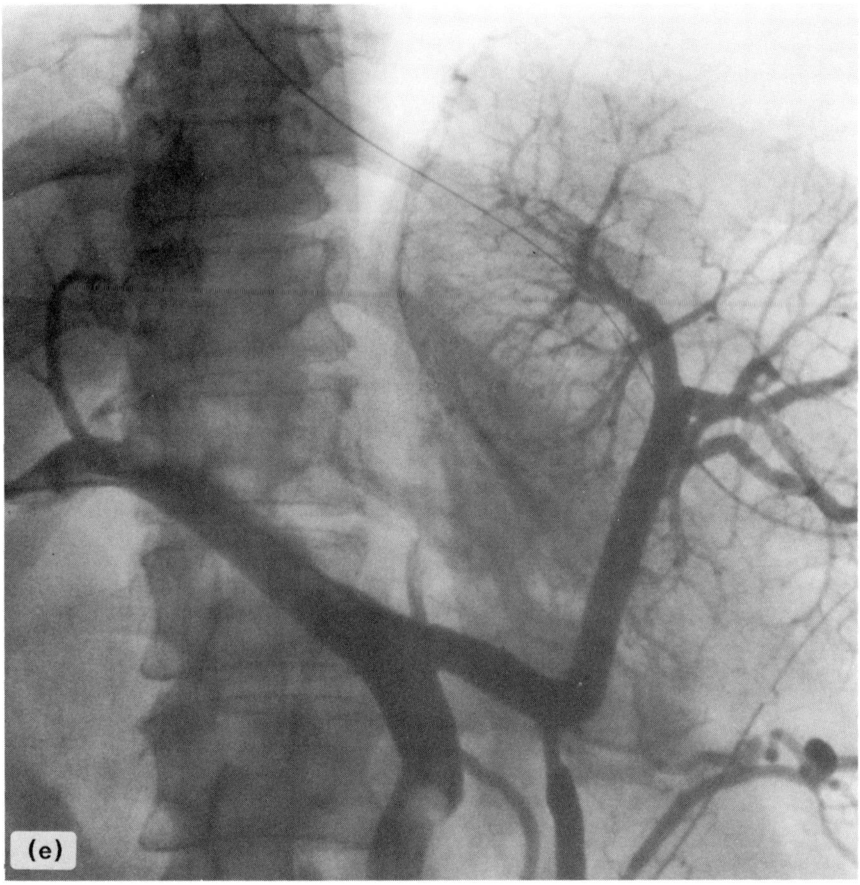

Fig. 5.2 (*e*) Veins feeding oesophageal varices are obliterated with Bucrylate. No filling of varices with contrast medium. Portal vein pressure 44 cm water.

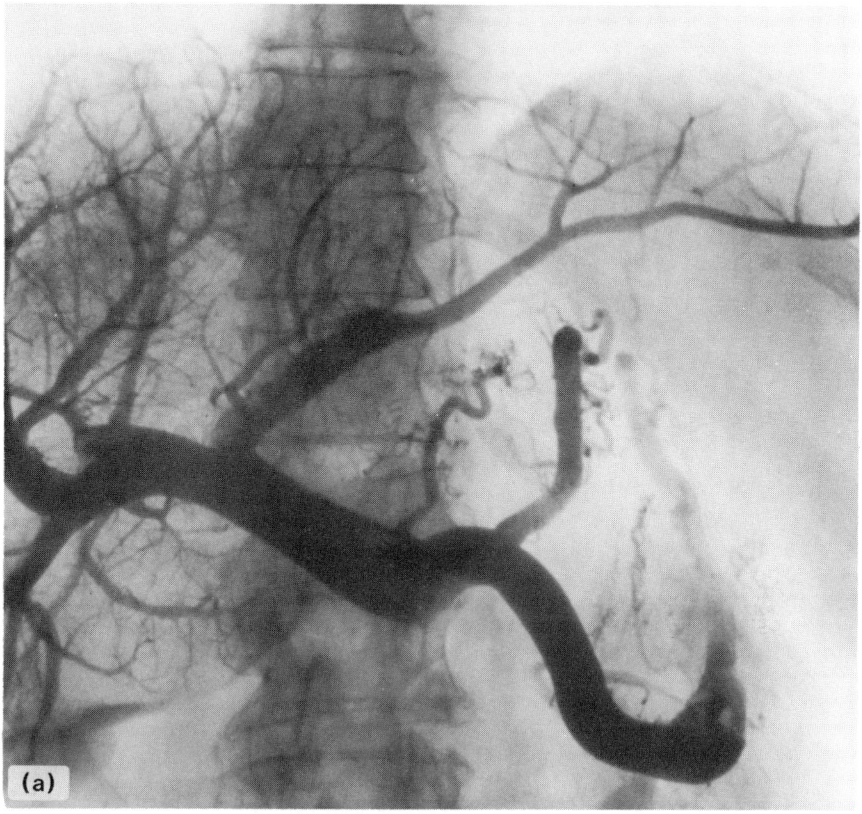

Fig. 5.3 (*a*, *b* and *c*) A 61-year-old woman with cirrhosis and bleeding oesophageal varices. Percutaneous transhepatic portography. (*a*) Portal vein pressure 39 cm water. One wide and one smaller vein extends towards the fundus of the stomach.

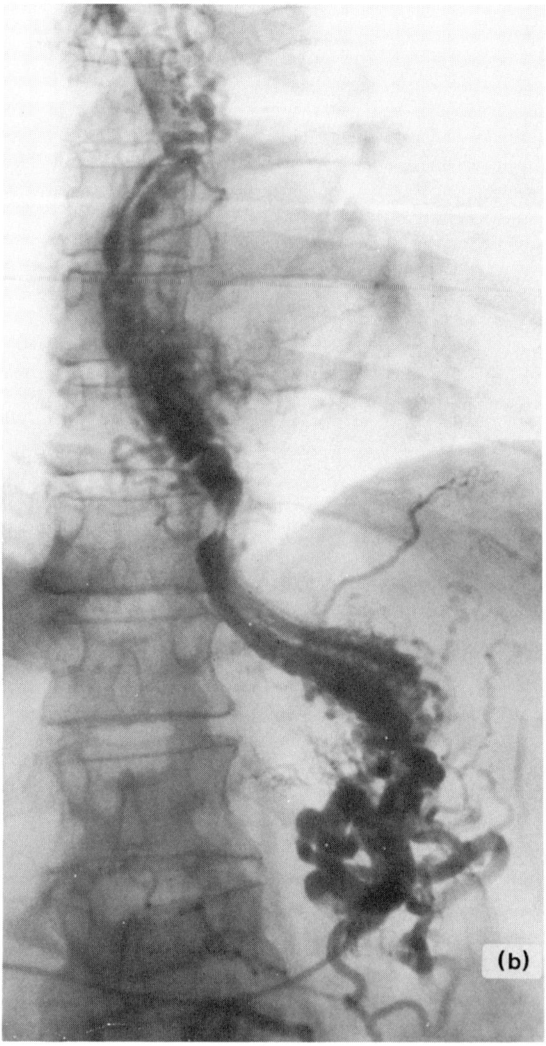

Fig. 5.3 (*b*) Selective catheterization of the wider vein which feeds large oesophageal varices.

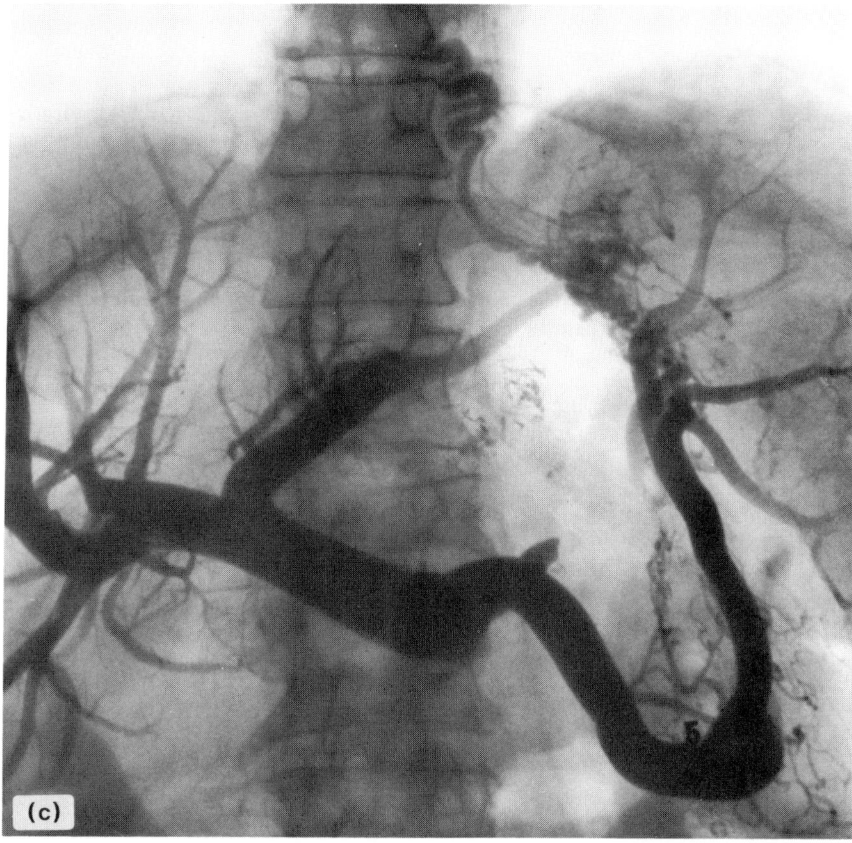

Fig. 5.3 (*c*) Portal vein pressure 39 cm water. Both the larger and smaller collateral seen in (a) are obliterated with Bucrylate. However, numerous small veins from upper hilum of spleen are still feeding the varices.

REFERENCES

Bengmark, S. *et al.* (1979). Obliteration of esophageal varices by PTP – a follow-up of 43 patients. *Ann. Surg.*, in press.

Freeny, P. C. and Kidd, R. (1979). Transhepatic portal venography and selective obliteration of gastroesophageal varices using isobutyl-2-cyanoacrylate (Bucrylate). *Dig. Dis. Sci.*, **24**, 321–30.

Goldman, M. L. *et al.* (1976). Transcatheter therapeutic embolization in the management of massive upper gastrointestinal bleeding. *Radiology*, **120**, 513–21.

Hoevels, J. *et al.* (1978). Percutaneous transhepatic portography. *Acta Radiol. Diagn.*, **19**, 643–55.

Johnson, W. C. *et al.* (1977). Control of bleeding varices by vasopressin: a prospective randomized study. *Ann. Surg.*, **186**, 369–76.

Lunderquist, A. and Vang, J. (1974). Transhepatic catheterization and obliteration of the coronary vein in patients with portal hypertension and esophageal varices. *New Engl. J. Med.*, **291**, 646–9.

Lunderquist, A. *et al.* (1977). Follow-up of patients with portal hypertension and esophageal varices treated with percutaneous obliteration of gastric coronary vein. *Radiology*, **122**, 59–63.

Lunderquist, A. *et al.* (1978). Isobutyl-2-cyanoacrylate (Bucrylate) in obliteration of gastric coronary vein and esophageal varices. *Am. J. Roentg.*, **130**, 1–6.

Orloff, M. J. *et al.* (1975). Portacaval shunt as emergency procedure in unselected patients with alcoholic cirrhosis. *Surg. Gynec. Obstet.*, **141**, 59–68.

Paquet, K. J. and Oberhammer, E. (1978). Sclerotherapy of bleeding esophageal varices by means of endoscopy. *Endoscopy*, **10**, 7–12.

Pereiras, R. *et al.* (1977). New techniques for interruption of gastroesophageal venous blood flow. *Radiology*, **124**, 313–23.

Resnik, R. H. *et al.* (1974). A controlled study of the therapeutic portacaval shunt. *Gastroenterology*, **67**, 843–57.

Rueff, B. *et al.* (1976). A controlled study of therapeutic portacaval shunt in alcoholic cirrhosis. *Lancet*, **1**, 655–9.

Terblanche, J., Saunders, S. J. and Louw, J. H. (1974). *Surgical Forum – The Liver* (ed. R. Smith), Butterworths, London.

Viamonte, Jr. M. *et al.* (1977). Transhepatic obliteration of gastroesophageal varices: results in acute and nonacute bleeders. *Am. J. Roentg.*, **129**, 237–41.

6 Achalasia

G. VANTRAPPEN and J. HELLEMANS

Typical achalasia may be defined as a disease of unknown aetiology, characterized by absence of peristalsis in the body of the oesophagus and failure of an often hypertensive gastro-oesophageal sphincter to relax normally in response to swallowing. Loss of the propulsive peristaltic contractions together with defective sphincter opening result in stasis of food in a progressively dilating gullet. This oesophageal stasis brings about most of the symptoms and complications.

6.1 SYMPTOMS AND SIGNS

Dysphagia is present in nearly all patients (Fig. 6.1), 70% of the patients having more trouble with solids than with fluids (Vantrappen *et al.*, 1971). The degree of swallowing difficulty varies from day to day, especially in the initial stage of the disease. Many patients admit they have more trouble when they are rushed or nervous.

Regurgitation is the second most common symptom (Sanderson, Ellis and Olsen, 1970). Active prandial or postprandial regurgitation occurs in 91% of patients, whereas regurgitation in the recumbent position is present in later stages of the disease. This results in nocturnal coughing spells in 30% of the patients and in bronchopulmonary complications in 5% (Sanderson, Ellis and Olsen, 1970) to 7.5% of the patients (Vantrappen *et al.*, 1971). Substernal pain was experienced by 60% of our patients at some time during the course of the disease. Attacks of cramp-like substernal pain not related to meals, often radiating to the neck or the back, may mimic angina pectoris or even myocardial infarction. Pain occurs especially in the initial stage of the disease and in cases of vigorous achalasia (Olsen, Holman and Anderson, 1953).

The degree of weight loss is related to the severity of the dysphagia. Anaemia has been observed (Olsen, Holman and Anderson, 1953), but haemorrhage is a rare symptom, occurring in 2.5% of the patients (Olsen, Holman and Anderson, 1953). Although it may be due to oesophagitis, it should particularly raise the suspicion of carcinomatous change.

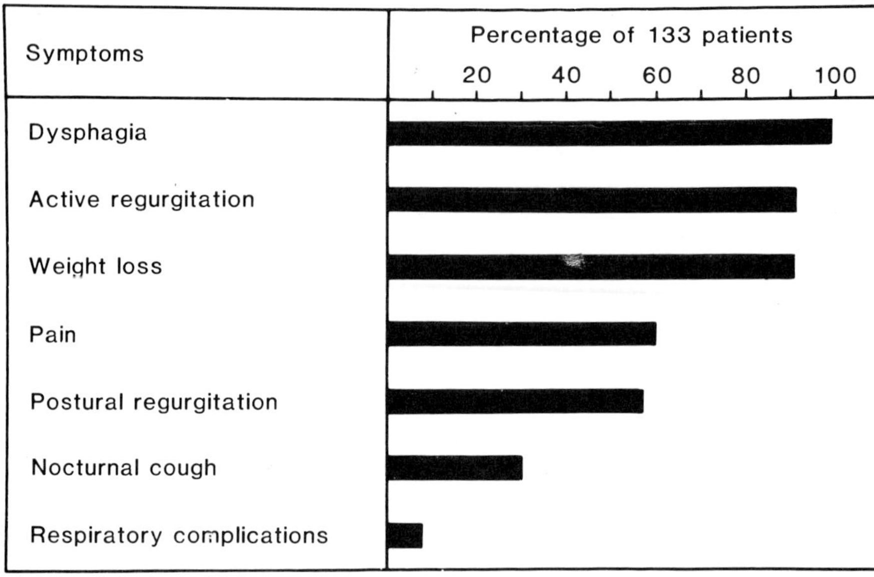

Fig. 6.1 Symptoms of achalasia.

In infants and children achalasia often goes unrecognized (Moersch, 1929). The respiratory symptoms of achalasia in childhood are particularly important. Nocturnal regurgitation is extremely common and the condition may be mistaken for chronic pulmonary infection.

6.2 DIAGNOSIS

The diagnosis of achalasia can be made by radiological and manometric examination of the oesophagus but it is wise always to perform endoscopy in order to exclude organic stenosis caused by benign or malignant lesions.

6.2.1 **Radiological appearance**

In the initial stage the oesophagus still has its normal calibre, there is little or no stasis of food, and the gastro-oesophageal sphincteric segment opens insufficiently. Later, retention occurs and the oesophagus becomes dilated over its full length. In the final stages the oesophageal body is wide and elongated, resulting in a tortuous, sigmoid-shaped gullet. In contrast, the terminal segment is narrow. The calibre of the oesophagus is seen to taper down gradually and terminate in a string-like passage into the stomach. The transition is usually smooth but in about 20% the lower narrow segment shows a symmetrical or asymmetrical dilatation, delineated proximally by a constriction and gradually tapering down distally (Van Goidsenhoven *et al.*, 1963) (Fig. 6.2). When the pouching effect is unilateral it may be mistaken for an ulcer. Irregularities in the outline of this segment, or an abnormal mucosal pattern always suggests a carcinoma. Amyl nitrate or an effervescent powder may help to differentiate achalasia from organic stenosis of the cardia, but endoscopy and bougienage are indispensable.

On fluoroscopy in the recumbent position the barium is seen to pass into the stomach with great difficulty or not at all. In the upright position, the oesophageal lumen fills until the weight of the barium opens the sphincter wide enough for a small amount of barium to spurt into the stomach. There is no peristalsis; simultaneous or unco-ordinated contractions progressively disappear as the oesophagus becomes more distended. After administration of a cholinergic drug the unco-ordinated

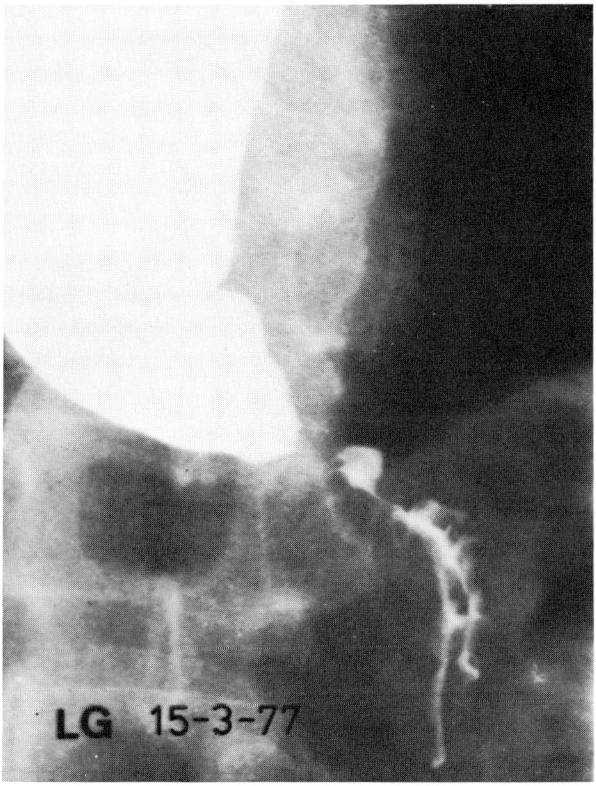

Fig. 6.2 A pseudoulcer niche is found in about 20% of patients with achalasia.

activity increases, the calibre of the oesophagus decreases due to a massive contraction and the barium is usually regurgitated.

6.2.2 **Manometric examination**

This is the best method for demonstrating the motility disorder in achalasia. Typical cases of achalasia are characterized by deglutitive pressure peaks occurring simultaneously over the entire length of the gullet, by abnormalities or absence of gastro-oesophageal spincter relaxation, by normal to high pressures in this sphincter and by high resting pressure in the body of the oesophagus (Butin *et al.*, 1953; Vantrappen *et al.*, 1963; Cohen, 1965). The differential diagnosis of achalasia and diffuse oesophageal spasm, another primary oesophageal motility disorder, can best be made by manometry. On manometry typical diffuse oesophageal spasm is characterized by non-sequential, frequently repetitive pressure peaks of high amplitude and long duration on deglutition (Creamer, Donoghue and Code, 1958; Bennett and Hendrix, 1970; Roth and Fleshler, 1964; Vantrappen and Hellemans, 1976). Usually the oesophagus retains some peristalsis, particularly in its upper third. A minority of patients have impaired lower oesophageal sphincter relaxation with or without an increased spincter pressure, but most patients have normal and complete relaxation (DiMarino and Cohen, 1974).

Twenty-four percent of our patients with primary oesophageal motility disorders which caused such a severe degree of dysphagia that treatment by pneumatic dilatation was necessary, did not fit well into the two classical disease entities, diffuse oesophageal spasm and achalasia (Vantrappen *et al.*, 1979). These patients presented either with complete absence of peristalsis and presence of (at least some) normal lower oesophageal sphincter relaxation or with some degree of peristalsis and complete absence of normal sphincter relaxation. These motor disorders constitute intermediate forms between the two classical disease entities. These observations suggest that primary oesophageal motility disorders constitute a spectrum of motor disorders composed of achalasia, diffuse oesophageal spasm, and related or intermediate types (Vantrappen *et al.*, 1979; Castell, 1976) (Fig. 6.3). It is important to characterize the motility disorder as precisely as possible because the results of treatment of typical cases of diffuse oesophageal spasm are markedly less favourable than those of other primary motility disorders.

Oesophagogastroscopy with biopsy is desirable, in order to exclude carcinomatous change in the oesophageal body, to differentiate achalasia from carcinoma of the cardia or the gastric fundus, and to establish the degree of stasis oesophagitis.

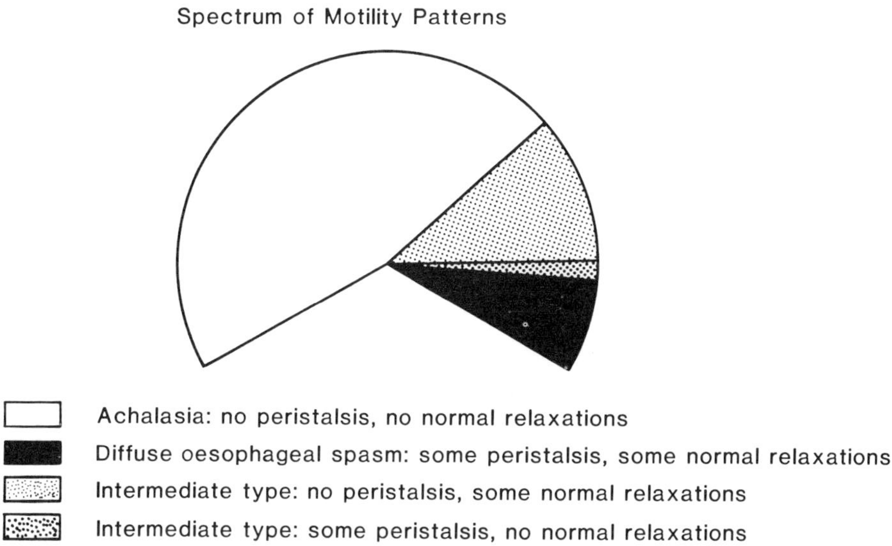

Fig. 6.3 Severe primary motility disorders of the oesophagus constitute a spectrum of motility patterns.

6.3 COMPLICATIONS

The incidence of carcinoma developing in an achalasic oesophagus is about 4%, which is clearly higher than its incidence in the general population (Vantrappen and Hellemans, 1974). Cancer develops mostly in patients with a long history of achalasia. Oesophagitis due to stasis does not seem to be the major cause, because even patients who undergo an early and successful myotomy may develop cancer. Moreover, cancers can develop at any level in the oesophagus. The most common tumour is a squamous cell carcinoma. Such cancers cause late symptoms when they are located in a wide oesophagus. The diagnosis must be suspected particularly when weight loss, dysphagia, continuous discomfort or regurgitation recur some time after an initially successful treatment; also when there is haematemesis. On radiological examination the diagnosis is easily missed. Oesophagoscopy is indicated whenever malignant change is suspected.

6.4 TREATMENT

The current methods of treatment aim to improve the passage of food into the stomach by weakening the insufficiently relaxing sphincter. This can be achieved by stretching it forcefully (dilatation) or by dividing the circular muscle (cardiomyotomy). Theoretically, it should be possible to decrease the resistance of the sphincter by medication but current medical therapy can offer at most temporary symptomatic relief. Whatever treatment is chosen the sphincteric function should be preserved sufficiently to prevent reflux.

6.4.1. **Dilatation**

Temporary relief of the dysphagia can be obtained by passing a mercury bougie, an olive dilator, or an oesophagoscope through the cardia. The relief is temporary and incomplete, yet real. To obtain good, long-term results a forceful dilatation of the sphincter is necessary. Several methods are currently available.

The *Starck dilator* is a device with expanding metal arms. The expanding part is introduced to the level of the cardia and the sphincter is dilated manually. The advantage of the system is that one can feel the moment the sphincter yields. Its disadvantages are that the diameter of the dilator is not exactly known, and that the rigidity of the instrument precludes its use in treatment of the elongated sigmoid-shaped oesophagus (Starck, 1924; Crump, Flood and Hennig, 1952; Schindler, 1956).

The *Negus hydrostatic dilator* (Thomson, Negus and Bateman, 1955) is introduced through a large oesophagoscope into the cardia, where the balloon is expanded.

The *Plummer system* (Plummer, 1908) has been used extensively by the Mayo group. The instrument consists of a stomach tube with side openings. Three bags are mounted over the end of the tube: an inner rubber, a middle silk and an outer rubber bag. The silk bag limits the maximal diameter of the dilator to 3.6 cm. A flexible whale-bone staff is passed through the rubber tube and a 41 F olive-tipped metal bougie is attached to the threaded end of the whale-bone staff. The dilator is passed over a previously swallowed thread to avoid perforation. The correct position is determined in advance, not by fluoroscopy, but by measuring the distance between upper incisors and cardia by means of a 41 F olive-tipped bougie attached to a whale-bone. Once positioned in the cardia, the dilator is connected to a water source and pressure gauge. The bag is slowly filled until a pressure of 18–22 feet of water is reached.

The *Tucker bag* (Tucker, 1939) and the *Browne–McHardy bag* (Browne and McHardy, 1939) are cylindrical balloons consisting of silk and rubber bags coated with radio-opaque material. The maximal diameter is 3 cm. The Tucker instrument is a mercury filled rubber tube on which the bag is mounted. The balloon is inflated to a pressure at which the constriction at the level of the cardia disappears. The high pressure is maintained for 30–60 s and then released. A few moments later the bag is reinflated. Disappearance of the constriction at 300 mm Hg or less is taken as evidence of successful dilatation. If necessary the procedure is repeated a second time during the same session (Bennett and Hendrix, 1970). The Brown–McHardy bag is almost the same instrument but it contains a mercury-filled tip.

The *Mosher bag* (Mosher and McGregor, 1928) has a maximum diameter of 3.6 cm, but as used by Nanson (Nanson, 1962) is inflated only to 15 psi which does not expand it fully. It may be difficult to introduce these instruments into the cardia when the oesophagus is widely dilated and sigmoid-shaped. Bergan (Bergan, 1952; Sakai *et al.*, 1979) overcame this problem by mounting the bag around an oesophagoscope.

Endoscopic pneumatic dilator. A pneumatic balloon fitted over a fibreoptic endoscope has recently been described (Witzel and Schilt, 1980). This allows positioning of the balloon under direct endoscopic vision.

For many years we have been using a pneumatic system with a *Sippy type dilator* (Vantrappen *et al.*, 1971). The dilator is assembled and thoroughly tested before each dilatation (Fig. 6.4). Two latex balloons (condoms), one inside the other, surrounded by a nylon bag, are mounted on a metal spiral terminated by an olive bougie (1) (Mueller,

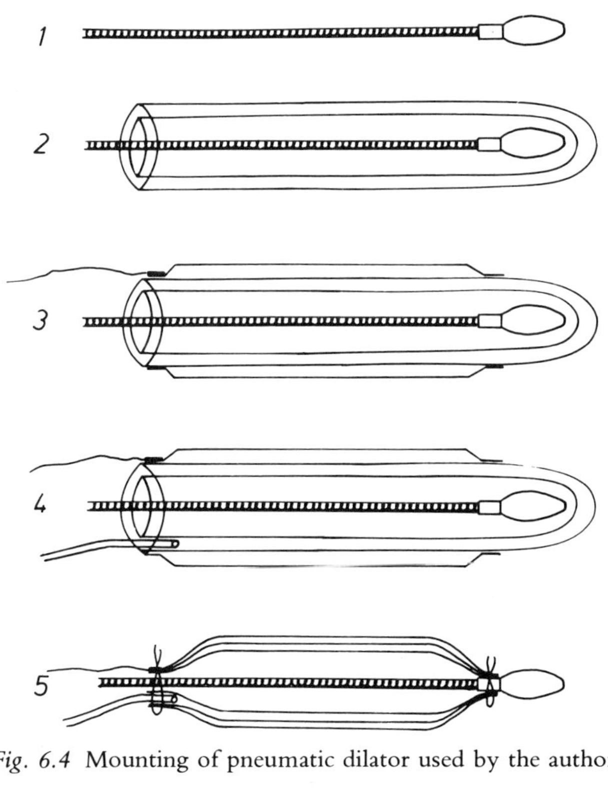

Fig. 6.4 Mounting of pneumatic dilator used by the authors.

Chicago). The nylon bags (2) have a length of 15 cm and a diameter of 3–5 cm, depending upon the bag selected. At both ends the diameter of the bag tapers down to about 1.5 cm. A 50-cm nylon ribbon is sewn on to the proximal end of the bag (3). On this ribbon a mark is made which indicates the 40 cm distance from the middle of the bag. It also helps to ensure that the entire dilator, bag and spiral, stay together when the dilator is pulled back at the end of the procedure. A polyvinyl tube with a non-compressible end (the tubing from an IV infusion set) is inserted between the balloons (4). When balloons and bags are ligated at both extremities (5), insufflation of air through the polyvinyl tube produces a cylinder, the diameter and shape of which are determined by the nylon bag. The pressure in the balloon can be measured by connecting the polyvinyl tube to a sphygmomanometer. To facilitate the introduction of the dilator a latex balloon is mounted around the nylon bag. The day before dilatation the patient swallows a string (Mersilene No. 1) weighted by a mercury filled bag. The string becomes anchored in the small bowel and acts as a guide for the dilator. If the oesophagus is markedly widened and sigmoid-shaped the mercury-filled bag may fail spontaneously to pass into the stomach. It may be possible to introduce it into the stomach with the help of a fibre-endoscope, or a Seldinger catheter may gently be passed under fluoroscopic control into the stomach and used instead of the Mersilene string as a guide for the dilator. Before introducing the balloon a metal wire with an eye at the end is threaded over the string into the stomach, providing a rigid guide which ensures safe introduction of the dilator. If it is not possible to pass this rigid wire over the string, a more flexible wire should be used. If even such a flexible wire fails to enter deep enough into the stomach, the dilator may be passed directly over the Mersilene string. The dilator is pushed down until the middle of the balloon reaches the level of the cardia (about 41 cm from the incisor teeth). The correct position of the balloon is always checked by fluoroscopy. In most cases an indentation on the left lateral aspect of the inflated balloon indicates the level of the diaphragm. Sometimes it is difficult to keep the balloon in the correct position because it is pushed upwards or downwards quite forcefully. Therefore, the dilator is fixed between the eye at the distal end of the wire and forceps placed on the wire immediately above the proximal end of the spiral. In this way the position of the balloon can be adjusted under fluoroscopic control. The balloon is then insufflated to a pressure of 200 mm Hg for the first minute, then to 300 mm Hg for an additional minute. Initially a balloon with a diameter of 3 cm is used; at each subsequent session the calibre of the dilator is increased. Nylon bags with a diameter of 3 cm, 3.5 cm, 3.8 cm, 4.2 cm, 4.5 cm and exceptionally 5 cm should be available. Three to four dilatations are performed in most patients until the criteria for adequate dilatation are met. These include disappearance, or substantial reduction, of the pressure in the lower oesophageal sphincter and, on fluoroscopy, easy emptying of the oesophagus and widening of the previously narrow lower oesophageal segment.

Important points in this method are the relatively low pressure (300 mm Hg) which is used to inflate the balloon and the fact that the procedure is spread over several sessions, using progressively larger balloons. The treatment is guided by the result of manometric and fluoroscopic examinations carried out after each procedure. The diameter of the balloon, and hence the distending force, can be adapted to each patient. In addition the method has the advantage that a flexible instrument is used, passed over a guide wire, so that it can be used even when the oesophagus is tortuous.

Before dilatation is performed an organic obstruction at the cardia must be excluded by oesophagoscopy or by passing a 41 F metal olive bougie into the stomach. A liquid diet is given for a couple of days and the oesophagus is evacuated before the first dilatation in order to prevent aspiration pneumonia. The dilatation is performed with the patient in the upright position (standing or sitting) to avoid aspiration of secretions into the airways. If pain becomes severe, the dilatation is stopped. If the patient fails to co-operate sufficiently because of youth or mental disease, dilatation is abandoned. Usually pain disappears or diminishes considerably within two minutes after the dilatation ends. Analgesics are not given. A small amount of blood on the dilator as it is removed is normal and does not indicate a complication. Patients must refrain from drinking or eating for two hours after dilatation. If pain persists longer, a perforation must be suspected. In that case, it is of the utmost importance that the patient does not take anything by mouth and is given antibiotics as soon as possible. If the patient's condition is good two hours after the dilatation no other measures are necessary.

6.4.2 **Complications of dilatation**

The major *immediate complication* of dilatation is perforation of the oesophagus at the cardia. Up to 1979 we had treated 537 patients and performed usually three or four pneumatic dilatations per patient. Perforation occurred in 13 patients (2.6% of the patients; 0.7% of the dilatations). A diagnosis of perforation was made whenever extravasation of contrast material could be demonstrated radiologically.

It is very important after each dilatation to observe the patient carefully for possible complications. A perforation must be suspected if the pain does not diminish 30–60 min after dilatation or if it becomes worse. Cramp-like pains similar to the attacks the patient experienced spontaneously before the treatment may be expected. However, if the pain radiates to the back or left lower thorax, or if respiration becomes painful, perforation must be suspected. After a few hours the breath sounds may diminish and there may be epigastric tenderness. A radiograph may show blurring of the left costophrenic angle or a pleural effusion. Hydropneumothorax occurred only once in our series and was associated with air in the mediastinum. According to Ellis and Olsen (1969) subcutaneous emphysema is frequently observed after perforation of the oesophagus. In our series we noticed it only in the one patient who had a perforation at the level of the hypopharynx. Within a few hours of perforation the patient develops fever and leucocytosis and looks severely ill.

Whenever a patient experiences prolonged or abnormally severe pain after dilatation, oral feeding is stopped and parenteral treatment with broad spectrum antibiotics is started. The next day a radiographic examination with gastrografin is performed to check whether there is a perforation. If not, oral feeding is resumed as soon as the fever has passed. If there is a perforation, broad spectrum antibiotics, analgesics and parenteral feeding are continued. Pleural aspiration or suction drainage are sometimes indicated. The majority of these patients improve considerably after about three days of conservative therapy. After that, food may be administered through a gastric tube, but this is not started immediately as it may cause vomiting. If a surgical repair of the perforation is deemed necessary it is best to perform it shortly after the accident. Residual abscesses of mediastinum or pleural cavity may require subsequent surgical drainage.

Most authors consider oesophageal perforation an indication for immediate surgical intervention, but it is our experience that perforation of the cardia, caused by pneumatic dilatation, can usually be successfully treated conservatively. Ten of the 13 patients with proven perforation healed completely after parenteral alimentation and broad spectrum antibiotics for one or two weeks. In four of them a pleural effusion was aspirated. Two other patients had to be treated by surgical drainage of the mediastinum. (One had active Hodgkin's disease, the other had eaten normally before the perforation was recognized.) Only one of the 537 patients died, a woman of 83 years to whom food was given by mistake, in spite of a radiologically demonstrated perforation.

Other complications, such as prolonged pain, a peak of fever or a sterile pleural effusion, were observed in 10 other patients, which brings the complication rate to 4.3%, similar to that in other large series. (Olsen *et al.*, 1951: 2.2% perforation and 4.6% other complications in 452 patients; Sanderson, Ellis and Olsen, 1970: 2.4% perforations and 2% other complications in 408 patients.)

Late complications are rare after pneumatic dilation. In our experience symptomatic reflux occurred in less than 1% of 455 patients.

6.4.3 **Results of dilatation**

In the 20 years 1957–1977 we treated 455 patients by this method of pneumatic dilatation. The *immediate results* were excellent. After the first dilatation there was considerable improvement of the dysphagia. By the end of the treatment all patients stated that they were able to eat without distress. Regurgitation also had disappeared completely. Attacks of substernal pain did not always disappear immediately; in some cases it took several weeks before relief was obtained, although the cramp-like pain was less severe than before dilatation. Most patients gained weight rapidly.

The *late results* could be evaluated for 424 (93%) of the patients; 21 of these patients, suffering from diffuse oesophageal spasm, will be considered separately. The duration of follow-up ranged from 1–20 years (mean 7.8 years). The clinical evaluation of these patients was based upon the incidence and degree of dysphagia, retrosternal pain, regurgitation and weight loss. They were subdivided into four groups according to the following criteria. Group I (excellent results) includes those patients who are completely free of symptoms. Group II (good results) consists of those patients who experience dysphagia or pain of short duration only occasionally: less than once a week there is a hesitancy of food retrosternally, lasting from a few seconds to a couple of minutes, and disappearing on drinking some fluid; there is no weight loss and no regurgitation. Group III comprises the moderate results. These patients experience dysphagia at least once a week. The sensation of food sticking in the oesophagus does not last longer than a few minutes and does not prevent the patient from finishing his meal. It is not accompanied by regurgitation and weight loss. The patients are markedly improved as compared with the pretreatment situation. Group IV comprises the poor results. These patients have frequent dysphagia, regurgitation or weight loss, or daily retrosternal pain.

At the time of evaluation, 77% of the patients had good or excellent results, 8.7% had moderate results and 14.4% had poor results; 93% of the patients were significantly improved by the treatment. Symptoms recurred and more than one series of dilatations had to be performed in 41 of these patients. About half of them got excellent or good results when dilatation was repeated, but the overall results were not as good as in the whole group. In contrast with many other published reports, a good result did not mean that the symptoms had improved, nor a poor result that there was no improvement or worsening of the condition. Several patients were classified in the group of poor results, in spite of considerable subjective improvement, because there was weight loss or regurgitation.

The results of pneumatic dilatation in patients with diffuse oesophageal spasm are less satisfactory. We treated 18 patients with severe symptoms of diffuse oesophageal spasm and evaluated the results, after a follow-up period of 1–6 years. Excellent or good results were obtained in only 45%. Patients with intermediate types of primary motility disorders (in whom either some degree of normal sphincteric relaxation or of normal peristalsis is preserved), or patients with vigorous achalasia, respond to pneumatic dilatation in the same way as do patients with typical achalasia.

Radiological examination before, immediately after and late after treatment indicated that dilatation resulted in an immediate and sustained reduction in the diameter of the oesophagus. A return to normal was observed only if the oesophageal diameter before treatment was not larger than 70 mm. The mean maximal diameter of the lower oesophageal sphincter increased from 2 mm before to 9 mm late after treatment. Some patients denied dysphagia in spite of considerable stasis of food residue after an overnight fast on radiological examination.

A gastric air bubble was absent in 86% of the patients before treatment, but in only 8.4% later after treatment. The best results were obtained in patients over the age of 45 years, in patients with a history of more than five years' duration, and in patients with a moderately dilated gullet.

6.4.4 **Results of myotomy**

The Heller procedure yields 'good results' in 64% to 88% of patients (Vantrappen and Hellemans, 1974). Persistent dysphagia, not relieved by the myotomy, is mostly due to incomplete section of the circular muscle or, more rarely, to restoration of continuity of the myotomized muscle by scar formation. The major late complications of surgical treatment of achalasia are gastro-oesophageal reflux, oesophagitis and peptic stricture. The incidence of gastro-oesophageal reflux after a Heller procedure varies considerably from one surgeon to another, but amounts on average to 18% of the patients, whereas peptic oesophagitis rises from about 5% in the early postoperative period to about 10% late postoperatively and peptic stricture is reported in 3.4% of 1045 cases collected from the literature (Vantrappen and Hellemans, 1974; Hollender *et al.*, 1977). The value of combining an antireflux procedure with the Heller myotomy is still a matter of controversy.

6.5 CONCLUSION

We consider pneumatic dilatation the treatment of choice for most patients with achalasia. It is a safe procedure in experienced hands and can be used even when the oesophagus is widened and tortuous or when the patient is cachectic. A previous unsuccessful Heller operation is not a contraindication to pneumatic dilatation, if an organic obstruction can be ruled out. The immediate and long-term results compare favourably with those of surgery, and stenosing reflux oesophagitis is rare after pneumatic dilatation. We agree with Castell (Castell, 1976) that surgery is to be preferred: 1) after several unsuccessful attempts at pneumatic dilatation, 2) when oesophageal carcinoma cannot be excluded and 3) in children and psychiatric patients who are unable to co-operate. Patients with an epiphrenic diverticulum should be treated surgically because of the risk of perforation by dilatation.

REFERENCES

Bennett, J. R. and Hendrix, T. R. (1970). Diffuse esophageal spasm: a disorder with more than one cause. *Gastroenterology,* **59**, 273–9.

Bergan, F. (1952). Discussion. *Acta Chir. Scand.,* **103**, 464–6.

Browne, D. C. and McHardy, G. (1939). A new instrument for use in esophagospasm. *J. Am. Med. Ass.,* **113**, 1963–4.

Butin, J. W. *et al.* (1953). A study of esophageal pressures in normal persons and patients with cardiospasm. *Gastroenterology,* **23**, 278–93.

Castell, D. O. (1976). Achalasia and diffuse esophageal spasm. *Arch. Intern. Med.,* **136**, 571–9.

Cohen, B. R. (1965). 'Cardiospasm' in achalasia: demonstration of an abnormally elevated esophagogastric sphincter pressure with partial relaxation on swallowing (abstract). *Gastroenterology,* **48**, 864.

Creamer, B., Donoghue, F. E. and Code, C. F. (1958). Pattern of esophageal motility in diffuse spasm. *Gastroenterology,* **34**, 782–96.

Crump, A. C., Flood, C. A. and Hennig, G. C. (1952). Results of medical treatment of idiopathic cardiospasm. *Gastroenterology*, **20**, 30–38.

DiMarino, A. J. and Cohen, S. (1974). Characteristics of lower esophageal sphincter function on symptomatic diffuse esophageal spasm. *Gastroenterology,* **66**, 1–6.

Ellis, F. H., Jr. and Olsen, A. M. (1969). Achalasia of the esophagus. In: *Major Problems in Clinical Surgery*, **IX**, (Ellis, F. H. and Olsen, A. M., eds.), W. B. Saunders Co., Philadelphia, London and Toronto.

Goidsenhoven, G. E. Van *et al.* (1963). Treatment of achalasia of the cardia with pneumatic dilatations. *Gastroenterology,* **45**, 326–34.

Hollender, L. F. *et al.* (1977). L'opération de Heller dans le traitement du méga-oesophage idiopathique. *Méd. Chir. Dig.,* **6**, 89–94.

Moersch, H. J. (1929). Cardiospasm in infancy and in childhood. *Am. J. Dis. Child.,* **38**, 294–8.

Mosher, H. P. and McGregor, G. W. (1928). A study of the lower end of the esophagus. *Ann. Otol. Rhinol. Lar.,* **37**, 12–70.

Nanson, E. M. (1962). Treatment of cardiospasm by the expanding bag technique. *Can. Med. Ass. J.,* **86**, 1107–11.

Olsen, A. M. *et al.* (1951). The treatment of cardiospasm: analysis of a twelve-year experience. *J. Cardiovasc. Surg.,* **22**, 164–87.

Olsen, A., Holman, C. and Anderson, H. (1953). The diagnosis of cardiospasm. *Dis. Chest*, **23**, 477–98.

Plummer, H. S. (1908). Cardiospasm: a report of 301 cases. *J. Am. Med. Ass.*, **51**, 549–54.

Roth, H. P. and Fleshler, B. (1964). Diffuse esophageal spasm. Clinical, radiological and manometric observations. *Ann. Intern. Med.*, **61**, 914–23.

Sakai, P. *et al.* (1979). Treatment of megaesophagus with forced dilatation of cardia through hydrostatic balloon attached to a fiberesophagoscope. *Endoscopy*, **2**, 116–20.

Sanderson, D. R., Ellis, F. H., Jr. and Olsen, A. M. (1970). Achalasia of the esophagus: results of therapy by dilation, 1950–1967. *Chest*, **58**, 116–21.

Schindler, R. (1956). Observations on cardiospasm and its treatment by brusque dilatation. *Ann. Intern. Med.*, **45**, 207–15.

Starck, H. (1924). Die Behandlung der spasmogenen Speiseröhrenerweiterung. *Münch. Med. Wschr.*, **71**, 334–6.

Thomson, S., Negus, V. E. and Bateman, G. H. (1955). Disease of the nose and throat. In: *A Textbook for Students and Practioners*, Cassel, London, p. 776.

Tucker, G. (1939). Cardiospasm: a pneumatic mercury dilator. *Ann. Otol. Rhinol. Lar.*, **48**, 808–16.

Vantrappen, G. *et al.* (1971). Treatment of achalasia with pneumatic dilatations. *Gut*, **12**, 268–75.

Vantrappen, G. *et al.* (1963). Manometric studies in achalasia of the cardia, before and after pneumatic dilations. *Gastroenterology*, **45**, 317–25.

Vantrappen, G. *et al.* (1979). Achalasia, diffuse esophageal spasm, and related motility disorders. *Gastroenterology*, **76**, 450–7.

Vantrappen, G. and Hellemans, J. (1976). Diffuse muscle spasm of the oesophagus. *Clin. Gastroent.*, **5**, 59–72.

Vantrappen, G. and Hellemans, J. (1974). Achalasia. In: *Diseases of the Esophagus*. (Vantrappen, G. and Hellemans, J., eds.) Springer Verlag, Berlin, pp. 287–354.

Witzel, L. and Schilt, W. (1980). Treatment of achalasia with a new pneumatic dilator attached to a gastroscope. *Abstr. IV Eur. Congr. Gastrointest. Motility*, Georg Thieme Verlag, Stuttgart, New York.

7 Foreign bodies of oesophagus and stomach

K. F. R. SCHILLER

Mary had a little watch,
She swallowed it one day.
Now she's taking Cascarets
To pass the time away.
(Eldridge, 1961)

Of all the many types of foreign bodies which may enter the stomach and oesophagus, some may cause serious complications while many are harmless. A large majority are passed spontaneously. In this chapter no attempt will be made at a comprehensive approach to the subject of upper gastrointestinal foreign bodies. The emphasis will be on the role of endoscopy, with particular reference to fibre-endoscopy. Nevertheless, it is necessary to describe the types of foreign bodies that have been found in the oesophagus and stomach, how they got there, how their presence was established, the indications for their attempted removal, and methods used in their removal. That the subject is not without its lighter aspects should not divert the gastroenterologist from his serious responsibilities in this field. Indeed, his interest will be heightened by the opportunity for inventiveness and manipulative skill which the challenge of a foreign body presents.

7.1 FOREIGN BODIES FOUND IN THE UPPER GASTROINTESTINAL TRACT

It is convenient to classify such foreign bodies arbitrarily into four groups: swallowed foreign bodies, bezoars, retained surgical suture material and a group of miscellaneous foreign bodies.

7.1.1 **Swallowed foreign bodies**

(a) *Types of swallowed foreign bodies*

A large variety of swallowed objects has been reported, and any classification or list of such objects must be selective and arbitrary (Table

Table 7.1 Types of swallowed foreign bodies.

Personal effects	coins, keys, razor blades, dentures, hairgrips
Writing utensils	pencils, ball-point pens
Sewing equipment	buttons, needles, safety pins
Cutlery	knives, forks, spoons
Miscellaneous household effects	paper clips, drawing pins, paper knife, pull-tabs, torch batteries, assorted tools, wire, ball-bearings, nails, glass fragments
Articles of food	chicken and fish bones, fruit stones, fruit pulp, meat bolus
Medication	methylcellulose and antacid tablets
Medical equipment	pieces of tubing, hypodermic needles, dental reamer, thermometer
Worms and insects	*Anasakis* larvae, yellow-jacket

7.1). It is not so much the type of foreign body swallowed as the possible consequences which make this subject clinically important.

(b) *Who swallows foreign bodies?*
Children, especially those under the age of five, are fond of putting objects to their mouths, and consequently form the largest group of patients presenting with ingested foreign bodies. Patients with mental disturbance, on the other hand, present with the largest number of foreign bodies per patient (Eldridge, 1961; Bitar and Holmes, 1975). Prisoners are fond of swallowing foreign bodies (Manegold, 1973) but, since most of these can now be extracted easily, the fashion is waning. As a group, normal free adults are least likely to ingest foreign bodies. Mainly at risk are the elderly, the edentulous, the inebriated and the careless. The subject was fully reviewed, prior to the advent of fibre-endoscopy, by Jackson and Jackson (1937).

(c) *What happens to swallowed foreign bodies?*
Most ingested foreign bodies are passed spontaneously without complications; McCafferey and Lilley (1975) quote a figure of 90%. Eldridge (1961), from his experience of mental patients, believes that almost all ingested foreign bodies are eventually passed, and mentions one of his previous papers (no reference given) entitled 'The intelligent neglect of foreign bodies in the gastrointestinal tract'.

In the normal upper gastrointestinal tract many foreign bodies are likely to be held up at the level of cricopharyngeus, the oesophagogastric junction, the pylorus and the duodenojejunal flexure. They may also be held up at points of abnormal narrowing, e.g. where a paraoesophageal hernia presses on the oesophagus (Pillari *et al.*, 1979), in diverticula (Munsell and Walker, 1972; Armengol-Miro *et al.*, 1977), above strictures, rings, webs, a narrowed pylorus or tumours (Kassner *et al.*, 1975).

According to Earlam (1976) coins are second only to bones with regard to sticking in the oesophagus: 75% lodge just below the cricopharyngeal sphincter, the rest lower.

(d) *Complications (Table 7.2)*

Oedema or occlusion of the upper airways may be caused by damage during ingestion. A foreign body may abrade the upper gastrointestinal tract; the author has performed an oesophagoscopy on a patient who had experienced severe pain after swallowing a piece of apple. A 10 cm tear of the oesophageal wall was seen, but the patient made a good recovery.

A sharp foreign body may penetrate the wall of the oesophagus or stomach causing it to be retained and requiring removal, e.g. a dental reamer penetrating the antral wall, as described below. A foreign body may even perforate the wall of an organ without clinical evidence of peritonitis (Sartory and Trabant, 1978). When a foreign body has caused a silent perforation, it may migrate and present itself elsewhere in the body. The author has seen a swallowed hairgrip in a child eventually presenting with haematuria due to migration to the right kidney. Abscess formation is a well known complication, and mediastinal abscesses have involved the aorta, with fatal results.

Perforation is a serious complication of the ingestion of foreign bodies. Ashby and Hunter-Craig (1967) described 11 patients with gastrointestinal perforation, and concluded that chicken and fish bones were especially prone to cause perforation, sharp metallic foreign bodies less so. In 313 cases seen by Savary and Miller (1978) there were 17 perforations, all in adults; 15 of these were due to ingested bone fragments. In Miller's series (1975) the frequency of perforation was equally distributed between stomach and duodenum, small bowel, appendix and caecum, and colon and rectum. Norberg and Reyes (1975) described the tragic case of a child sustaining severe colonic complications following the ingestion of glass Christmas tree lights. Perforation may also be due to local pressure necrosis, and revealed only when the foreign body is extracted (Classen *et al.*, 1976). The mortality is appreciable: according to Goff (1968) 1865 citizens died on inhaled or ingested foreign bodies in the United States in 1964; 61% were children under the age of four. In 1506 cases the foreign body was an article of food.

Table 7.2 Hazards of foreign body ingestion.

Respiratory problems	Perforation
Abrasion	Abscess formation
Retention	Haemorrhage
Penetration	Migration

Finally, impaction of a foreign body may cause obstruction of oesophagus, pylorus or, rarely, small or large intestine.

(e) *Diagnosis and management*

Usually the patient is known or witnessed to have swallowed a foreign body. On other occasions this may be suspected, for example in a mentally disturbed patient given to repeated episodes of this type of behaviour. An ingested foreign body may be responsible for a new symptom such as dysphagia even when the episode of swallowing the foreign body cannot be remembered (Banks and Potsic, 1978). Metal-containing objects will be relatively radio-opaque, but non-ferrous metal objects, e.g. aluminium pull-tabs from metal beverage cans (Burnington, 1976), may be difficult to demonstrate radiologically. Radiolucent foreign bodies may be shown as filling defects during contrast studies, especially in the oesophagus. In the radiological search for an ingested foreign body, soft tissue techniques and special views may be necessary. Endoscopy may be useful for diagnosis, as well as therapy.

Diagnosis becomes additionally difficult if only part of the ingested foreign body is radio-opaque and the foreign body splits into its radio-opaque and radiolucent portions. A patient seen by Zeegen and Lance (1979) swallowed a small metal paperknife. Endoscopy revealed a flat object which, after endoscopic retrieval, was found to be a flat plastic toy soldier, part of the handle of the knife. It proved necessary to remove the second half of the handle and the knife itself surgically.

As the majority of ingested foreign bodies are excreted uneventfully without the need for medical intervention, it is usual to advise a 'wait-and-see' policy, unless there are specific indications for immediate treatment, such as impaction. In general terms foreign bodies that are both long and sharp, or very bulky, will eventually require removal. Immediate removal, impaction apart, is recommended for objects that have points at both ends, are hooked, or have a sharp edge. If observation is decided on, frequent radiological monitoring is advised: if, even in the absence of symptoms, the foreign body appears not to progress down the gastrointestinal tract, removal should be considered (Swarbrick *et al.*, 1972), though a conservative policy may be best in disturbed or attention-seeking patients.

Non-endoscopic treatment must be considered. Enzymatic dissolution is sometimes appropriate (see below). Pillari *et al.* (1979) described the use of glucagon with a barium-containing contrast medium: glucagon selectively relaxes the lower oesophageal sphincter while preserving oesophageal peristalsis, and the weight of the barium suspension helps to propel an impacted bolus into the stomach.

Treatment involving endoscopy is discussed later in this chapter.

7.1.2 **Bezoars**

Bezoar is derived from the Arabic *badzehr*, the Persian *padzahr* and the Turkish *panzehir*, each of which means antipoison or antidote (DeBakey and Ochsner, 1938). Thus bezoars derived from the entrails of animals were believed to have useful properties in, for example, the treatment of weakness of the heart and loss of sexual powers (Elgood, 1935). Murdock (1934) further expands on the magical property of bezoars and comments on their use by Queen Elizabeth I.

(a) *Trichobezoars*
A trichobezoar is a hairball made up of swallowed strands of hair. Trichobezoars are uncommon and may be asymptomatic for many years. They are found in younger patients, mainly women, who indulge in trichophagia. There is no medical or endoscopic treatment, and if removal is indicated on symptomatic grounds this must be by surgical means.

(b) *Phytobezoars*
Plant bezoars are composed of leaves, roots, skins, pulp and other plant residue. They occur most commonly in patients with disturbed gastric motility or after partial gastrectomy. Of special interest is the phytobezoar caused by the ingestion of persimmons; these bezoars occur in subjects with normal stomachs; 14% of the pulp of this fruit is made up of pectin and gum (Murdock, 1934); gastric acidity causes a coagulum to form. In the series of phytobezoars reported by DeBakey and Ochsner (1938 and 1939) those derived from persimmons accounted for 73%. Symptoms may include dyspepsia, nausea, vomiting, ulceration and obstruction. The diagnosis may be confirmed radiologically or by endoscopy. Enzymatic dissolution has been described (Dann *et al.*, 1959; Pollard and Block, 1968), but surgery may be indicated. Endoscopic methods of treatment include the instillation of cellulase into the bezoar (Gold *et al.*, 1976), fragmentation of the bezoar using biopsy forceps (Lukash, Fornes and Johnson, 1970; McKechnie, 1972; Brady, 1978) and removal of the bezoar (Munsell and Walker 1972; McLoughlin *et al.*, 1979). Armengol-Miro *et al.* (1977) describe removal of a prepapillary intradiverticular bezoar which had caused obstructive jaundice. Yeast bezoars occur not uncommonly in Scandinavia (Bong *et al.*, 1966; Perttala *et al.*, 1975).

7.1.3 **Retained surgical suture material**

Retained non-absorbable sutures are usually asymptomatic, but are thought by some to cause suture line ulcer leading to 'a needless cause of pain, dyspepsia and bleeding' (Small *et al.*, 1968), though Hoare and Alexander-Williams (1977) doubt that sutures actually cause ulcers, or that their removal is of any value. However, Belber (1978) quotes a patient where a single suture had 'transfixed an artery and for many months had acted as a wick which led to severe chronic blood loss'. Diagnosis is by endoscopy. Retained sutures can usually be removed endoscopically, and excision of the suture line should not be necessary.

7.1.4 **Miscellaneous foreign bodies**

Gallstones may be passed into the bowel and cause intestinal obstruction (Tongerson *et al.*, 1979). Other concretions may be made up, for example, of medication conglomerates (Townsend *et al.*, 1973); concretions have weighed 4 lb (2 kg approx.) or more and may require surgical removal (DeBakey and Ochsner, 1938).

Worms and insects could be categorized as unusual foreign bodies. The vagaries of *Ascaris lumbricoides* are well known, though obstruction of a gastrojejunostomy is uncommon (Lefton, 1976). Less is known of the genus *Anisakis*, larvae of which may be ingested in areas where there is a predilection for raw fish (Marsden, 1978). Anisakiasis may now be managed endoscopically (Akasaka *et al.*, 1979). The consequences of the inadvertent ingestion of a yellow-jacket are the subject of a report by Houston (1975).

Even more unusual is the appearance of a foreign body in the gastrointestinal tract years after a war injury. Weithofer *et al.* (1977) described the emergence of a rifle bullet in the duodenum 32 years after wounding in the back. The bullet was seen endoscopically to be entering the duodenal wall but was passed spontaneously before endoscopic removal could be arranged.

Of unusual foreign bodies it may be appropriate finally to quote Lehrer's remark that 'these are the only ones of which the news has come to Harvard/And there may be many others but they haven't been discovered'.

7.2 ENDOSCOPIC TREATMENT OF FOREIGN BODIES

In this section instrumentation, patient preparation, general points of technique, and complications of foreign body extraction will be discussed, and selected examples of methods employing fibre-endoscopy will be presented. The emphasis will be on fibre-endoscopic methods.

According to Manegold (1977) laparotomy for the removal of ingested foreign bodies is now hardly ever indicated; every swallowed foreign body which at the time of diagnosis lies proximal to the duodenojejunal junction can be endoscopically removed if it has not altered its shape and has not caused a perforation. Even when partial perforation has occurred endoscopic removal may be possible (Schiller and Salmon, 1973; Honaas and Shaffer, 1977; Sartory and Trabant, 1978).

7.2.1 **Instrumentation**

The traditional rigid oesophagoscope, long used for the extraction of oesophageal foreign bodies, requires no further description. It is increasingly being replaced by the fibreoptic endoscope used in the ways described below. The various sizes and models of fibreoptic endoscopes are described in Chapter 1.

Standard biopsy forceps are usually unsuitable, as it is difficult to obtain a grip on the foreign body with these, especially if they possess a central spike or thorn. Several specially designed devices are now commercially available (Fig. 7.1). There are various types of toothed forceps, graspers, suture cutting devices, snares of different shapes and sizes, Dormia baskets and Fogarty catheters. The ingenuity of endoscopists has added other items not primarily designed for the extraction of foreign bodies, e.g. condoms (Wren and Cockel, 1978), to this list. It is advised that any hospital offering a gastrointestinal endoscopy service equip itself with a range of extraction devices, so as to be prepared to intervene quickly if required.

7.2.2 **Preparation of the patient**

In general, there is no need to employ a general anaesthetic for the extraction of foreign bodies. The decision may be more difficult in children, in patients already on psychotropic medication, and where the extraction procedure may be prolonged and difficult. In other respects patient preparation is as for routine endoscopy with regard to obtaining informed consent, a preceding period of starvation, the use of a local anaesthetic and an atropine-like substance, and the choice of tranquillizer or analgesic.

7.2.3 **General points of technique**

Whenever possible prior radiographic confirmation of type, site and size of the foreign body will have been obtained. Special risk factors such as sharpness, impaction or even perforation will have been noted, and the devices most likely to be required for extraction or other endoscopic treatment prepared. It is expedient to perform a dummy run with the extraction device on an object similar to that to be removed. After introduction of the most suitable available endoscope the foreign body will be identified. Attempts at manipulation or extraction may well require the cooperation of more than one endoscopist, as well as full support from an endoscopy nurse assistant. These helpers must be able to see what the senior endoscopist sees: a teaching side arm is of help, closed circuit television is better.

Unless the foreign body to be extracted is fixed by wedging, impaction or penetration, or lies conveniently in a diverticulum, it is often necessary to prevent its moving every time it is touched with the extraction device. Coins in the stomach are particularly difficult to secure if they are entirely free lying. Thus it is advisable to wedge the foreign body as appropriate, e.g. in the antrum. It may also be useful in this connection to change the patient's position on the endoscopy table, or to apply external pressure. On occasions the author has passed a second, small diameter, endoscope in parallel with the first, and has used this as a prop for holding the foreign body in a suitable position.

A larger foreign body should be grasped or otherwise secured so that during extraction its long axis lies in the line of extraction, otherwise it will be impossible to pull it into the oesophagus. Similarly, it is essential that sharp foreign bodies should be extracted with their sharp points caudad rather than cephalad for fear of impaction or perforation during extraction. For long and sharp foreign bodies the sheathing tube methods described by Witzel *et al.* (1974) and later by Rogers (1979), and Martin *et al.* (1979) are particularly recommended.

The extraction of foreign bodies is usually simple, safe and quick, but may sometimes be difficult or complicated. Other methods of treating foreign bodies, e.g. enzyme treatment of bezoars or the piecemeal removal of an impacted food bolus, may be a lengthy procedure. Experience and skill is required when any of these manoeuvres are undertaken. The management of foreign bodies in the upper gastrointestinal tract is not for the tyro endoscopist.

7.2.4 **Examples of methods employing fibre-endoscopy**

The methods described below are among the more important in the literature; no attempt has been made to present a comprehensive review of all published methods.

(a) *Simple grasping forceps*

One of the commonest foreign bodies ingested is a coin. It is not usually possible to grasp a foreign body firmly using normal biopsy forceps, especially if such forceps have a central spike or thorn. Miederer (1977) has devised a special snare for smooth coins, i.e. coins without a raised rim, but it is likely that toothed forceps (Fig. 7.1(*a*)) will suffice in most cases. The coin is manoeuvred into the best position, firmly gripped by the jaws of the grasping forceps, and removed (Fig. 7.2). Grasping forceps are invaluable for the removal of a variety of foreign bodies. The author has successfully removed a number of coins including a Victorian gold half-sovereign, a bunch of keys and a dental reamer, as well as

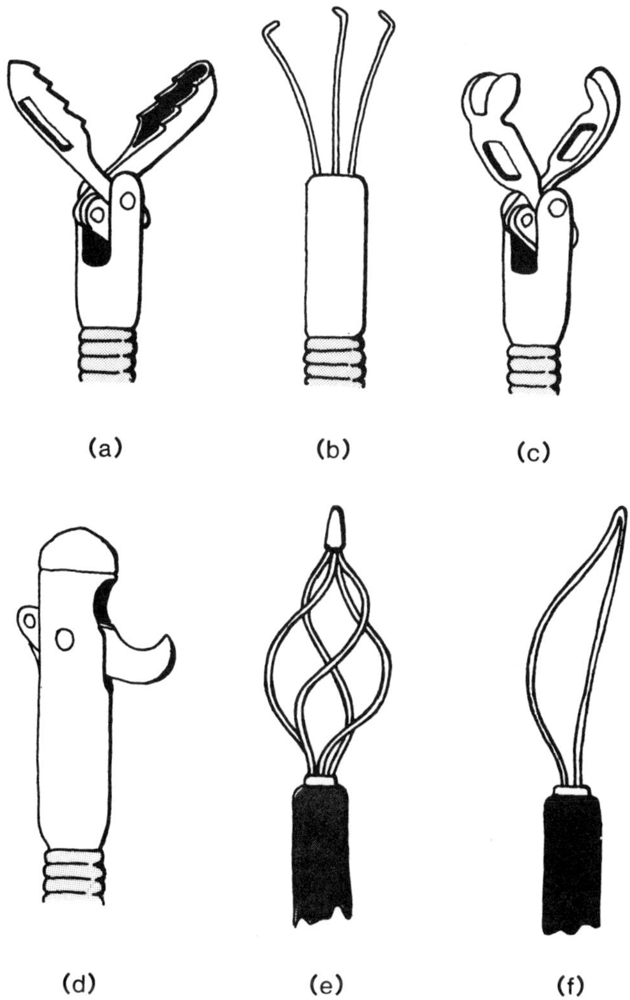

Fig. 7.1 A selection of grasping forceps and other extraction devices. (a) Alligator jawed forceps. (b) Three-nail grasping forceps. (c) Rat-tooth forceps. (d) Suture cutting forceps. (e) Dormia basket. (f) Wire snare.

retained sutures on several occasions. More unusual objects removed using forceps include the larvae of *Anisakis* from the gastric wall (Akasaka *et al.*, 1979), and a species of *Ascaris lumbricoides* from a gastrojejunostomy (Lefton, 1976).

(b) *Forceps as an expanding extraction device*
Certain ingested foreign bodies have an orifice through which biopsy forceps can be passed and then opened, the diameter of the opened forceps being greater than that of the orifice 'cannulated', enabling the

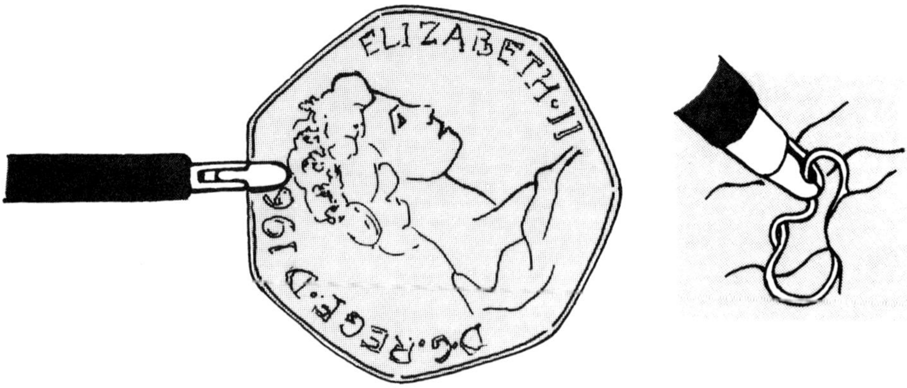

Fig. 7.2 Toothed forceps grasping a coin.

foreign body to be extracted. Manegold (1973) successfully removed a knife blade by this method (Fig. 7.3). An ingested piece of plastic tubing was removed by Gupta, Ricca and Ingegno (1977), biopsy forceps having been passed through the lumen of the tubing (Fig. 7.4).

(c) *Mobilization and removal*

Certain foreign bodies may have to be mobilized prior to attempted removal, for example because of impaction or penetration of the organ wall. The author (Schiller and Salmon, 1973) removed a dental reamer which was embedded in the antral wall, but without evidence of perforation (Fig. 7.5). There is a report of this unusual foreign body being extracted from the bronchus, using a fibre-endoscope (Papamichael, 1976).

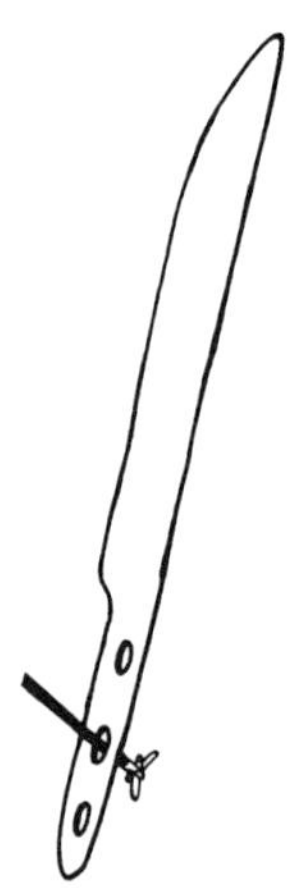

Fig. 7.3 Extraction of knife blade using biopsy forceps (after Manegold, 1973).

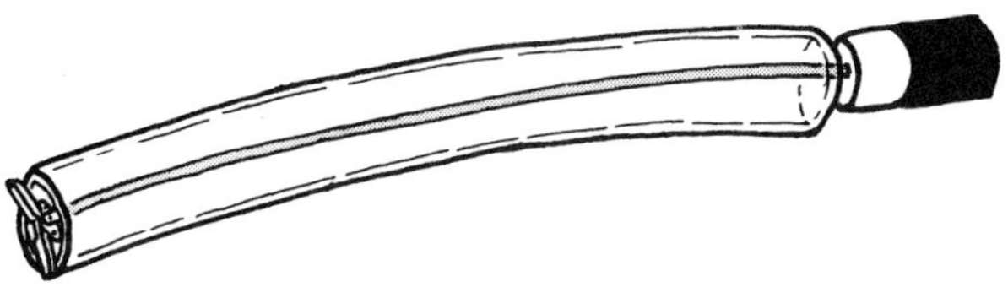

Fig. 7.4 Extraction of plastic tubing using biopsy forceps (after Gupta, Ricca and Ingegno, 1977).

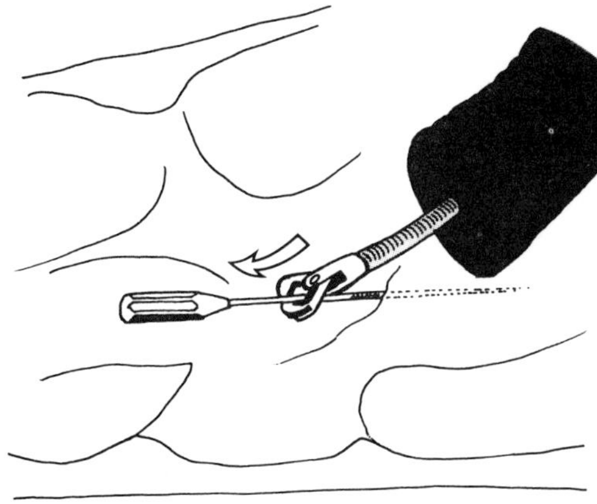

(a)

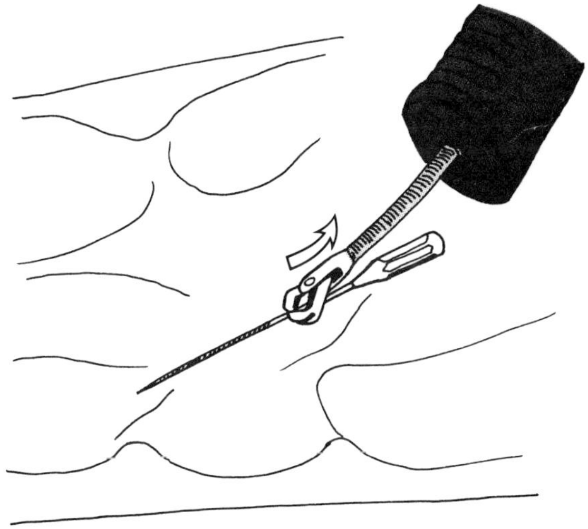

(b)

Fig. 7.5 Extraction of dental reamer using toothed forceps.

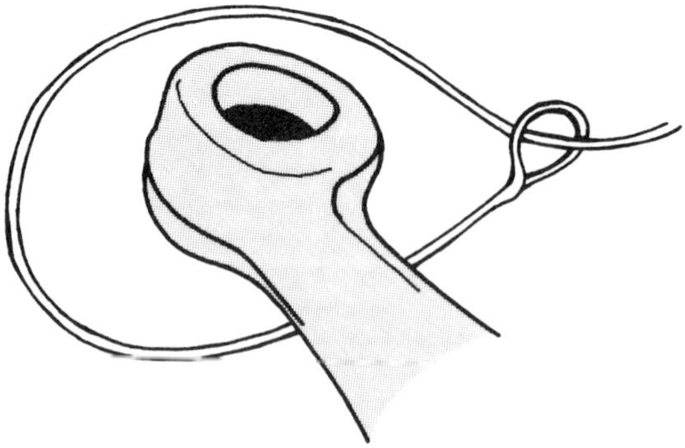

Fig. 7.6 Attempted extraction of toothbrush using nylon snare.

(d) *Simple snaring*

A polypectomy snare is so designed that, by pulling the wires back into the covering insulating sheath, the loop size is reduced. This makes polypectomy snares of various sizes and design well suited for the extraction of ingested foreign bodies (e.g. DeGerome, 1973; Kline, 1974; Olsen, Lawrence and Bernstein, 1974; Roesch *et al.*, 1974; Van Thiel and Stefan, 1974; McCafferey and Lilley, 1975; Waye, 1976; Miederer, 1977; Lux *et al.*, 1978). Griffiths *et al.* (1979) described the uneventful removal of a collection of ballpoint pens and paintbrushes from a patient, but Schiller and Salmon (1973), using a snare, failed to remove a toothbrush because it lay across the fundus (Fig. 7.6).

(e) *Snare closure of an open safety pin*

Open safety pins may be removed from the oesophagus (Barlow, 1960; Griswold, Haislip and Gardiner, 1973) but it is preferable to close the safety pin prior to extraction. Altman and Gottfried (1978) describe a method by which an open safety pin in the stomach was endoscopically snared and closed by tightening of the snare, after which it was safely extracted (Fig. 7.7).

(f) *Foley catheters and Dormia baskets*

Foley catheters have been passed beyond impacted foreign bodies which have then been mobilized and removed (Bigler, 1966). Similarly, small foreign bodies may be trapped in an endoscopically passed Dormia basket. These methods are of special value following endoscopic papillotomy where stones may be retrieved from the biliary tree or the duodenum (see Chapter 12).

(g) *Large diameter sheathing tubes*

Ségal (1960) and Boros (1961) described the insertion of plastic tubes into the oesophagus, enabling rigid endoscopes to be passed through these

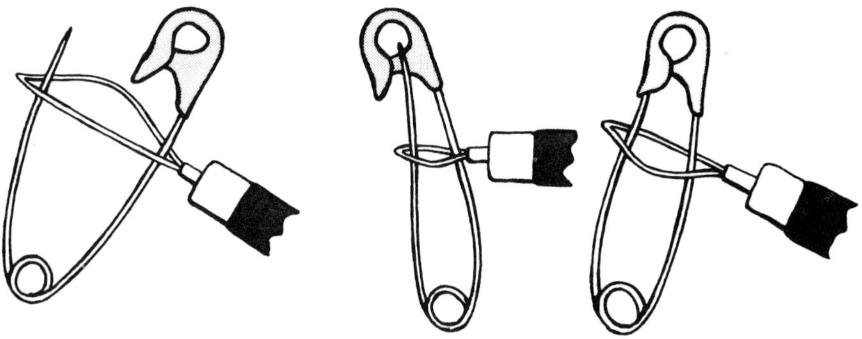

Fig. 7.7 Closure and removal of safety pin using snare (after Altman and Gottfried, 1978).

tubes. Witzel *et al.* (1974) modified this method and applied it to the problem of removing ingested razor blade segments. A plastic tube (80 cm long, inner diameter 15 cm) was slipped over the distal tip of a fibre-endoscope, and the assembly introduced into the stomach. Six razor blade fragments were in turn seized by means of a polypectomy snare and withdrawn, together with the endoscope, while the plastic tube was left *in situ* (Fig. 7.8). Martin *et al.* (1979) slid a colonoscopy stiffening tube over an upper gastrointestinal fibre-endoscope into the oesophagus. Two long foreign bodies (a pencil and a ballpoint pen), were then pulled one at a time into the stiffening tube and safely extracted (Fig. 7.9). The sheath used for oesophageal varices injection (Chapter 3) may be used for the same purpose.

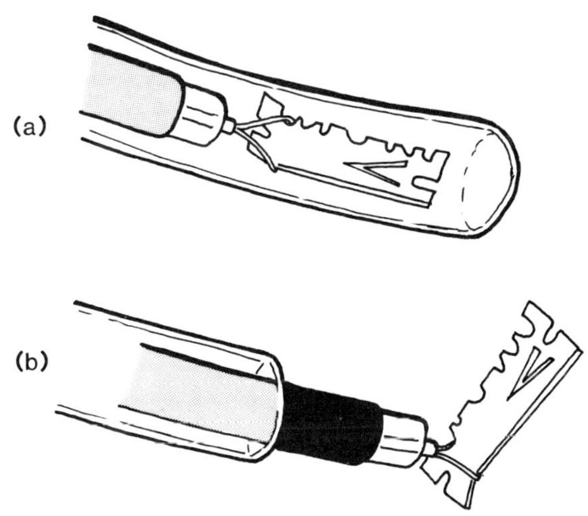

Fig. 7.8 Extraction of broken razor blade with snare using overtube method (after Witzel *et al.*, 1974).

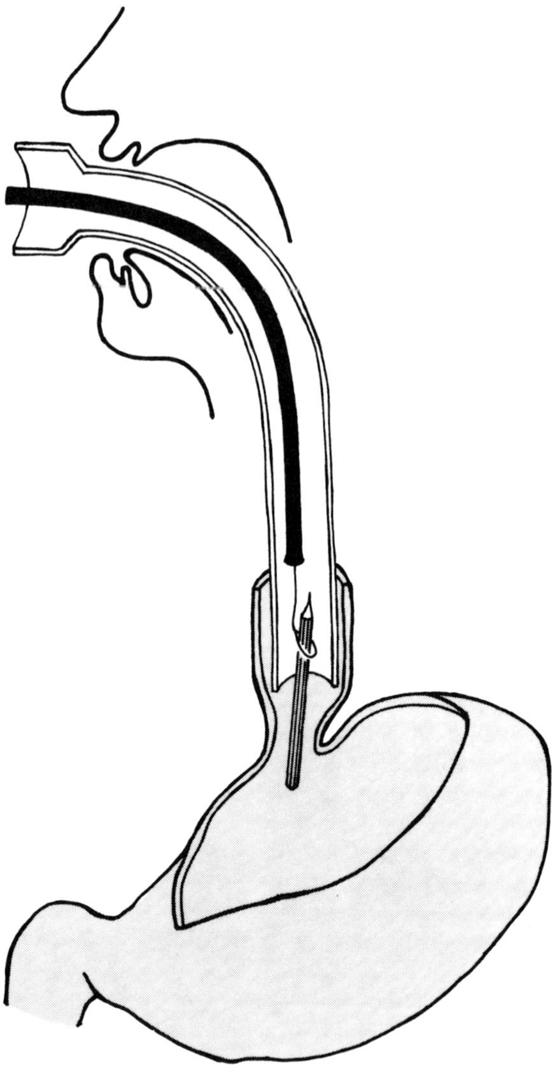

Fig. 7.9 Extraction of pencil with snare using colonic stiffening tube method (Martin *et al.*, 1979).

(h) *Cutting and removing retained suture material*
Gear and Dowling (1970) and Roesch (1970) reported simple endoscopic removal of retained sutures. Sutures may however prove difficult to remove by attempting simply to pull, using forceps. Seifert (1973) designed an endoscopic cutting device (Fig. 7.1(*d*)) for use in such patients, while Classen and Roesch (1974) have cut such sutures with a diathermy snare.

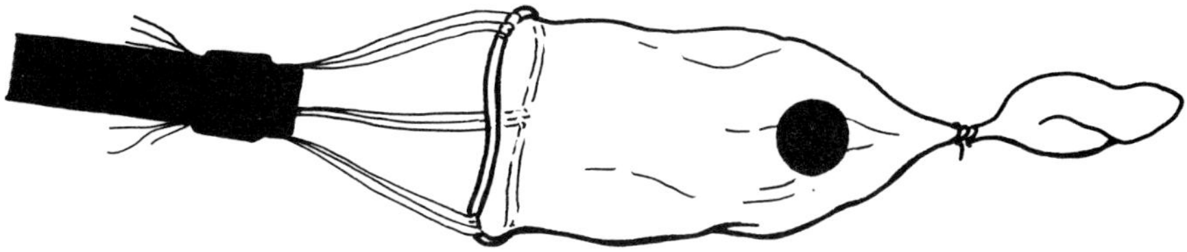

Fig. 7.10 Extraction of ballbearing, using a modified condom (after Wren and Cockel, 1978).

(i) *Trawling*
The method described by Wren and Cockel (1978) is mentioned because of its ingenuity. A steel ball-bearing, 17 mm in diameter, was swallowed by a four-year-old boy and retained in the stomach for six weeks. A latex contraceptive condom (Fig. 7.10) was attached by three cotton ties to the tip of an Olympus GIF D2 endoscope, the detachable hood being used to anchor the threads. The ball-bearing was easily made to roll into the self-opening 'trawl net', and safely removed. Mainguet (1978) has constructed an endoscopic trawl net from nylon stocking.

(j) *Loop technique*
Middleton and Nava (1978) describe an ingenious technique for the removal of a large rubber tube. A silk suture was tied to the tip of a nasogastric tube which was passed into the stomach. The suture was grasped tightly by endoscopic forceps, trapping the rubber tube (which had been retained in the stomach postoperatively) and thus removing it successfully (Fig. 7.11). Dunkerley *et al.* (1975) used a loop of umbilical tape passed by the endoscopist to retrieve a swallowed ring.

(k) *Mobilization: pushing a food bolus from oesophagus into stomach*
In the 'steak house syndrome' a large bolus of meat may be held up in the oesophagus. Provided there is nothing to suggest an obstructive lesion below the bolus, the tip of the fibre-endoscope may be used to push the bolus into the stomach (Roesch *et al.*, 1974). Endoscopy may be helpful even in the presence of a lesion: Graham *et al.* (1978*b*) described an instance where 'the endoscope was used as a bougie to guide a hot dog through an oesophageal stricture'.

(l) *Mechanical fragmentation of a bezoar*
A bezoar may lend itself to disruption under fibre-endoscopic control using biopsy forceps (McKechnie, 1972; Lukash, Fornes and Johnson, 1970; Brady, 1978).

(m) *Fragmentation combined with mobilization*
A potentially harmless foreign body such as an oesophageal meat bolus

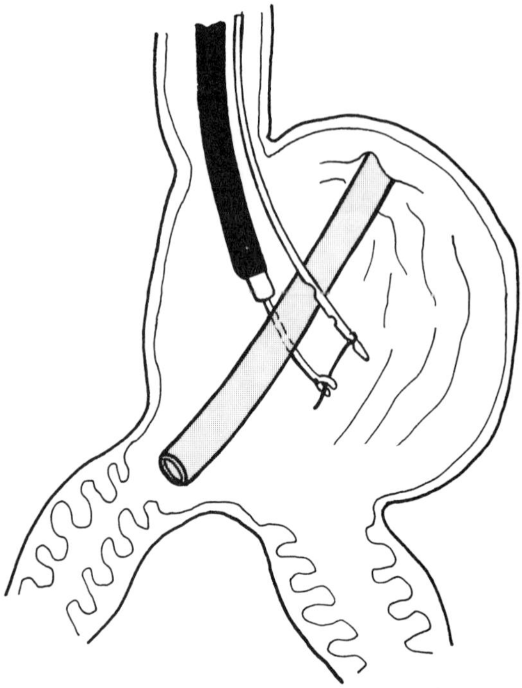

Fig. 7.11 Extraction of tubing by the loop technique (after Middleton and Nava, 1978).

can sometimes be pushed into the stomach if previously made smaller by the method described by Rogers (1979). This entails the use of an overtube method (Witzel *et al.*, 1974). The meat bolus is broken up in stages using a four-pronged grasper, and finally pushed into the stomach.

(n) *Dissolution of a bezoar*

As mentioned above, various enzymatic methods of inducing dissolution of bezoars have been described. Gold, Patteson and Green (1976), using the endoscope, injected cellulase directly into a bezoar with success.

(o) *Endoscopy under gnotobiotic conditions*

Graham *et al.* (1978*a*) described the mobilization of an ingested coin impacted in the oesophagus of a 6-year-old child suffering from severe combined immune deficiency. The procedure was undertaken without general anaesthesia, the child lying in a plastic bubble equipped with the necessary number of entry ports for the endoscope and the required manipulations. No significant complication ensued. This illustrates that the endoscopic management of ingested foreign bodies can be successfully accomplished even under difficult circumstances.

7.2.5 **Complications**

Any of the recognized complications of upper gastrointestinal fibre-endoscopy (Schiller and Prout, 1976; Mandelstam *et al.*, 1976) may occur during foreign body extraction. According to Classen *et al.* (1978) the particular complications of attempted endoscopic removal include perforation, haemorrhage, incomplete extraction, impaction of the foreign body and pulmonary aspiration of the object. In a previous series (Classen *et al.*, 1976) there was one patient with oesophageal perforation, but this was thought to have been due to pressure necrosis caused by the impacted object rather than attempts at removal. The use of enzymatic methods but softening and dissolving bezoars has already been mentioned, but Holsinger, Fuson and Sealy (1968) reported an oesophageal perforation following the therapeutic ingestion of papain to treat an impacted meat bolus.

ACKNOWLEDGEMENTS

My thanks are due to my colleague, Dr. John Patten, who kindly prepared the line drawings, and my secretary, Mrs. Ann Terry, for her help with the text.

REFERENCES

Akasaka, Y. *et al.* (1979). Endoscopic management of acute gastric anisakiasis. *Endoscopy*, **2**, 158.

Altman, A. R. and Gottfried, E. B. (1978). Intragastric closure of an ingested safety pin. *Gastrointest. Endosc.*, **24**, 294.

Armengol-Miro, J. R. *et al.* (1977). Prepapillary intradiverticular bezoar as cause of obstructive jaundice. *Endoscopy*, **9**, 247.

Ashby, B. S. and Hunter-Craig, I. D. (1967). Foreign body perforation of the gut. *Br. J. Surg.*, **54**, 382.

Banks, W. and Potsic, W. P. (1978). Unsuspected foreign bodies of the aerodigestive tract. *Ann. Oto. Rhinol. Lar.*, **87**, 515.

Barlow, D. (1960). Device for removing an open safety pin from oesophagus or bronchial tree. *Lancet*, **1**, 208.

Belber, J. P. (1978). Gastroscopy and duodenoscopy. In: *Gastrointestinal Disease* (ed. M. H. Sleisenger and J. S. Fordtran), W. B. Saunders Co., Philadelphia, London, Toronto.

Bigler, F. E. (1966). The use of a Foley catheter for removal of blunt foreign bodies from the esophagus. *Thorac. Cardiovasc. Surg.*, **51**, 759.

Bitar, D. E. and Holmes, T. W. (1975). Polybezoar and gastrointestinal foreign bodies in the mentally retarded. *Am. Surg.*, **41**, 497.

Bloomfield, D. A. (1978). The nonsurgical retrieval of intracardiac foreign bodies – an international survey. *Cath. Cardiovasc. Diag.*, **4**, 1.

Bong, I. *et al.* (1966). Massive growth of yeasts in resected stomach. *Gut*, **7**, 244.

Boros, E. (1961). Esophageal intubator – its use in esophagoscopy. *Am. J. Gastroent.*, **35**, 326.

Brady, P. G. (1978). Gastric phytobezoars consequent to delayed gastric emptying. *Gastrointest. Endosc.*, **24**, 159.
Burnington, J. D. (1976). Aluminium 'pop tops' – a hazard to child health. *J. Am. Med. Ass.*, **235**, 2614.
Classen, M. and Roesch. W. (1974). Endoscopic cutting of persisting suture material. *Gastrointest. Endosc.*, **20**, 130.
Classen, M. *et al.* (1976). Endoskopische Fremdkoerperentfernung aus den oberen Verdauungstrakt. *Dt. Aert.*, **73**, 1969.
Classen, M. *et al.* (1978). Operative and therapeutic techniques, In: *Clinics in Gastroenterology. Endoscopy*, **7** (3), (ed. K. F. R. Schiller), W. B. Saunders Co. Ltd., London, Philadelphia, Toronto.
Dann, S. *et al.* (1959). The successful medical management of a phytobezoar. *Arch. Intern. Med.*, **103**, 598.
DeBakey, M. and Ochsner, A. (1938). Bezoars and concretions. *Surgery*, **4**, 934.
DeBakey, M. and Ochsner, A. (1939). Bezoars and concretions. *Surgery*, **5**, 132.
DeGerome, J. M. (1973). Snare extraction of foreign body. *Gastrointest. Endosc.*, **19**, 73.
Dehler, J. R. *et al.* (1979). Endoscopic identification and removal of unusual symptomatic colonic foreign body. *Dig. Dis. Sci.*, **24**, 237.
Dunkerley, R. E. *et al.* (1975). Fiber endoscopic removal of large foreign bodies from the stomach. *Gastrointest. Endosc.*, **21**, 196.
Earlam, E. (1976). *Clinical Tests of Oesophageal Function*, Crosby Lockwood Staples, London.
Eldridge, W. W. (1961). Foreign bodies in the gastrointestinal tract. *J. Am. Med. Ass.*, **178**, 665.
Elgood, C. (1935). A treatise on the bezoar stone. By the late Mahmud bin Masud the Imad-ul-din, the Physician of Ispahan. *Ann. Med. Hist.*, **7**, 73.
Gear, M. W. L. and Dowling, B. L. (1970). Suture-line ulcer after gastric surgery caused by non-absorbable suture materials. *Br. J. Surg.*, **57**, 356.
Goff, W. F. (1968). What to do when foreign bodies are inhaled or ingested. *Postgrad. Med.*, **44**, 135.
Gold, M. H., Patteson, T. E. and Green, G. I. (1976). Cellulase bezoar injection. A new endoscopic technique. *Gastrointest. Endosc.*, **22**, 200.
Graham, D. Y. *et al.* (1978*a*). Endoscopy under gnotobiotic conditions. *Gastrointest. Endosc.*, **24**, 298.
Graham, D. Y. *et al.* (1978*b*). Value of fibreoptic gastrointestinal endoscopy in infants and children. *South. Med. J.*, **71**, 558.
Greenwood, A. G. and Wild, D. (1977). Fibreoptic gastroscopy in a grey seal, *Halichoreus grypus*. *Aquat. Anim.*, **5**, 67.
Greenwood A. G. *et al.* (1978). Fibreoptic gastroscopy in dolphins. *Vet. Rec.*, **102**, 495.
Griffiths, W. J. *et al.* (1979). Fiberoptic endoscopic retrieval of swallowed intragastric foreign objects. *J. Oklahoma St. Med. Ass.*, **72**, 67.
Griswold, F. C., Haislip, C. E. and Gardner, R. J. (1973). Removal of an intragastric foreign body using the flexible fiberoptic esophagoscope. *Gastrointest. Endosc.*, **19**, 194.
Gupta, J. K., Ricca, J. J. and Ingegno, A. P. (1977). Removal of inadvertently swallowed endotracheal tube from the stomach through an esophagostomy stoma with the fiberoptic endoscope. *Gastrointest. Endosc.*, **23**, 31.
Hoare, A. M. and Alexander-Williams, J. (1977). Thread ulcers seen on gastroscopy: do they cause ulcers or indigestion? *Br. Med. J.*, **2**, 996–7.
Holsinger, J. W., Fuson, R. L. and Sealy, W. C. (1968). Esophageal perforation following impaction and papain ingestion. *J. Am. Med. Ass.*, **204**, 188.

Honaas, T. O., and Shaffer, E. A. (1977). Endoscopic removal of a foreign body perforating the duodenum. *Can. Med. Ass. J.*, **116**, 164.

Houston, H. E. (1975). Unusual esophageal foreign body: dead or alive. *Arch. Surg.*, **110**, 1516.

Jackson, C. and Jackson, C. L. (1937). *Diseases of the Air and Food Passages of Foreign Body Origin*, W. B. Saunders Co., Philadelphia.

Kassner, E. G. *et al.* (1975). Retention of small foreign objects in the stomach and duodenum. *Radiology*, **114**, 683.

Kline, M. M. (1974). Endoscopic snare in removal of an esophageal foreign body. *Gastrointest. Endosc.*, **20**, 165.

Lefton, H. B. (1976). Endoscopic discovery and removal of *Ascaris lumbricoides*. *Gastrointest. Endosc.*, **22**, 87.

Lukash, W. M., Fornes, M. F. and Johnson R. B. (1970). Gastric bezoars. *Gastroenterology*, **58**, 1070.

Lux, G. *et al.* (1978). Gastrointestinal fiberoptic endoscopy in pediatric patients and juveniles. *Endoscopy*, **10**, 158.

McLoughlin, J. C. *et al.* (1979). Intact removal of phytobezoar using fibreoptic endoscope in patient with gastric atopy. *Br. Med. J.*, **2**, 1466.

McCafferey, T. D. and Lilley, J. O. (1975). The management of foreign bodies of the gastrointestinal tract. *Am. J. Dig. Dis.*, **20**, 121.

McKechnie, J. C. (1972). Gastroscopic removal of a phytobezoar. *Gastroenterology*, **62**, 1047.

Mainguet, P. (1978). Personal communication.

Mandelstam, P. *et al.* (1976). Complications associated with esophogastro-duodenoscopy and with esophageal dilatation: an analysis of the 1974 ASGE survey. *Gastrointest. Endosc.*, **22**, 16.

Manegold, B. C. (1973). Fiberendoskopische Fremdkoerperextraktion aus Magen und Duodenum. *Chirurg*, **44**, 523.

Manegold, B. C. (1977). Endoskopische Fremdkoerperextraktion und intra-operative Endoskopie. *Lang. Arch. Chir.*, **345**, 299.

Manialawi, M. *et al.* (1978). Endoscopic examination of Egyptian mummies. *Endoscopy*, **10**, 191.

Marsden, P. D. (1978). Other nematodes. In: *Clinics in Gastroenterology, Intestinal Parasites*, **7**, (1), (ed. P. D. Marsden), W. B. Saunders Co. Ltd., London, Philadelphia, Toronto.

Martin, W. C. *et al.* (1979). Fiberendoscopic removal of long foreign bodies from the stomach using a colon stiffening tube as a protection sheath. *Am. J. Gastroent.*, **71**, 505.

Middleton, P. E. and Nava, H. (1978). Retrieval of a large rubber tube from the stomach by a loop technique. *Gastrointest. Endosc.*, **24**, 295.

Miederer, S. E. (1977). A snare for the endoscopic extraction of coins. *Endoscopy*, **9**, 99.

Miller, S. F. (1975). Foreign body ingestion. *J. Am. Fam. Physician*, **11**, 123.

Munsell, J. and Walker, P. (1972). Persimmon bezoar in an epiphrenic esophageal diverticulum with endoscopic removal. *Gastrointest. Endosc.*, **18**, 163.

Murdock, H. (1934). Persimmon bezoars occurring around Tulsa, Oklahoma. *J. Oklahoma St. Med. Ass.*, **27**, 442.

Norberg, H. P. and Reyes, H. M. (1975). Complications of ornamental Christmas bulb ingestion. *Arch. Surg.*, **110**, 1494.

Olsen, H., Lawrence, W. and Berstein, R. (1974). Fiberendoscopic removal of foreign bodies from the upper gastrointestinal tract. *Gastrointest. Endosc.*, **20**, 58.

Papamichael, E. E. (1976). Removal of foreign bodies from subsegmental bronchi with the fiberbronchoscope. *Endoscopy*, **8**, 192.

Perttala, Y., *et al.* (1975). Yeast bezoar formation following gastric surgery. *Am. J. Roentg.*, **125**, 365.
Pillari, G. *et al.* (1979). Meat bolus impaction of the lower esophagus associated with a paraesophageal hernia. *Am. J. Gastroent.*, **71**, 287.
Pollard, H. B. and Block, G. E. (1968). Rapid dissolution of phytobezoar by cellulase enzyme. *Am. J. Surg.* **116**, 933.
Roesch, W. (1970). Suture material and suture-line ulcer following gastric surgery. *Endoscopy*, **2**, 237.
Roesch, W. *et al.* (1974). Operative endoscopy of the upper gastrointestinal tract. *Gastrointest. Endosc.*, **20**, 108.
Rogers, B. H. R. (1979). A new method for extraction of impacted meat from the esophagus using a flexible fiberoptic endoscope and an overtube. *Gastrointest. Endosc.*, **25**, 47.
Sartory, A. and Trabant, G. (1978). Endoscopic extraction of a perforating paperclip from the stomach. *Endoscopy*, **10**, 217.
Savary, M. and Miller, G. (1978). *The Esophagus: Handbook and Atlas of Endoscopy.* Gassmann, Solothurn.
Schiller, K. F. R. and Prout, B. J. (1976). Hazards. In *Modern Topics of Gastrointestinal Endoscopy* (ed. K. F. R. Schiller and P. R. Salmon), Wm. Heinemann Medical Books, London.
Schiller, K. F. R. and Salmon, P. R. (1973). Extraction of foreign bodies utilizing fibre-endoscopy. *Gut*, **14**, 920.
Ségal, S. (1960). In: *Traite Pratique de Photographie et de Cinematographie Medicales*, (ed. P. Mantel), Paris. (see Witzel, 1974).
Seifert, E. (1973). Appliances for surgical endoscopy. *Endoscopy*, **5**, 96.
Small, W. P. *et al.* (1968). Suture-line ulcer following gastric surgery. *Am. J. Surg.*, **115**, 477.
Swarbrick, E. T. *et al.* (1972). Removal of a darning needle with a fibreoptic gastroscope. *Br. Med. J.*, **3**, 470.
Tongerson, S. A. *et al.* (1979). Gallstone obstruction of duodenal cap (Bouveret's syndrome) diagnosed by endoscopy. *Am. J. Gastroent.*, **72**, 165.
Townsend, C. *et al.* (1973). Intestinal obstruction from medication bezoar in patients with renal failure. *New Eng. J. Med.*, **288**, 1058.
Van Thiel, D. H. and Stefan, N. J. (1974). Removal of soft foreign bodies from the esophagus using a flexible instrument. *Gastrointest. Endosc.*, **20**, 163.
Waye, J. D. (1976). Removal of foreign bodies from the upper intestinal tract with fiberoptic instruments. *Am. J. Gastroent.*, **65**, 557.
Weithofer, G. *et al.* (1977). Spontaneous expulsion of a migrating infantry missile impacted in the duodenum and the common bile duct 32 years after wounding. *Endoscopy*, **9**, 106.
Wirtschafter, M. Z. (1977). Successful recovery of a foreign body from the forestomach of a dolphin by peroral endoscopy. *Gastrointest. Endosc.*, **23**, 156.
Witzel, L. *et al.* (1974). Removal of razorblades from the stomach with fibreoptic endoscope. *Br. Med. J.*, **2**, 539.
Wolf, L. and Geraci, K. (1978). Colonoscopic removal of balloons from the bowel. *Gastrointest. Endosc.*, **24**, 41.
Wren, C. and Cockel, R. (1978). Endoscopic removal of a swallowed ballbearing from stomach of a four year old child. *Br. Med. J.*, **2**, 252.
Zeegen, R. and Lance, P. (1979). Personal communication.
Zipkin, B. and Rosenfeld, D. L. (1979). Hysteroscopic removal of a Heyman radium capsule. *J. Reprod. Med.*, **22**, 133.

8 Gastroduodenal haemorrhage – lasers

P. R. SALMON

8.1 INTRODUCTION

Non-operative methods for controlling gastro-intestinal haemorrhage have been the goal of gastroenterologists for many years, but it is only since the advent of fibre-optic endoscopy that this has become possible. The diagnostic accuracy of endoscopy in upper alimentary haemorrhage has now been established, but current interest has centred on an additional therapeutic role whereby the endoscope is employed as a delivery system for haemostatic devices. Most of these systems require tissue contact, but non-contact methods have also been developed (see Chapter 9). Of these the most interesting at present is the use of a laser beam focused into the end of a flexible fibre, which is itself passed down the operating channel of a fibre-optic endoscope. The laser beam can be focused to give a high power density over a small area and will produce a sharply defined area of thermal coagulation. The word laser is an acronym for Light Amplification by the Stimulated Emission of Radiation; coherent mono-chromatic light with a very small divergent angle is produced so that high energies are emitted. The principle of laser light, first enunciated by Einstein, was put into practice as recently as 1960 by Maiman, whilst the first trial of lasers in gastroenterology was the use of the CO_2 laser transmitted through a hollow rigid endoscope to coagulate bleeding superficial lesions in the dog stomach (Goodale *et al.*, 1970). Since then there has been considerable experimental work designed to evaluate the effects of lasers in normal tissues and the haemostatic action of lasers. In this chapter discussion will centre around the types of laser in use, their comparative roles in producing haemostasis and the problems involved in clinical application of laser photocoagulation.

8.2 LASER SOURCES

Two types of laser are currently in use for the endoscopic control of alimentary haemorrhage; the argon ion laser which is a gas laser, and the

Nd-YAG (Neodymium Yttrium Aluminium Garnet) laser which is a solid state laser. These lasers have different wavelengths and therefore different absorption patterns in living tissue. These are currently the only lasers whose beams can be transmitted via flexible fibres, although a fibre is being developed that will transmit a CO_2 laser beam.

The argon laser emits light in the green region of the spectrum (varying between 452.5 and 514.5 nm) whilst the Nd-YAG laser emits in the invisible near infra-red region (1060 nm).

8.3 PENETRATION OF LASER BEAMS INTO TISSUE

Whilst penetration (Transmission) of the laser beam into tissues is an important phenomenon, both for the therapeutic action of photocoagulation, and for considerations of safety (i.e. perforation), other tissue interactions occur and may be of considerable importance in the overall understanding of haemostasis by laser photocoagulation. Fig. 8.1

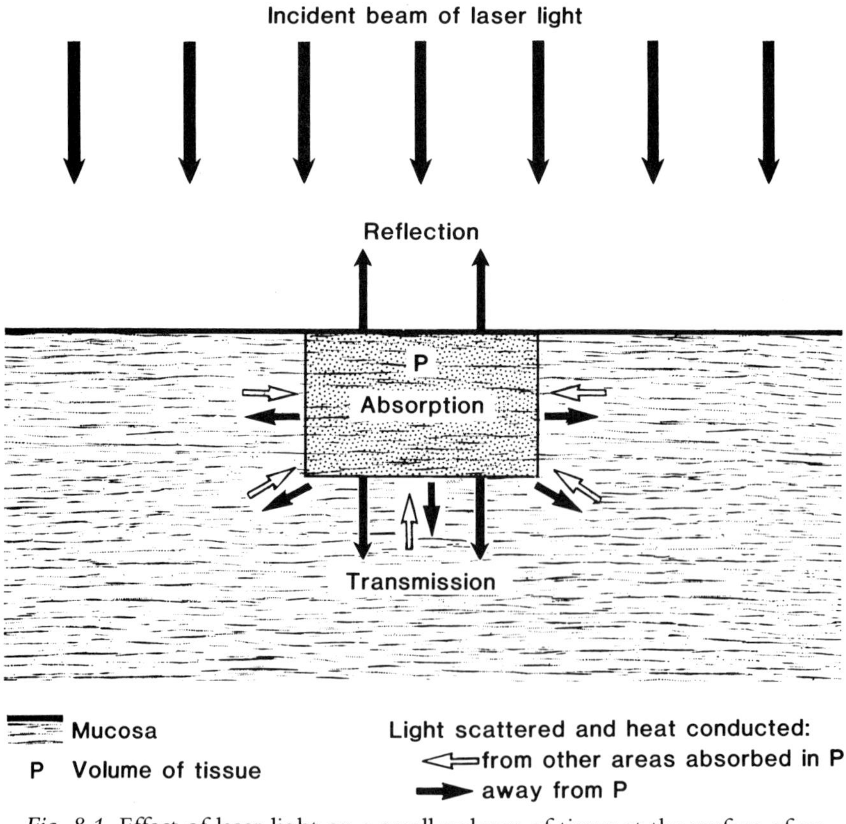

Fig. 8.1 Effect of laser light on a small volume of tissue at the surface of an area of mucosa [reproduced, with permission, from *Gut* (1979), **20**, 680–687].

demonstrates four possible physical effects that may occur when a laser beam is incident on living tissue. The penetration depth of a laser beam depends on the absorption coefficient of the tissue which is itself dependent on the wavelength of the laser beam. Table 8.1 demonstrates this relationship for liver tissue.

The effect of tissue penetration and therefore tissue damage (coagulation) that occurs depends not only on the depth of penetration but also on the thermal conductivity of the tissue and the quantity of applied energy which is itself dependent on the exposure time and the laser power.

Reidenbach *et al.* (1975) have shown in experiments with thin layers of blood (10 μm to 300 μm) that increased optical absorption can be observed below a wavelength of 600 nm. This explains why the argon-ion laser with wavelengths between 454.5 nm and 514.5 nm is particularly suitable for photocoagulation (Table 8.2).

8.4 LASER SYSTEMS FOR CLINICAL USE

In order to employ a laser beam for photocoagulation of bleeding lesions in humans the laser output must be coupled to a flexible fibre which is itself passed down the operating channel of a fibre-optic endoscope. Considerable research has been performed on the types of fibre that can

Table 8.1 Penetration depth in liver.

Laser	*Penetration depth (mm) for liver*
CO_2 (10 600 nm)	0.05
Nd-YAG (1060 nm)	0.8
Argon (500 nm)	0.2

(From Kiefhaber, Moritz and North, 1974)

Table 8.2 Haemostatic effect of argon-ion photocoagulation.

Power (W)	*Ulcers No.*	*Ulcers Haemostasis*	*Average blood loss*	
2–5	6	2	0.1	N.S.
7–9	23	22	<0.05	$P < 0.001$
12	5	2	>0.05	N.S.

(From Bown *et al.*, 1979)

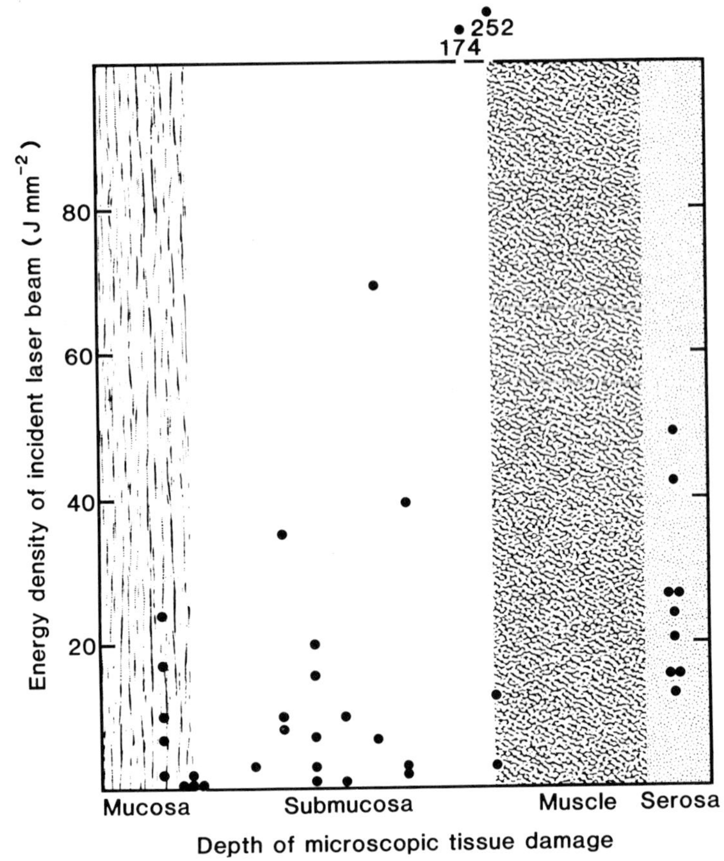

Fig. 8.2 Normal gastric mucosa – acute lesions [reproduced, with permission, from *Gut* (1979), **20**, 680–687].

be employed for laser beam transmission. An endoscopic light transmission system should meet the following requirements:

(a) Have high light transmission.
(b) Have low optical attenuation.
(c) Have sufficiently low beam divergence at the distal end.
(d) Have a small fibre diameter.
(e) Be flexible.
(f) Be robust.
(g) Be thermally and chemically stable.

Research has been directed essentially into either plastic or quartz light guides.

Work on plastic light guides (Reidenbach *et al.*, 1975; Reidenbach and Bodem, 1975a and b) has employed core-cladding combinations such as polystyrene–polymethyl methacrylate (Ps–PMMA) and polymethyl methacrylate–fluorine copolymer (PMMA-F-cop). 1.5 mm plastic fibres between 1.5 m and 3 m long have been found to be suitable. Beam divergence from the distal end of these fibres varied between 14° and 28°. The optical transmission of these plastic fibres is inferior to that of quartz fibres which will transmit 90% of either Nd-YAG or argon-ion laser beams. For this reason, in spite of the greater expense, quartz fibres have now largely replaced plastic light guides. It was thought at first that beam divergence was an important factor in reducing tissue effects due to the expression $B = P/F\Omega$ (were B = brightness of the laser, F = beam cross sectional area, Ω = solid angle of beam divergence) so that at a given distance of the transmitting fibre from the tissues, if the beam divergence was relatively high the power density on the tissues would be unacceptably low. Because of this a special triconic quartz fibre (Fig. 8.2) was developed by Kiefhaber *et al.* (1977). This fibre is 3 m in length, having a transmission of 90%. It consists of a wide proximal end, allowing entry of the laser beam, followed by a more flexible narrow section (diameter $\simeq$ 300 μm) reducing further to about 200 μm before widening at the distal end. This fibre has a beam divergence of only 4.2° (full angle). This fibre is no longer justified due to its high cost and the fact that coaxial gas flow is not possible as the fibre itself must be protected by a quartz window (involving modification of the endoscope). Also, recent work shows that the mean energy required for haemostasis is in fact lower when employing the much cheaper single filament 600 μm quartz fibre which allows coaxial gas flow (Table 8.1 and Fig. 8.2).

8.5 ARRANGEMENT OF LASER FOR ENDOSCOPIC PHOTOCOAGULATION

The laser beam is focused onto the end of a single filament quartz fibre (Fig. 8.3). This is effected by the fibre, which is held in a clamp, being moved by micrometer adjustments across the laser beam until maximum transmission occurs. 200, 400 or 600 μm quartz fibres of 4 m length are available. The free end of the fibre is passed down a 2 mm diameter 3 m catheter through a connecting box which allows CO_2 gas to be blown coaxially with the laser fibre (Silverstein *et al.*, 1978). The tip of the fibre is adjusted to lie several millimetres inside the distal end of the catheter which protects it. The catheter and fibre are then passed down the biopsy channel of a standard endoscope. The coaxial CO_2 is employed as a slow continuous background flow serving to keep the fibre tip clear of blood and to prevent backflow of secretions into the catheter. A higher flow rate can be activated by a footswitch prior to photocoagulation in order to blow blood away from the bleeding site, both for identification of the bleeding site and to prevent blood from absorbing the laser power.

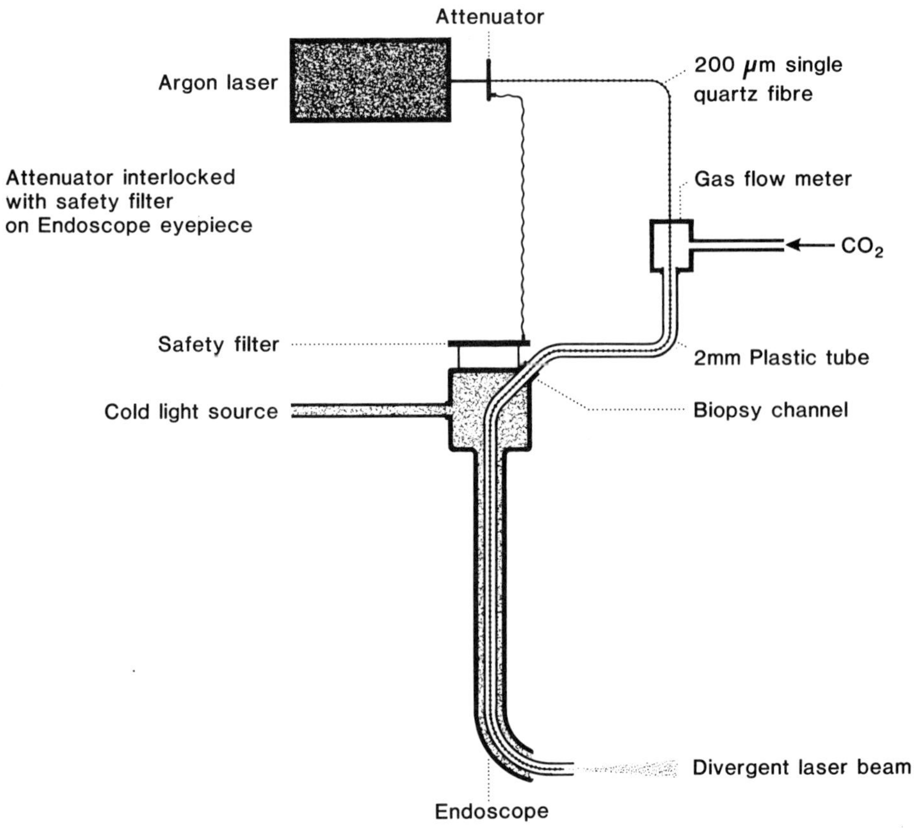

Fig. 8.3 Endoscopic photocoagulation – experimental arrangement of laser [reproduced, with permission, from *Gut* (1979), **20**, 680–687].

Gas flow rates may be pre-set. The footswitch control keeps an attenuator across the laser beam until full power is required so that only about 0.1% of peak power is initially allowed down the fibre. This small amount is sufficient to serve as an aiming beam. In the case of the Nd-YAG laser which emits in the invisible near infra-red spectrum, a low power Helium–Neon laser is employed which produces a red light. Full power is applied by activating the footswitch which moves the attenuator out of the main laser beam. This attenuator is interlocked with a safety filter which passes across the endoscope eyepiece, in order to protect the endoscopist's eye. In open animal experiments safety goggles of a type suitable for the laser which is to be employed, must be worn.

8.6 EXPERIMENTAL WORK WITH LASERS

Animal experiments have concentrated on the effects of lasers (chiefly the Argon and Nd-YAG lasers) on normal living tissues and the effect of

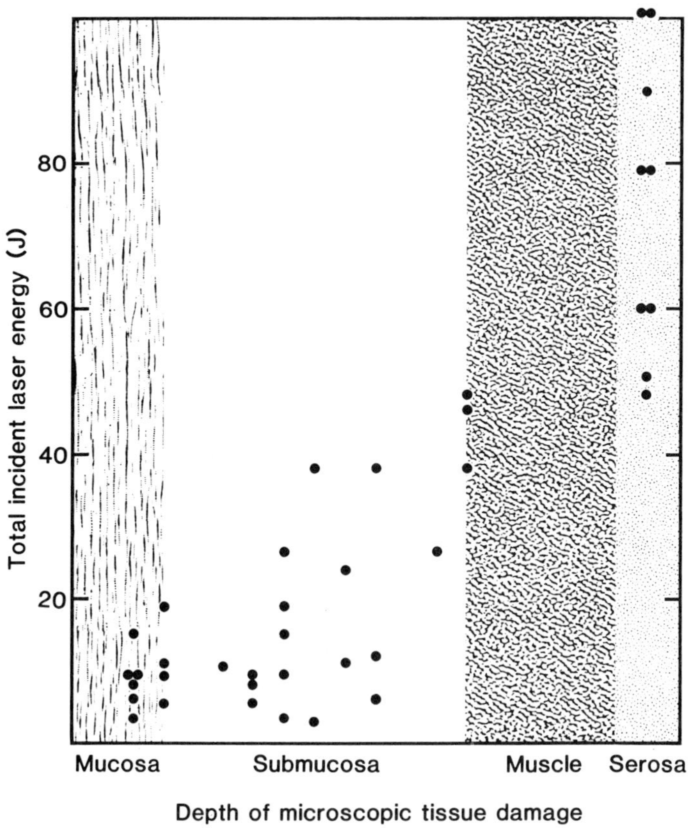

Fig. 8.4 Normal gastric mucosa – acute lesions [reproduced, with permission, from *Gut* (1979), **20**, 680–687].

each laser on inducing haemostasis in experimental lesions. Studies on the normal dog stomach (Bown *et al.*, 1979) have shown that the depth of tissue damage depends on the total incident laser energy on any one spot rather than the energy density, and that below 50 J the risk of perforation is low. Figs. 8.2 and 8.4 show the effect of energy density and total energy on the depth of histological damage in acute lesions produced by the argon laser. Fig. 8.2 demonstrates that, whilst there is a general tendency for the depth of damage to increase with the energy density, there are anomalies (e.g. 174 and 252) where with high energy densities full thickness damage does not occur, yet there are instances of full thickness damage at low energy densities. These data should be contrasted with Fig. 8.4 where there is a much closer correlation between total energy and tissue damage with a critical energy in the dog stomach of about 50.5.

These results are power dependent and require powers of 4 W and above (Argon laser). Similar results were obtained in chronic studies and

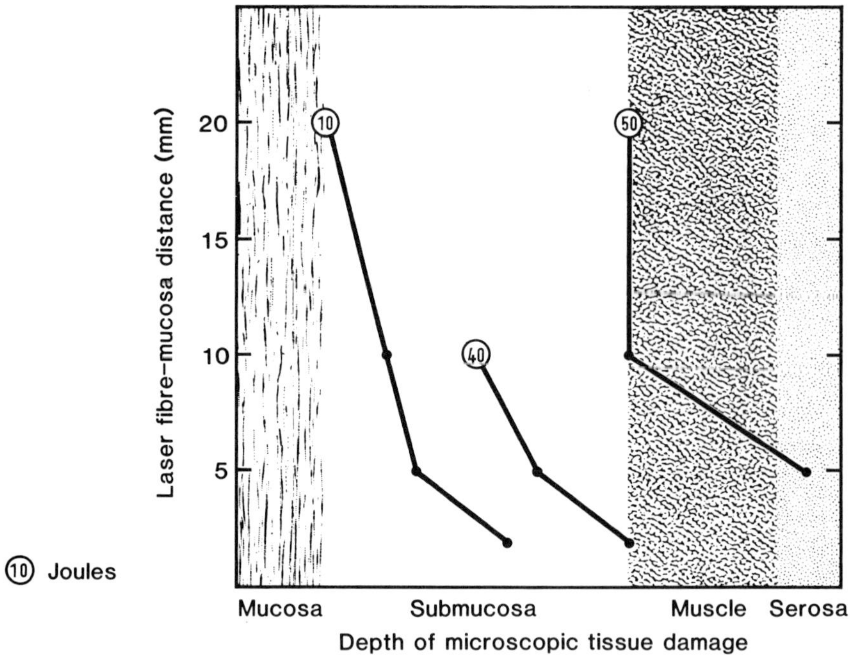

Fig. 8.5 Normal gastric mucosa – acute lesions [reproduced, with permission, from *Gut* (1979), **20**, 680–687].

also for the Nd-YAG laser. Fig. 8.5 demonstrates how the depth of damage varies with the energy density at three values of total energy. Fig. 8.6 shows the much closer correlation between total energy and depth of damage which is independent of energy density, since the lines for three values of energy density cross each other.

Experimental bleeding has usually involved use of the Beagle dog in which blood loss from experimental gastric ulcers is measured at gastrotomy, and haemostasis is assessed after laser photocoagulation. Ulcers are made with the Quinton ulcer maker (Protell *et al.*, 1976). This produces ulcers of a standard depth thus enabling any laser induced damage to be readily assessed. Experiments have been performed on heparinized animals to produce a clotting time of at least three times that of controls (Silverstein *et al.*, 1977; Bown *et al.*, 1979). Blood loss has been quantified by collection in wide mouth vials from the edge of each ulcer. Studies have compared both the triconic and single filament fibre and have investigated the efficacy of haemostasis at different energy levels (energy = power × time).

With the Argon laser at 7–9 W twenty-two out of twenty-three ulcers (96%) stopped bleeding in one study (Bown *et al.*, 1979) (Table 8.2). This supports earlier work by Silverstein *et al.* (1977). With the Nd-YAG laser, powers of 45 W or more achieved haemostasis in all ulcers treated

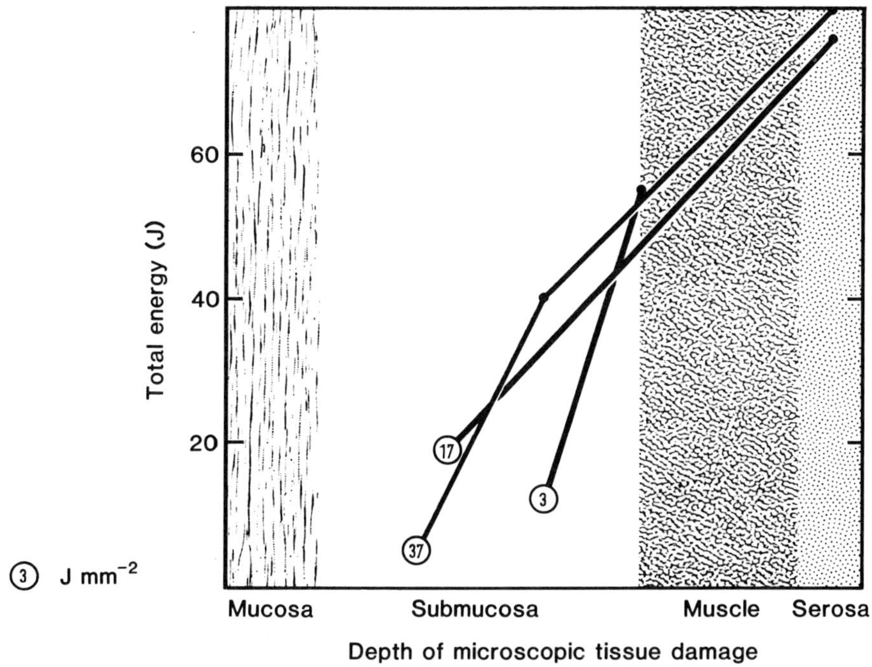

Fig. 8.6 Normal gastric mucosa – acute lesions [reproduced, with permission, from *Gut* (1979), **20**, 680–687].

(Table 8.3). Table 8.3 shows that the average energy (power × average no. of pulses required) with the triconic fibre is higher than with the 600 μm fibre at comparable power levels, this probably being partly due to the beneficial effect of coaxial gas blowing blood from the lesion in the case of the 600 μm fibre. The average energy required for haemostasis decreased as the laser power increased, so that with powers above 66 W haemostasis is achieved with exposure times below 1 s. This important finding shows that pulses of fractions of one second at the highest

Table 8.3 Photocoagulation of experimental ulcers.

Fibre	*Power (W)*	*No. of ulcers*	*Mean no. of pulses for haemostasis*	*Range in no. of pulses*	*Mean energy required for haemostasis (J)*
Triconic	47	6	21	11–32	990
Triconic	66	6	11	4–31	730
600 μm	26	5	25	8–53	650
600 μm	43	6	13	6–30	560
600 μm	53	5	6	4–11	320

powers available (>90 W with the Nd-YAG laser) may be sufficient to induce haemostasis, thus lowering the average energy required for coagulation (Bown *et al.*, 1980). Since the extent of damage to tissues is dependent chiefly on the total energy applied, this means haemostasis may be achieved well within the safety limits imposed by the critical energy for each tissue (that energy required to produce full thickness damage).

Other factors are those imposed by the size of blood vessels. In experimental studies the upper limit for coagulation by the YAG laser was 3 mm diameter (Leheta and Gorisch, 1975).

8.7 CLINICAL STUDIES

Since the first clinical report of laser photocoagulation (Frühmorgen *et al.*, 1975) in which some colonic haemangiomata and a bleeding gastric ulcer were successfully treated, there have been numerous reports of successful photocoagulation of bleeding and non-bleeding lesions, chiefly in the upper alimentary tract. Reports have been anecdotal but enthusiastic with both the Argon and the Nd-YAG lasers.

Both lasers require a 3-phase electric power supply, and water for cooling. In addition to this there are local safety regulations involving safety interlocking circuits and safety switches. Misalignment of the laser, which reduces its efficiency, is common and the user must work closely with a medical physics department and have a clear understanding of the system.

Care of the fibre tip is crucial for achieving optimum power levels at the tissues, so some device for scrupulous cleaving of the fibre tip (should it become damaged) is essential. The importance of an inert (CO_2) gas stream to allow a clear field of view for aiming the laser beam has been stressed already, but a return pathway for the gas is also necessary. This can be achieved either by employing a two-channel endoscope so that the gas is vented via the second channel, or by the use of a specially designed closed-circuit system. Use of a standard single channel endoscope is feasible if a thin naso-gastric tube is strapped to the endoscope in order to vent the gas. At present there are no reports of a completed randomized study of the use of lasers in patients with alimentary bleeding although one is in progress in the U.S.A. and in the U.K.

Uncontrolled studies (Frühmorgen *et al.*, 1978; Brunetaud *et al.*, 1980; Lawrence *et al.*, 1980) demonstrate encouraging results with the Argon laser whilst equally good results are reported with the Nd-YAG laser (Kiefhaber *et al.*, 1977).

In one study (Brunetaud *et al.*, 1980), 54 out of 71 ulcers showing evidence of active bleeding were successfully treated following Argon laser photocoagulation. Sixty stopped bleeding following laser therapy, but 6 re-bled within 7 days. Reasons for failure include inability accurately to identify the bleeding point, scarring of the duodenal bulb making accurate aiming of the laser beam difficult and some failures in spite of apparently accurate and adequate photocoagulation (10%). Haemostasis is probably effected by thermal contraction of the walls of the vessels and surrounding tissues. In the case of varices, which are large, unsupported thin-walled vessels, it is difficult to understand the apparently high success rates reported by some groups. It would seem likely that laser photocoagulation would be less successful in these cases and could even exacerbate bleeding by burning a hole in a varix.

The future of laser photocoagulation in controlling alimentary haemorrhage depends on the results of a sufficiently large randomized controlled trial of photocoagulation. The optimum energy requirements for producing defined controlled lesions with high safety are now defined and should help to clarify the role of laser photocoagulation in this important clinical area. If this accuracy can be refined and can be shown to achieve good and predictable control of haemorrhage, then later photocoagulation will justify the high cost of the equipment compared with other methods of coagulation described in Chapter 9.

REFERENCES

Bown, S. G. *et al.* (1979). Argon laser photocoagulation in the dog stomach. *Gut*, **20**, 680–7.

Bown, S. G. *et al.* (1980). Pulsed Nd YAG laser photocoagulation in the dog stomach. *Eur. Endosc. Cong. Hamburg* (Abstract to be published in *Endoscopy*).

Brunetaud, J. M. *et al.* (1980). Argon laser photocoagulation – the current situation. *Eur. Endosc. Cong. Hamburg* (Abstract to be published in *Endoscopy*).

Frühmorgen, P. *et al.* (1975). The first endoscopic laser coagulation in the human GI tract. *Endoscopy*, **7**, 156–7.

Goodale, R. L. *et al.* (1970). Rapid endoscopic control of bleeding gastric erosions by laser radiation. *Arch. Surg.*, **101**, 211.

Kiefhaber, P., Moritz, K. and North, G. (1974). First laser endoscopy with a flexible fibreoptic delivery system. *Prog. 3rd Int. Congr. Gastrointest. Endosc.*, Mexico City, Mexico.

Kiefhaber, P., North, G. and Moritz, K. (1977). Endoscopical control of massive gastrointestinal haemorrhage by radiation with a high power Neodymium-YAG laser. *Prog. Surg.*, **15**, 140–55.

Lawrence, B. H. *et al.* (1980). Endoscopic laser photocoagulation for bleeding peptic ulcers. *Lancet*, 124–5.

Leheta, F. and Gorisch, W. (1975). Coagulation of blood vessels by means of Argon-ion & Nd-YAG laser radiation. *Proc. 1st Int. Symp. Laser Surg., Israel Nov. 1975*, Jerusalem Academic Press, pp. 178–84.

Maiman, T. H. (1960). Stimulated optical radiation in Ruby. *Nature*, **187**, 433.

Protell, R. L. *et al.* (1976). A reproducible animal model of acute bleeding ulcer – the ulcer maker. *Gastroenterology*, **71**, 961–4.

Reidenbach, H. D. and Bodem, G. (1975a). Optical transmission of bulk plastic material and plastic light guides at high optical powers. *Optics Laser Tech.*, **7**, 131.

Reidenbach, H. D. and Bodem, F. (1975b). Investigations of various transmission properties and launching techniques of plastic optical fibres suitable for transmission of high optical powers. *Opt. quant. Electron.*, **7**, 355.

Reidenbach, H. D. *et al.* (1975). The plastic lightguide in endoscopic laser photocoagulation. *Endoscopy*, **7**, 196–201.

Silverstein, F. E. *et al.* (1977). Endoscopic laser treatment. 2. Comparisons of the efficacy of high and low power photocoagulation in control of severely bleeding experimental ulcers in dogs. *Gastroenterology*, **73**, 481–6.

Silverstein, F. E. *et al.* (1978). Endoscopic laser treatment 3. Development and testing of a gas-jet-assisted Argon laser wareguide in control of bleeding experimental ulcers. *Gastroenterology*, **74**, 232–9.

9 Gastroduodenal haemorrhage – other endoscopic techniques

R. L. PROTELL, F. E. SILVERSTEIN
and D. A. GILBERT

Upper gastrointestinal bleeding is a commonly encountered problem in clinical medicine. The purpose of this chapter is to discuss haemostatic methods which can be delivered via a fibreoptic endoscope. Techniques of therapeutic endoscopy can be divided into those that require tissue contact and those that do not. Contact methods include mono- and bipolar electrocoagulation, the heater probe, injection techniques and the placement of haemostatic clips. The non-contact methods include laser photocoagulation, haemostatic sprays of tissue adhesives or clotting factors and electrofulguration. In this chapter methods other than laser photocoagulation will be discussed. Animal studies will be reviewed as will be the reported clinical experience. Some of the advantages and disadvantages of each technique will be considered.

9.1 ENDOSCOPIC ELECTROCOAGULATION

9.1.1 **Monopolar electrocoagulation**

Monopolar electrocoagulation has been used in surgery for over 50 years (McLean, 1929). In this technique current passes from a small active electrode through the patient to a wide dispersal plate. Coagulation occurs because of the heat produced at the area of high energy density at the small active electrode (Fig. 9.1).

An electrosurgical generator can produce two wave forms: coagulating current or cutting current. In the latter, a continuous sine wave current causes rapid tissue heating and vaporization which favours tissue incision. In the former, repeated short bursts of high voltage favour tissue desiccation and coagulation without vaporization or cutting. The coagulating wave form is most commonly used in clinical work and was utilized in all the studies to be described.

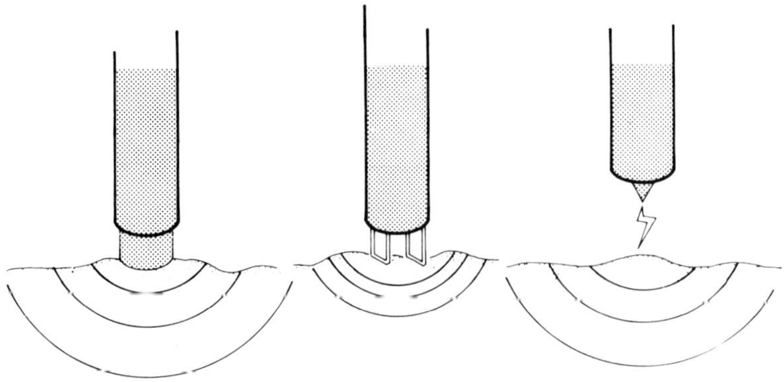

Fig. 9.1 Diagram of the three types of electrocoagulation. In monopolar the electrode tip contacts the tissue; the circuit is completed through the patient to a large dispersal plate. In bipolar, the current path is between the two closely opposed electrodes. In fulguration, a spark travels across a gap between the electrode and the tissue. Current pathways, represented by arcing lines in the tissue, are theoretically more localized for bipolar electrocoagulation.

In 1974, Blackwood *et al.* reported using a ball-tipped monopolar electrode to produce standard-sized lesions in canine intestinal tissue. The authors found that the diameter of the white mucosal electrocoagulation defect was directly related to the depth of tissue necrosis. Papp *et al.* (1975, 1976) also studied the effect of experimental monopolar electrocoagulation on the oesophageal, gastric and duodenal mucosa of dogs. They concluded that the tissue damage produced by endoscopic monopolar electrocoagulation was directly related to the duration and pressure of electrode application. In contrast to Blackwood *et al.*, Papp found no evidence that the diameter of mucosal blanching correlated with the depth of tissue necrosis. Neither group of authors was able precisely to control or monitor the pressure or duration of electrode application. Nor were they able to measure the total energy delivered to the tissue. Different electrosurgical generators of the same model, from the same manufacturer, have different power outputs at identical dial settings (Ellefson, 1978). In addition, current density at the monopolar electrode tip, which may affect tissue damage, is dependent on the shape of the electrode and the area in contact with the mucosa. This variable was not standardized in the above studies.

In order to overcome these difficulties, Piercey *et al.* (1978) developed an analogue computer for use in experimental electrocoagulation. This computer interfaces with a standard electrosurgical generator (Valley Lab., SSE2-K, Boulder, Colorado) and is capable of monitoring the power, energy and duration of electrode application. Alternatively, the computer can deliver a predetermined amount of energy by continuously adjusting the electrosurgical generator's voltage to compensate for changes in tissue impedance during electrocoagulation.

Using this computer a series of experiments was performed in heparinized dogs at laparotomy. A monopolar endoscopic electrode was modified to provide a reproducible area of electrode–tissue contact and a hand-held gauge ensured a reproducible electrode application pressure. In randomized controlled animal studies, using a standard-sized bleeding acute gastric ulcer model (Protell *et al.*, 1976), monopolar electrocoagulation was found to be haemostatically effective, but unpredictable with respect to tissue necrosis produced. In all 56 treated acute gastric ulcers, monopolar electrocoagulation stopped bleeding after a mean of 11 0.6-sec applications of approximately 22 joules per application. In studies performed to assess the maximal tissue damage produced by monopolar electrocoagulation, 71 standard-sized gastric ulcers were treated in dogs at sterile laparotomy. The animals were allowed to recover and were sacrificed at intervals up to 28 days. There were three full-thickness injuries to the gastric wall with a mean damage to the muscularis externa of 44%. The extent of tissue necrosis following monopolar electrocoagulation of these experimental ulcers did not correlate with the number of electrode applications, joules per application or the total joules per ulcer.

Despite the unpredictable tissue damage produced by experimental monopolar electrocoagulation, uncontrolled clinical experience with this technique has been modestly successful. Papp (1976), Sugawa *et al.* (1975), Gaisford (1979) and Volpicelli *et al.* (1978) all report successful endoscopic monopolar electrocoagulation of bleeding upper gastrointestinal lesions in patients. They report 87–96% success rate in stopping bleeding with no complications. This contrasts with a survey of German endoscopists showing 81–95% successful endoscopic monopolar electrocoagulation with a 1.8% perforation rate (Stadelmann *et al.*, 1977).

In summary, endoscopic monopolar electrocoagulation is a relatively inexpensive, available endoscopic technique. Although it has been successfully employed in uncontrolled non-randomized clinical series, proper controlled trials are required before this technique can be considered sufficiently safe for widespread clinical use.

9.1.2 **Monopolar electrofulguration**

In electrofulguration the monopolar electrode does not contact the target tissue. Instead, once the electrode is in close proximity to the tissue, a spark jumps across a small gap to the surface being coagulated (Fig. 9.1). Thermal energy may be deposited more superficially than with other electrocoagulative techniques because of the absence of physical contact.

Using the previously described analogue computer (Piercey *et al.*, 1978), electrofulguration was studied by Dennis (1980) in a canine laparotomy model of acute gastric ulcer bleeding. In controlled laparotomy studies in seven heparinized foxhounds, monopolar electrofulguration therapy of bleeding acute gastric ulcers was compared at three different settings of the electrosurgical generator. During electrofulguration a jet of CO_2 gas was employed to blow away obscuring blood. In acute studies to assess the effectiveness of electrofulguration at three generator settings, all 32 treated ulcers stopped bleeding. When treated ulcers were examined after seven days to determine the depth of tissue damage, the mean injury to the muscularis externa was approximately 30%. The same workers then performed an experiment to attempt to reduce the depth of injury. Because the fulguration spark is produced by ionization of the gas between the electrode and the tissue, argon, a more easily ionizable gas than CO_2, was studied. This allowed the generation of a spark using less power, which theoretically might reduce tissue damage during electrofulguration. A study was done of electrofulguration, comparing CO_2 gas with a 50/50 mixture of CO_2 and argon. Both produced effective haemostasis. However, when treated ulcers were examined after seven days to determine the maximal tissue damage produced, there was no significant reduction in the extent of injury (mean injury to muscularis externa was 29% with CO_2/argon and 41% with CO_2). Tissue damage was not related to the number of joules per ulcer or to the number of electrode applications.

The authors concluded from these animal studies that electrofulguration is effective, but the tissue damage produced is unpredictable and deeper than that with other endoscopic methods. Electrofulguration is not currently being considered for clinical use.

9.1.3 **Bipolar electrocoagulation**

Bipolar electrocoagulation uses two active electrodes in close apposition (<3 mm for endoscopic use), both of which touch the tissue (Fig. 9.1). This theoretically provides more localized current pathways and is the basis for the hypothesis that bipolar electrocoagulation may cause less tissue damage.

All published reports of endoscopically deliverable bipolar electrocoagulation use the Medi-tech electrode. In 1978 Moore *et al.* evaluated the effect of bipolar electrocoagulation on normal canine gastric mucosa, canine gastric mucosa ulcerated three days earlier, and on standard sized acute gastric ulcers made at laparotomy in heparinized dogs. Pressure of electrode application and the irrigant flow rate from the central channel of the bipolar electrode were not controlled. Furthermore, the energy delivered to the tissue was not quantified. Only two full-thickness injuries to the gastric wall were observed in 87 lesions treated with bipolar electrocoagulation. This group also performed uncontrolled non-randomized experimental endoscopic comparisons of bipolar electrocoagulation with monopolar electrocoagulation which showed that monopolar electrocoagulation produced deeper tissue damage.

The endoscopic research group at the University of Washington used the analogue computer to study the efficacy and resultant depth of tissue damage from endoscopically deliverable bipolar electrocoagulation (Protell *et al.*, 1978*a*). The previously described acute bleeding ulcer model was used at laparotomy in heparinized foxhounds. Pressure, duration of electrode application and energy per application were controlled. In acute experiments all 27 treated ulcers stopped bleeding while the 14 untreated controls did not. Chronic experiments performed to assess histologically the depth of tissue damage following bipolar electrocoagulation showed that six of 24 treated ulcers had full-thickness injury. This initial study concluded that bipolar electrocoagulation was effective but capable of producing deep tissue damage. The investigators are now comparing bipolar and monopolar electrocoagulation using the same ulcer model and the analogue computer.

A third study compared bipolar electrocoagulation with argon laser photocoagulation in the treatment of bleeding canine gastric ulcers (Johnston *et al.*, 1978). In randomized experiments at laparotomy, all ulcers treated with bipolar electrocoagulation or argon laser photocoagulation stopped bleeding. Chronic studies showed damage to the external muscle greater than 50% in 13 of the 27 bipolar-treated ulcers but only one of the 34 laser-treated ulcers. The coagulation setting, force and duration of electrode application, and irrigant infusion rate were controlled in this study, but the energy delivered to the tissue could not be monitored. These careful experiments suggested that both methods are effective in stopping experimental bleeding but that bipolar electrocoagulation produced more histological injury.

There are no reports of the clinical use of endoscopic bipolar electrocoagulation in man.

In summary, all three electrocoagulative techniques are haemostatically effective. However, the depth of tissue damage is unpredictable and more work is required before widespread clinical use of these methods can be endorsed. Only properly designed controlled clinical trials will firmly answer questions regarding the safety and efficacy of endoscopic electroagulation.

9.2 HEATER PROBE

The heater probe represents another way to use electricity for endoscopically delivered haemostasis. The heater probe allows the

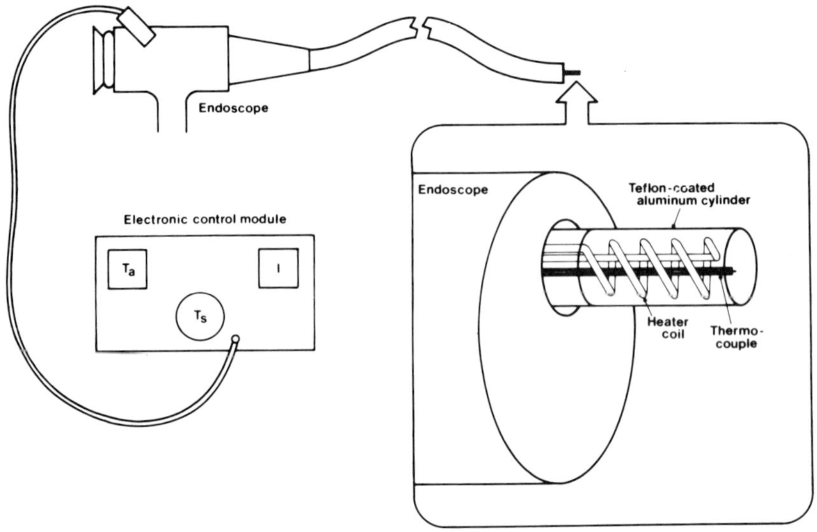

Fig. 9.2 Scheme of the heater probe, shown exiting an endoscopic biopsy channel (from Protell *et al.*, 1978*b* with permission of the publisher, the Williams and Wilkins Company).

simultaneous application of heat and pressure. An electrical resistance heater is embedded in a 10-mm long Teflon-coated aluminium capsule (Fig. 9.2). A central thermocouple element maintains any preset temperature by a servocontrol feedback loop. The first prototype heater probe was 6.4 mm in diameter; later models measure 3.2 mm in diameter. Studies of the heater probe at the University of Washington used both diameter prototypes (Protell *et al.*, 1978*b*). Pilot experiments with each probe showed that the most effective haemostasis with least tissue damage occurred with multiple one second probe applications at 150–160°C.

In randomized controlled laparotomy experiments in heparinized foxhounds, both the 6.4 mm and the 3.2 mm diameter heater probes were 100% effective in stopping acute gastric ulcer bleeding. Chronic studies were performed at sterile laparotomy in nine heparinized foxhounds to assess the tissue injury produced by the heater probe. The 6.4 mm diameter probe produced full-thickness injury in seven of 18 treated ulcers; the 3.2 mm diameter probe in only two of 30 treated ulcers.

The heater probe is an effective way of stopping gastrointestinal bleeding. However, in its present state the tissue damage produced is occasionally deep. The reasons for this are not yet clear, but may be related to the difficulty of accurately touching the bleeding vessel, and the inability precisely to control the pressure of application when the heater probe is used endoscopically. Newer generation probes may overcome these problems and this device may ultimately be useful clinically. No patients have been treated with the heater probe.

9.3 ENDOSCOPIC SPRAYS

Endoscopic sprays are a diverse group of compounds with two common characteristics: (1) they can be applied as a spray from a catheter not touching the mucosa; (2) they produce no thermal damage to the target tissue. Tissue adhesives, mixtures of clotting factors and an iron–oil mixture have been used experimentally to stop bleeding via the endoscope. Tissue adhesives have been studied in most detail and these substances will be emphasized in the following discussion.

9.3.1 **Endoscopic tissue adhesives**

Tissue adhesives were developed in the 1950s for battle field use (Matsumoto, 1972). Two types of these acrylic polymers have been used endoscopically.

Keller (1976) studied a preformed acrylic polymer of Carboset resins 514 and 525 B (B. F. Goodrich Chemical Co., Akron, Ohio) in a 25% solution in 95% alcohol. Twenty-four hours following the creation of gastric ulcers in pigs, acrylic polymer sprays were applied. The duration of faecal occult blood loss, changes in haematocrit and ulcer healing were measured in both untreated control and treated animals. In the polymer-treated animals ulcer healing appeared to be more rapid and the duration of detectable occult faecal blood was shorter. A single terminally ill patient with haemorrhage from a large gastric erosion was treated by spraying this compound at the bleeding lesion endoscopically (Keller and Logan, 1974). Transient haemostasis was observed but exsanguinating haemorrhage occurred several hours later.

The other class of acrylic polymers that have been considered for endoscopic haemostasis are the alkyl 2-cyanoacrylates. These compounds polymerize rapidly upon contact with water and degrade slowly at a rate inversely related to the length of the alkyl 2-side chain. The first alkyl 2-cyanoacrylate used was the methyl derivative. It produced local tissue necrosis and is not suitable for use in biological preparations. Two research groups, including our own, have studied the trifluoroisopropyl analogue (Flucrylate™; MBR-4197). This compound polymerizes in under 10 seconds, adheres to virtually all surfaces except Teflon and polyethylene, and can be applied as a spray.

Protell *et al.* (1978*c*) performed a series of experiments in dogs to test the efficacy of trifluoroisopropyl 2-cyanoacrylate in the standard canine model of acute bleeding ulcer. An endoscopic catheter was developed for use in these studies. 112 Ulcers were made in 13 foxhounds at laparotomy. In both heparinized and unheparinized animals the cyanoacrylate spray did not produce haemostasis of bleeding ulcers. Nor could it predictably stop haemorrhage from ulcers that had been partially treated with a heater probe to slow the bleeding to an ooze. Histological data suggested that bleeding continued in deeper tissue layers even when no external haemorrhage was detectable through the layer of polymer.

Martin and Silvis (1977) used a different animal model to test the haemostatic efficacy of this cyanoacrylate analogue. Gastric ulcers were made in 10 dogs with an endoscopic left-and-cut technique (Martin *et al.*, 1976). Animals were heparinized three days after the ulcer was made; anticoagulation was continued for four days. Endoscopy was performed and Flucrylate™ was sprayed over the healing ulcers on days 3, 5, 7 and 10. Haematocrits were compared in the treated and untreated animals. A significantly smaller drop in haematocrit was observed in the cyanoacrylate-treated dogs than in sham-treated controls.

Martin *et al.* (1977) have used Flucrylate™ to treat six critically ill patients with upper gastrointestinal haemorrhage. In three patients bleeding stopped following application of the tissue adhesive. In two others the bleeding slowed. A multicentre, prospective, randomized clinical trial of Flucrylate™ (MBR-4197) is now in progress.

9.3.2 **Endoscopic clotting factors**

Linscheer and Fazio (1979) have developed an endoscopic technique for spraying a thrombin-cryoprecipitate mixture on to a bleeding site. In canine studies using the standard acute gastric ulcer model haemostasis was effected by application of clotting factor spray. In both heparinized and unheparinized animals, the thrombin-cryoprecipitate spray significantly decreased the time of ulcer bleeding when compared with untreated controls. A pilot clinical trial in nine critically ill patients produced immediate haemostasis in all (Fazio and Linscheer, 1978). Continued animal studies with this technique are now in progress and a controlled clinical trial is being considered.

9.3.3 **Iron–oil mixture**

Smith *et al.* (1978) have developed a new haemostatic method using an iron–oil mixture. This mixture is sprayed directly on a bleeding site using an endoscopic wash catheter. An external electromagnet then holds the mixture against the bleeding tissue. Haemostasis has been observed in approximately 20 experimental canine ulcers thus far reported. Work with this method is just beginning and many questions must be answered. What is the toxicity of the iron–oil spray? Can the cumbersome equipment required be conveniently installed in a clinical unit? There are no reports of the clinical use of the iron–oil spray.

9.4 MISCELLANEOUS

In addition to the above haemostatic techniques, several authors have reported their experience with mechanical methods of stopping bleeding via the endoscope. Haemostatic clips are available which can be endoscopically applied to bleeding lesions (Katon, 1976). Also, endoscopic injection needles are now available, and these devices have been used to inject bleeding tissue with adrenaline in a small number of patients (Soehendra and Werner, 1976).

Another endoscopic injection technique, the sclerotherapy of oesophageal varices, is discussed in Chapter 4.

ACKNOWLEDGEMENT

This study was supported by United States Public Health Service Contract NO1-AM-2-2211 and Clinical Investigator Award No. 1 K08 AM 00406.

REFERENCES

Blackwood, W. D. and Silvis, S. E. (1974). Standardization of electrosurgical lesions. *Gastrointest. Endosc.*, **21**, 22–24.

Dennis, M. B. (1980). Evaluation of electrofulguration in control of bleeding experimental gastric ulcers. *Dig. Dis. Sci.* (in press).

Ellefson, D. M. (1978). Development of an analogue computing monitor for high frequency electrosurgery. Masters Thesis. University of Washington, March 15.

Fazio, T. L. and Linscheer, W. G. (1978). Control of upper gastrointestinal hemorrhage by endoscopic spraying of clotting factors, (abstract), *Gastroenterology*, **74**, 1122.

Gaisford, W. D. (1979). Endoscopic electrohemostasis of active upper gastrointestinal bleeding. *Am. J. Surg.*, **137**, 47–53.

Johnston, J. H., Jensen, D. M. and Mautner, W. (1978). A comparison of bipolar electrocoagulation and argon laser photocoagulation with coaxial CO_2 in the treatment of bleeding canine gastric ulcer, (abstract), *Gastrointest. Endosc.*, **24**, 200–1.

Katon, R. M. (1976). Experimental control of gastrointestinal hemorrhage via the endoscope: a new era dawns. *Gastroenterology*, **70**, 272–7.

Keller, R. T. and Logan, G. M. (1974). Treatment of hemorrhagic gastritis by the endoscopic application of acrylic polymer. *Gastrointest. Endosc.*, **21**, 75–6.

Keller, R. (1976). Carboset resins for hemostasis: animal trials. *Minutes of the AGA Workshop Towards Controlled Trials in Upper Gastrointestinal Bleeding.* Keystone, Colorado.

Linscheer, W. G. and Fazio, T. L. (1979). Control of upper gastrointestinal hemorrhage by spraying of clotting factors. *Gastroenterology*, (in press).

McLean, A. J. (1929). The bovie electrosurgical current generator: some underlying principles and results. *Arch. Surg.*, **18**, 1863–73.

Martin, T. R. and Silvis, S. E. (1977). The endoscopic control of GI blood loss with a tissue adhesive (MBR-4197). (abstract), *Gastroenterology*, **72**, 1098.

Martin, T. R., Onstad, G. R. and Silvis, S. E. (1977). Endoscopic control of upper gastrointestinal bleeding with a tissue adhesive (MBR-4197). *Gastrointest. Endosc.*, **24**, 73–76.

Martin, T. R. *et al.* (1976). Left and cut biopsy technique for submucosal sampling. *Gastrointest. Endosc.*, **23**, 29–30.

Matsumoto, T. (1972). *Tissue Adhesives in Surgery*. Medical Examination Publishing Co. Inc., Flushing, N.Y.

Moore, J. P., Silvis, S. E. and Vennes, J. A. (1978). Evaluation of bipolar electrocoagulation in canine stomachs. *Gastrointest. Endosc.*, **24**, 148–51.

Papp, J. P. (1976). Endoscopic electrocoagulation of upper gastrointestinal hemorrhage. *Am. Med. Ass.*, **236**, 2076–9.

Papp, J. P., Fox, J. M. and Walbandian, R. M. (1976). Experimental electrocoagulation of dog esophageal and duodenal mucosa. *Gastrointest. Endosc.*, **23**, 27–8.

Papp, J. P., Fox, J. M. and Wicks, H. S. (1975). Experimental electrocoagulation of dog gastric mucosa. *Gastrointest. Endosc.*, **22**, 27–28.

Piercey, J. R. A. *et al.* (1978). Electrosurgical treatment of experimental bleeding canine gastric ulcers. Development and testing of a computer control and a better electrode. *Gastroenterology*, **74**, 527–34.

Protell, R. L. *et al.* (1976). A reproducible animal model of acute bleeding ulcer – the 'ulcer maker'. *Gastroenterology*, **71**, 961–4.

Protell, R. *et al.* (1978*a*). Efficacy and safety of computer-controlled bipolar electrocoagulation in experimental acute gastric ulcer bleeding. (abstract), *Clin. Res.*, **26**, 151A.

Protell, R. L. *et al.* (1978*b*). The heater probe: a new endoscopic method for stopping massive gastrointestinal bleeding. *Gastroenterology*, **74**, 257–62.

Protell, R. L. *et al.* (1978*c*). Failure of cyanoacrylate tissue glue (Flucrylate^{TM}; MBR-4197) to stop bleeding from experimental canine gastric ulcers. *Am. J. Dig. Dis.*, **23**, 903–8.

Smith, F. W. *et al.* (1978). Use of strong magnet fields in the control of gastrointestinal bleeding. Presented at the Annual Meeting of the Western Gut Club, Carmel, California, February.

Soehendra, N. and Werner, B. (1976). New technique for endoscopic treatment of bleeding gastric ulcer. *Endoscopy*, **8**, 85–7.

Stadelmann, O., Weisbart, D. and Zeus, U. (1977). Blutende Lasionen im Gastrointestinaltrakt Elektrokoagulation. Paper presented at Symposium *Operative Endoskopie*, Erlangen.

Sugawa, C. *et al.* (1975). Electrocoagulation of bleeding in the upper part of the gastrointestinal tract: a preliminary experimental clinical report. *Arch. Surg.*, **10**, 975–8.

Volpicelli, M. A. *et al.* (1978). Endoscopic electrocoagulation. An alternative to operative therapy in bleeding peptic ulcer disease. *Arch. Surg.*, **113**, 483–6.

10 Gastroduodenal haemorrhage – radiological identification and therapy

CHARLES T. DOTTER, JOSEF RÖSCH and FREDERICK S. KELLER

Visceral angiography has become the cornerstone of the radiological diagnosis of acute *arterial* gastroduodenal bleeding (Athanasoulis *et al.*, 1974; Baum *et al.*, 1965, 1969; Frey *et al.*, 1970; Grace and Gold, 1978; Janicki and Alfidi, 1976; Keller and Rösch, 1979; Palmer, 1970; Rabin *et al.*, 1977; Ring *et al.*, 1974; Rosenbaum *et al.*, 1975; Wenz *et al.*, 1969). Barium studies no longer play a role in acute active bleeding, but are reserved for patients with chronic blood loss or in controlled but unlocalized bleeding. If unwisely resorted to in acute bleeding, barium obscures physical and roentgenological landmarks precluding angiographic identification of the bleeding site for at least 24 hours.

The radiologically guided catheter management of bleeding relies upon selective vasoconstrictor infusions and the selective, mechanical transcatheter occlusion of bleeding arteries or their feeders (Athanasoulis, 1976; *et al.*, 1974, 1976; Bookstein *et al.*, 1974; Carsen *et al.*, 1978; Eisenberg and Steer, 1976; Goldman *et al.*, 1976; Grace and Gold, 1978; Granmayeh *et al.*, 1979; Janicki and Alfidi, 1976; Kadir and Athanasoulis, 1977; Katzen and McSweeney, 1975; Kaufman *et al.*, 1978; Keller and Rösch, 1979; Merland *et al.*, 1978; Nusbaum *et al.*, 1972; Rabin *et al.*, 1977; Reuter *et al.*, 1975; Ring *et al.*, 1974; Rösch *et al.*, 1970, 1972*a*,*b*, 1976; Rosenbaum *et al.*, 1975; Twiford *et al.*, 1978; Wenz *et al.*, 1969; White *et al.*, 1974*a*,*b*, 1979; Wholey, 1977, *et al.*, 1970). When introduced during the 1960s these techniques were controversial. With time, they gained wider clinical use and now are accepted as useful tools for the identification and therapy of acute arterial gastroduodenal bleeding.

10.1 DIAGNOSIS

10.1.1 **The approach to diagnosis**

Indications for diagnostic angiography and its timing in acute gastrointestinal bleeding in general, and gastroduodenal bleeding specifically, have undergone numerous changes and still vary between individual institutions (Athanasoulis *et al*., 1976; Keller and Rösch, 1979; Rösch *et al*., 1976). At first we used angiography as the initial diagnostic procedure in most instances of acute gastrointestinal bleeding but as our experience increased we learned that this approach was unjustified (in that it led to an unduly high proportion of negative studies), costly and, most important, could endanger patients. Such an aggressive angiographic approach fails to take into account the fact in 40% to 80% of patients bleeding will stop with bed rest and medical therapy (Palmer, 1970). Bleeding may also stop before emergency angiography, sometimes as a result of hypotension due to blood loss (Rösch *et al*., 1976). Since angiography demonstrates the actual flow of blood into the gut, it follows that when this has stopped, even temporarily, angiography is likely to be unproductive.

Our experience with more than 300 patients with gastrointestinal haemorrhage has led us to rely on alimentary endoscopy as the primary diagnostic test (Fig. 10.1) (Hedberg, 1974; Katon and Smith, 1973; Keller and Rösch, 1979; Palmer, 1970). It either indicates the site or directly exposes the bleeding lesion. Depending on the type of lesion and the patient's condition, a trial of medical therapy is often undertaken, its duration depending on the type and severity of bleeding, the patient's

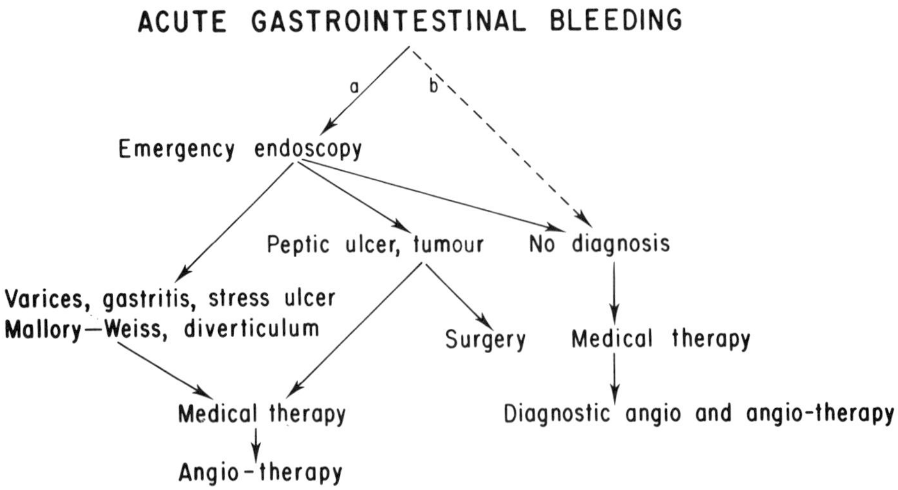

Fig. 10.1 An approach to acute gastrointestinal bleeding.

condition and his response to treatment (Keller and Rösch, 1979; Rösch *et al.*, 1976).

When medical therapy is unsuccessful, and the patient continues to bleed, we believe that angiography is then indicated. In those patients where emergency endoscopy has shown a bleeding site and/or diagnosed the responsible lesion (line *a*, Fig. 10.1), limited angiography keyed to an appropriate form of catheter therapy is done. In patients (line *b*, Fig. 10.1) where endoscopy is impossible or non-diagnostic, complete diagnostic angiography to find the bleeding lesion is performed, followed by catheter therapy when indicated.

10.1.2 **Technique**

Selective coeliac angiography is the basic diagnostic study in acute gastroduodenal bleeding. Selective superior mesenteric angiography is sometimes necessary to demonstrate bleeding from the distal duodenum. Such selective studies are ordinarily able to demonstrate bleeding at rates as low as 0.5 ml/min (Baum *et al.*, 1965). For precise localization of bleeding sites, especially in minor and multifocal bleeding, superselective catheterization of coeliac branches (particularly of the left gastric artery and occasionally the splenic, common hepatic and/or gastroduodenal arteries) is required. Superselective catheterization is essential in the catheter therapy of acute gastroduodenal bleeding (Athanasoulis, 1976; *et al.*, 1974, 1976; Carsen *et al.*, 1978; Goldman *et al.*, 1976; Kadir and Athanasoulis, 1977; Keller and Rösch, 1979; Raja Rao *et al.*, 1978; Ring *et al.*, 1974; Rösch *et al.*, 1970, 1976).

Angiographic examination is done under local anaesthesia with mild sedation. A transfemoral approach is used, the left transaxillary route being reserved for patients with prohibitive pelvic atherosclerosis or when the necessary superselective catheterization cannot be achieved from below. The tools and techniques of catheterization vary with individual angiographers. We use preshaped 6.5 French polyethylene catheters with an inner metal braid (Torcon, Cook), which give excellent torque control and make catheterization simple. Single curve catheters are used for simple selective studies. Superselective catheterization often requires double-curved catheters with the primary curve anterior (as for selective catheterization) and a secondary curve about 0.5 to 1.5 cm from the tip. The orientation of the secondary curve depends on the anatomy of the vessel to be catheterized; thus, the secondary curve for the left gastric artery is directed anteriorly. A simple external catheter tip deflector (Cook) helps to form the proper catheter shape in the distal thoracic aorta. Superselective catheterization is then accomplished by withdrawal and rotation of the catheter, allowing, not forcing, it to enter the desired artery (Dotter *et al.*, 1972).

High concentration contrast medium (Renograffin 76%, Squibb) is used for the injection, which usually lasts 4 seconds. The injected volume depends on the size and flow through the catheterized artery. In the coeliac and superior mesenteric arteries 8–10 ml are injected per second (32–40 ml total); in the common hepatic artery, 6–8 ml per second (24–32 ml total); in the left gastric and gastroduodenal arteries 2–4 ml per second (8–16 ml total).

The anteroposterior projection is normally used for the angiogram; additional oblique projections are sometimes needed. Serial films covering the arterial and early capillary phases are exposed at 1-second intervals (6–8 films) with an additional 5–6 films made at 2-second intervals.

The diagnosis of acute arterial bleeding is based on demonstrating extravasated contrast medium in the gut lumen. This is readily seen in patients with localized brisk bleeding from relatively large arteries,

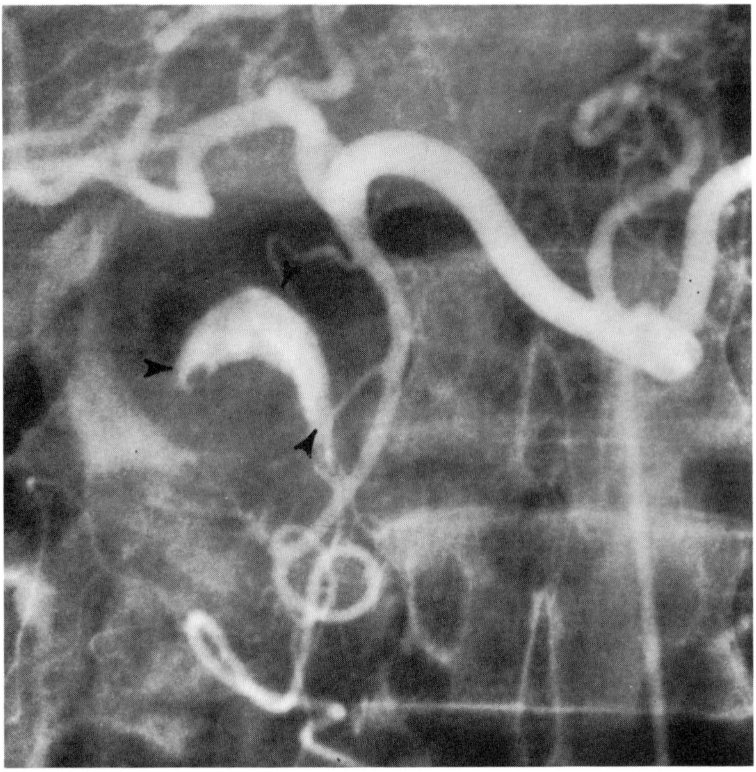

Fig. 10.2 Acute bleeding from a duodenal ulcer with extravasation of contrast medium (arrowheads) demonstrated on the coeliac angiogram.

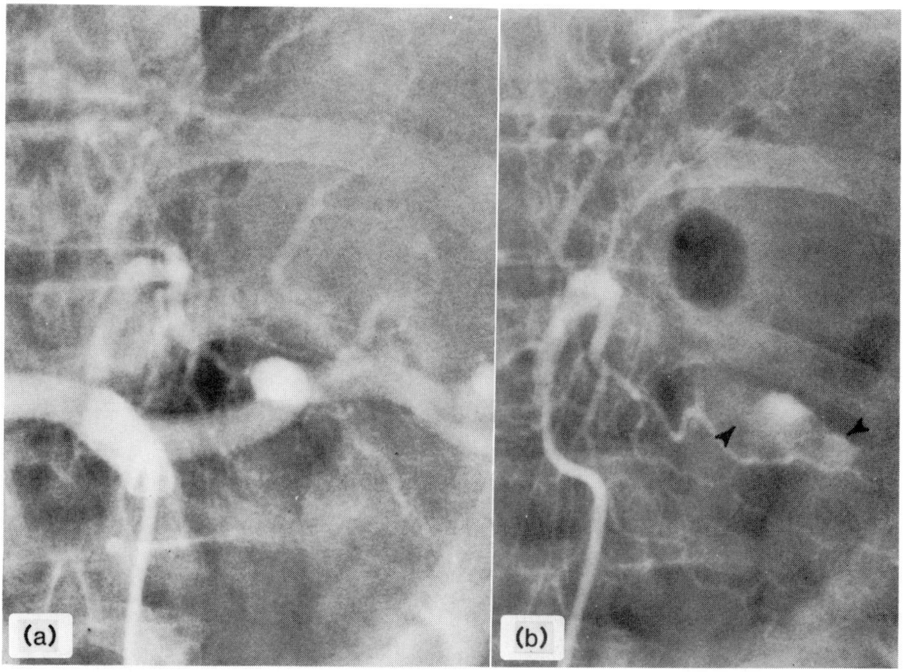

Fig. 10.3 Acute bleeding from a gastric ulcer in a 51-year old cirrhotic patient visualized by the left gastric angiogram only. (a) Coeliac angiogram does not show any extravasation. (b) Left gastric angiogram reveals a sizable extravasation of contrast medium (arrowheads).

particularly in peptic ulcers and often in Mallory–Weiss tears (Figs. 10.2, 10.3). In patients with minor bleeding or multiple capillary bleeding sites (as in erosive gastritis or stress ulcers) diagnosis is more difficult and superselective catheterization is necessary to show the extravasation (Fig. 10.4). Precise identification of the bleeding artery is needed for either surgical or catheter management by vasoconstriction or transcatheter occlusive haemostasis. Ulcers in the distal oesophagus, Mallory–Weiss tears and most lesions in the proximal stomach (including peptic and stress ulcers and erosive gastritis) bleed from the left gastric artery; some lesions in the upper stomach, however, may bleed from short gastric branches of the splenic artery (Fig. 10.5).

The right gastric or gastroepiploic artery often is the site of bleeding in lesions of the antrum and pylorus. The superior duodenal branch of the gastroduodenal artery is the commonest source of bleeding from a duodenal ulcer (Fig. 10.2); however, ulcers in the descending duodenum can also erode duodenal branches of the pancreaticoduodenal arcades. Erosion of an ulcer into the cystic artery and bleeding into the biliary

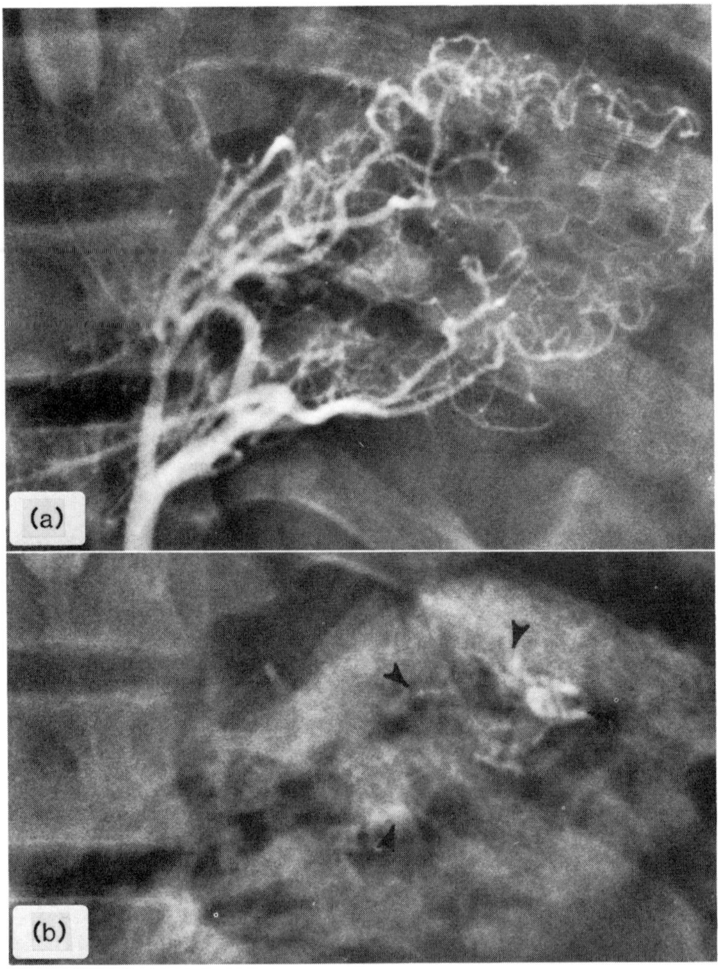

Fig. 10.4 Acute bleeding in an 18-year-old man with erosive gastritis. Left gastric angiogram. (a) Arterial phase demonstrates diffuse mucosal hypervascularity in the upper part of the stomach. (b) Capillary phase reveals multiple small extravasations of contrast medium (arrowheads).

tract are uncommon causes of gastroduodenal bleeding (Fig. 10.6). In postoperative bleeding from an anastomotic ulcer, one of the first jejunal branches can be the site of extravasation (Fig. 10.7).

The extravasation from an ulcer or a Mallory–Weiss tear usually forms a single pool of contrast agent in the gut lumen, a collection which persists for an appreciable time before its dilution by the arrival of

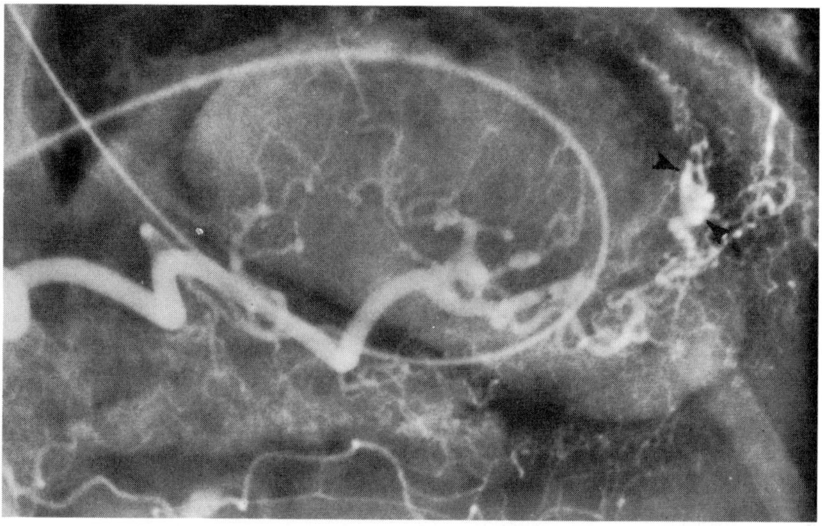

Fig. 10.5 Acute bleeding from a stress ulcer on the greater curvature of the gastric fundus with extravasation of contrast medium (arrowheads) from the short gastric arteries visualized on the splenic angiogram only.

unopacified blood. In bleeding from erosive gastritis and stress ulcers, films in the arterial phase may show only hypervascularity and early venous phases (Fig. 10.4).

10.1.3 **Complications**

The risk of diagnostic angiography is minimal (occlusion of the punctured artery in less than 0.5% and minor haematoma at the puncture site in 2–3% of cases), and is closely related to the radiologist's experience. In bleeding patients, however, the emergency procedure must go quickly with careful monitoring of the patient and replacement of blood. Close cooperation of angiographer and clinician is essential.

Atherosclerosis and hypertension increase the small risk of puncture site complications. Minor haematoma formation, of little importance in the femoral area, can lead to severe neurological consequences when the axillary artery is used for catheter introduction. The transaxillary approach should therefore be avoided in patients with severe hypertension or bleeding tendencies. After angiography, we keep patients in bed for six hours with a pressure bandage on the puncture site to prevent bleeding.

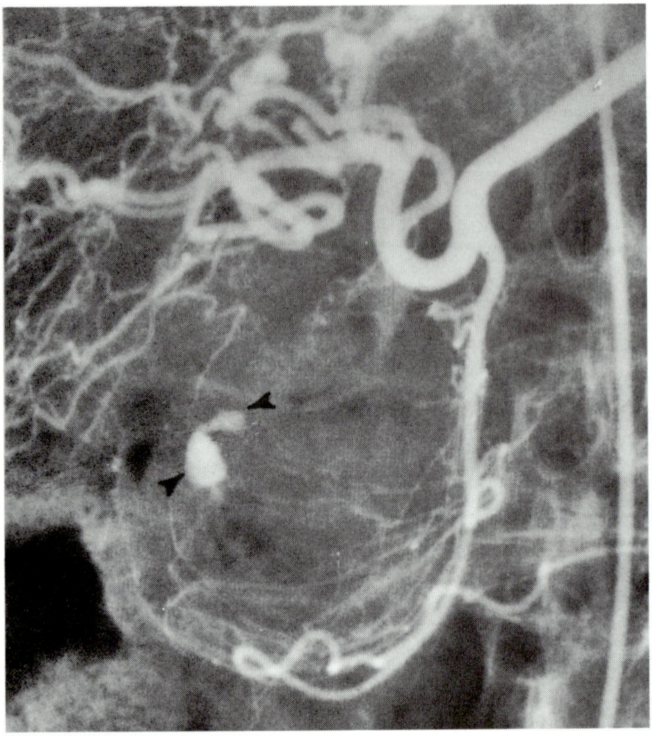

Fig. 10.6 Acute bleeding from a duodenal ulcer penetrating into the gallbladder. Common hepatic angiogram shows extravasation of contrast medium (arrowheads) on the lateral wall of the descending duodenum.

10.2 SELECTIVE VASOCONSTRICTION

The selective infusion of vasoconstrictors (vasopressin or adrenaline [epinephrine]) into the bleeding artery or its feeder is the older and more conservative method of radiological catheter therapy of acute gastroduodenal arterial bleeding. It is still useful on some occasions. Localized vasoconstriction, with temporary decrease or cessation of flow in the bleeding vessel, gives an opportunity for stable clot formation at the bleeding point(s) (Athanasoulis, 1976; *et al.*, 1974, 1976; Frey *et al.*, 1970; Grace and Gold, 1978; Janicki and Alfidi, 1976; Kadir and Athanasoulis, 1977; Keller and Rösch, 1979; Nusbaum *et al.*, 1972; Ring *et al.*, 1974; Rösch *et al.*, 1970, 1972*a*, 1976; Rosenbaum *et al.*, 1975). Selective vasoconstrictive infusion therapy, in our opinion, is primarily indicated in younger patients with good vascular reactivity and good haemocoagulation, who bleed from minor vessels and who are not acutely endangered by bleeding. In 80–95% of such patients,

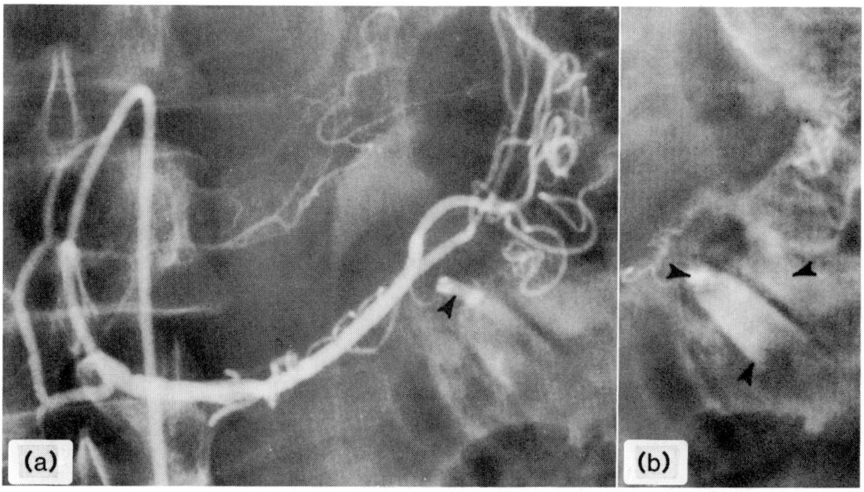

Fig. 10.7 Acute bleeding from an anastomotic ulcer in a 30-year-old man after partial gastrectomy and Bilroth II anastomosis. (a) The upper jejunal artery angiogram in the arterial phase shows extravasation of contrast medium (arrowhead) from a small jejunal branch. (b) Late capillary phase demonstrates increase and persistence of extravasation (arrowheads).

haemorrhage from Mallory–Weiss tears, diffuse erosive gastritis and stress ulcers can be controlled by selective vasoconstrictive infusion (Athanasoulis *et al.*, 1976; Kadir and Athanasoulis, 1977). On the other hand, this method has a low rate (40–50%) of success in bleeding from chronic peptic ulcers, where the bleeding artery is often fibrotic and does not constrict. Similar success rates have been reported by Athanasoulis: gastric mucosal lesions 80%, peptic ulcer 55%, diverticula 92%, angiomas 92%. Vasoconstrictive infusion therapy is the best method for bleeding following gastric surgery, where the ligation of collaterials substantially increases the risk of embolic vasoocclusive therapy (Bradley and Goldman, 1976). Vasoconstrictor therapy is also the only method to be used in patients where direct superselective catheterization of the bleeding vessel or its main feeder is technically impossible.

10.2.1 **Technique**

For optimal results in vasoconstrictive therapy, the catheter should be introduced into the bleeding vessel or its feeder; the left gastric artery is infused for bleeding from Mallory–Weiss tears and most upper gastric lesions (Figs. 10.8–10.10). Bleeding from short gastric arteries requires

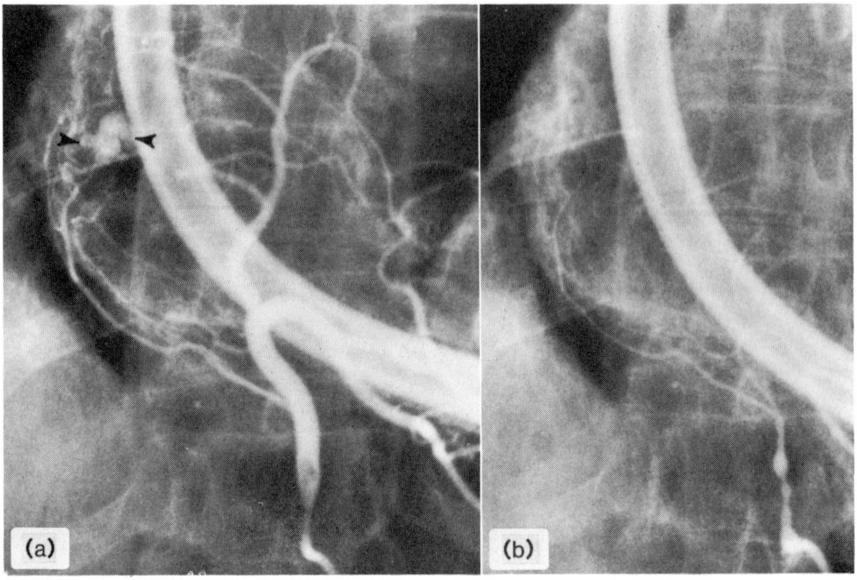

Fig. 10.8 Acute bleeding from a Mallory–Weiss tear in hiatal hernia successfully controlled with selective left gastric artery infusion of adrenaline. (a) Initial left gastric angiogram shows extravasation of contrast medium into a hiatal hernia (arrowheads). (b) Angiogram following 20-minute infusion of adrenaline (10 mg/min) demonstrates extensive vasoconstriction of the entire infused left gastric artery, including its main trunk, with no extravasation of contrast medium.

infusion into the splenic artery; the common hepatic artery is infused in lesions of the gastric antrum. Gastroduodenal artery infusions should be done in duodenal bleeding. Superselective catheterization with infusion of the bleeding jejunal artery offers good results in anastomotic ulcers following gastric resection. 'Superselectively' given vasoconstrictors are locally effective in low doses, so that systemic effects may be minimized or avoided. Infusions into the main coeliac and superior mesenteric arteries require higher doses to control bleeding. Furthermore, infusion into the coeliac artery is less likely to control upper gastric bleeding, since coeliac catheters tend to slip far into the coeliac trunk so that the injection is delivered beyond the orifice of the left gastric artery.

Vasopressin and adrenaline are the most commonly used agents for selective vasoconstrictive infusions. Vasopressin is a predominantly peripheral vasoconstrictor (Fig. 10.9), with a prolonged action which persists after the infusion and leads to no reactive increase in flow. Vasopressin constricts both the coeliac and mesenteric circulation, causing

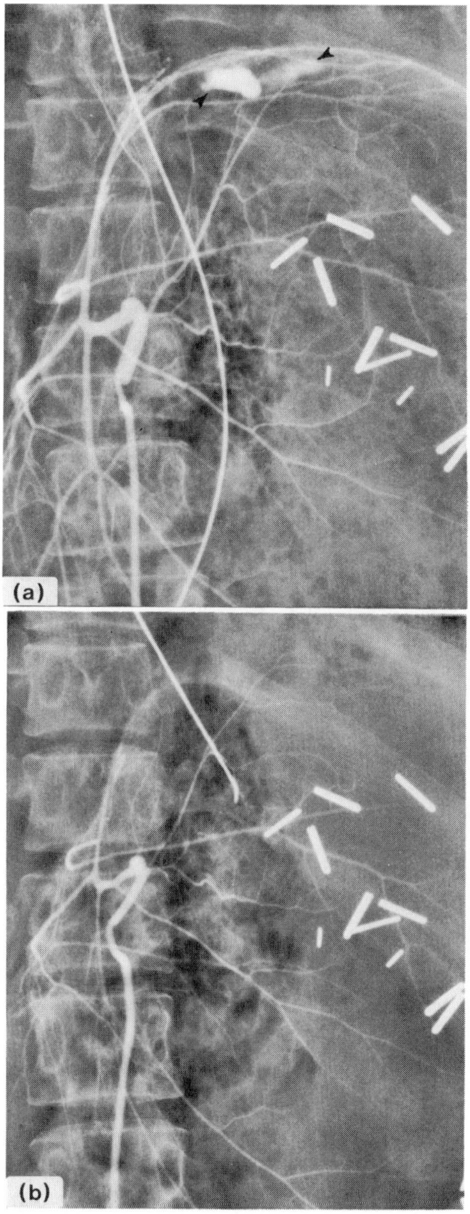

Fig. 10.9 Acute bleeding in a 23-year-old renal transplant patient from a fresh ulcer in the fundus of the stomach, successfully controlled by selective infusion of vasopressin. (a) Initial left gastric angiogram shows a sizeable extravasation of contrast medium (arrowheads). (b) After a 30-minute selective infusion of vasopressin (0.15 μg/min), the bleeding is no longer present and the left gastric circulation shows diffuse vasoconstriction, particularly in its medium-sized and peripheral branches.

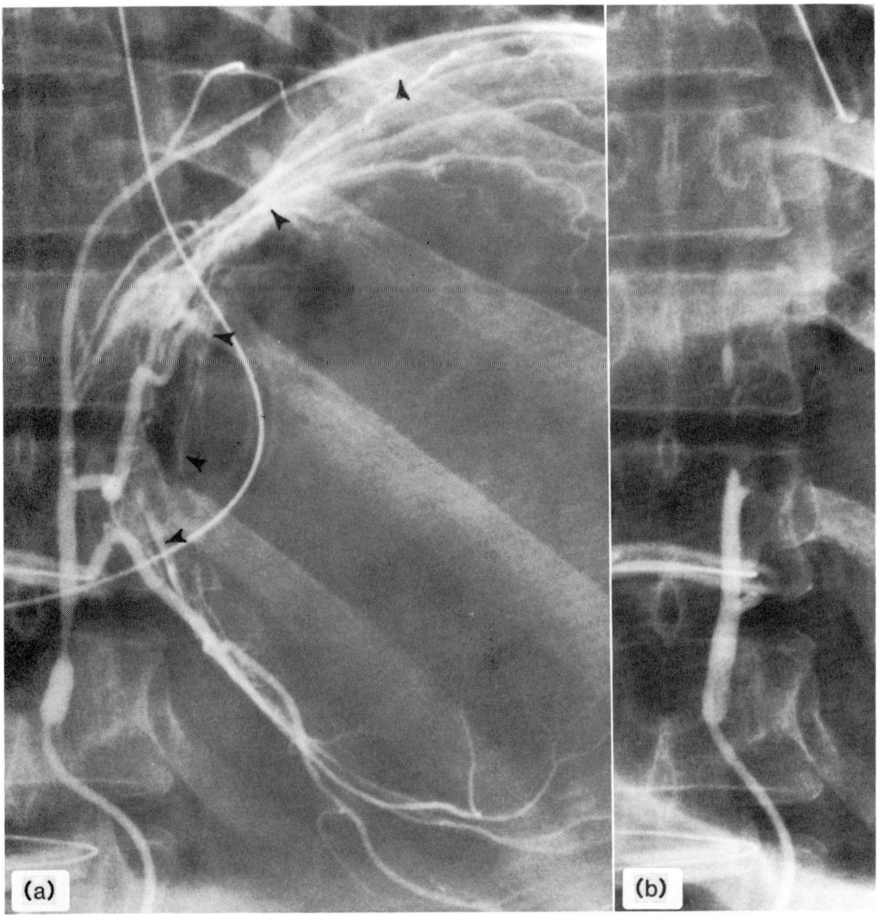

Fig. 10.10 Acute gastric bleeding in a 39-year-old man with several stress ulcers successfully controlled by infusion of adrenaline. (a) Initial left gastric angiogram demonstrates several extravasations of contrast medium (arrowheads) along the lesser curvature of the stomach, which is distended by blood. (b) Angiogram following 30-minute infusion of adrenaline (12 mg/min) reveals extensive vasoconstriction of the left gastric branches, with filling of the trunk of the left gastric artery only.

a 'paradoxical' vasodilatation of the hepatic arteries and increased arterial flow through the liver (Barr *et al.*, 1975). Adrenaline effectively constricts the coeliac artery branches, large and small (Figs. 10.8, 10.10); its effect, however, lasts only during the infusion, after which a brief (2–3 minute) period of reactive vasodilatation is followed by a return to normal flow. In the mesenteric circulation, adrenaline alone is not suitable, because it produces an undesirable beta-effect dilatation (Rösch *et al.*, 1970).

Dosage of the infused vasoconstrictor depends on the size of the catheterized vessel, and its response to an initial 5–10 minute infusion evaluated under fluoroscopy. A subsequent infusion with an adjusted dose is usually done in the ward. Dosages for individual vessels are shown in Table 10.1. Drugs are infused by a mechanical syringe pump; we use a Harvard pump.

The duration of infusion depends on the patient's response. In younger patients with good haemocoagulation, a 30-minute infusion is often enough. Older patients may require 2–3 hour infusions to control bleeding. After infusion, the catheter is left in position for 24 hours; should bleeding recur, another infusion may be done, or embolic vasoocclusion performed.

Risks associated with selective vasoconstrictive therapy of acute gastroduodenal bleeding approximate to those of diagnostic visceral angiography. A few patients experience abdominal cramps or minimal elevation of blood pressure; only rarely does spasm of the punctured femoral artery require catheter withdrawal. No instance of ischaemia or infarction of the stomach or duodenum has been reported in patients with acute gastroduodenal arterial bleeding treated with vasoconstrictive therapy (Athanasoulis *et al.*, 1974).

10.3 SELECTIVE VASOOCCLUSION

Selective vasoocclusion, mostly in the form of embolization of the

Table 10.1 Dosages of infused vasoconstrictors in selective vasoconstrictive therapy of acute gastroduodenal bleeding.

	Dose range per minute	
Site of injection	*Vasopressin (units)*	*Adrenaline (mg)*
Left gastric	0.05–0.1	8–10
Splenic	0.1 –0.3	10–16
Coeliac	0.3 –0.4	16–24
Common hepatic	0.2 –0.3	14–18
Gastroduodenal	0.05–0.1	8–10
Superior mesenteric	0.3 –0.4	—
Jejunal	0.5 –0.1	—

bleeding vessel or its feeder, is a newer, more aggressive method of therapy, which involves certain risks. The indications vary among angiographers. In our opinion, it should be reserved for patients where vasoconstrictive infusion has failed or appears unlikely to succeed because of faulty haemocoagulation or poor vascular reactivity. It is also indicated in patients with brisk bleeding who present too high a risk for vasoconstrictive therapy. *Direct superselective catheterization of the bleeding artery or its main feeder is a prerequisite for successful and safe vasoocclusive therapy in gastrointestinal bleeding.*

Vasoocclusive materials also vary with individual angiographers. In acute gastroduodenal arterial bleeding we prefer surgical gelatine (Gelfoam) (Athanasoulis *et al.*, 1974; Carsen *et al.*, 1978; Goldman *et al.*, 1976; Katzen and McSweeney, 1975; Keller and Rösch, 1979; Nusbaum *et al.*, 1972; Reuter *et al.*, 1975; Ring *et al.*, 1974; Rösch *et al.*, 1976). In the form of cut pieces or powder, mixed with contrast material, it is effective and easy to inject. Furthermore, the resulting occlusion is not permanent and recanalization occurs in a few days or weeks. Modified autologous clot with additives such as thrombin, oxidized cellulose (Oxycel), or aminocaproic acid (Amicar) are reported to be stable, firm and effective (Bookstein *et al.*, 1974; Eisenberg and Steer, 1976; Probst *et al.*, 1978; Rösch *et al.*, 1972*b*, 1976; White *et al.*, 1974*a*). Their preparation, however, may delay the procedure. Various types of microfibrillar collagen (Avitene, Lyodura), used with success in the obliterative therapy of cerebrofacial lesions, have not yet found wide use in gastroduodenal arterial bleeding, but appear promising (Kaufman *et al.*, 1978), as do detachable balloons (White *et al.*, 1979). Isobutyl-2-cyanoacrylate (Bucrylate), a fast polymerizing adhesive, causes permanent occlusion, and is indicated only under special circumstances, mainly in bleeding malignancies (Dotter *et al.*, 1975; Goldman *et al.*, 1976). Simple balloon catheters have been used to produce temporary occlusion in major bleeding as an adjunct to surgical intervention (Wholey, 1977; *et al.*, 1970).

Gelfoam powder is used for bleeding from small peripheral vessels in erosive gastritis, stress ulcers or peripherally located peptic ulcers. Gelfoam powder is mixed with Renografin 76% in an apple-sauce-like mixture, and the amount of embolic material injected is determined under fluoroscopic monitoring; 1–5 ml of the mixture usually suffice. Occasionally, Gelfoam powder is used in small vessel bleeding from Mallory–Weiss tears (Fig. 10.11). As well as the bleeding vessels, some non-bleeding gastric vessels will also be obstructed (Figs. 10.11, 10.12). In the stomach this causes no problem because of its rich collateral circulation. Embolization of the liver, spleen or pancreas by reflux of Gelfoam, however, should be carefully avoided by slow injection under fluoroscopic control. A special catheter with a balloon about 2–3 cm

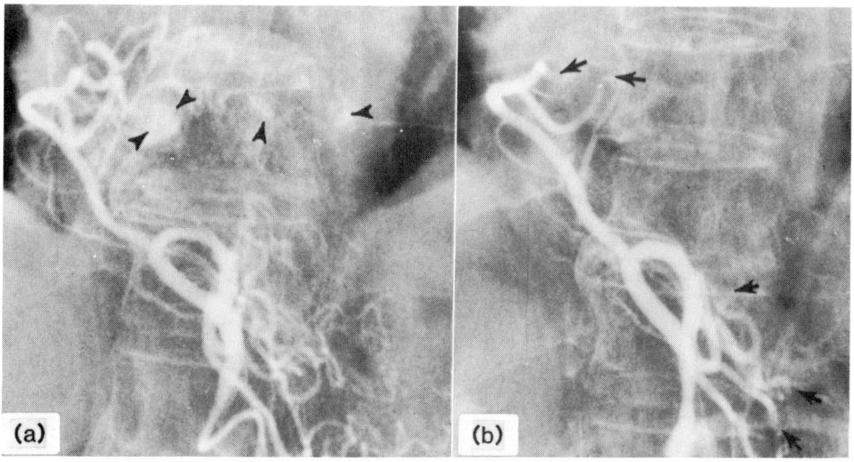

Fig. 10.11 Acute bleeding from Mallory–Weiss tears in hiatal hernia successfully controlled by embolization of Gelfoam powder. (a) Initial left gastric angiogram shows hiatal hernia with multiple bleeding points from several small vessels (arrowheads). (b) Follow-up angiogram after injection of 2 ml of Gelfoam powder demonstrates occlusion of most small and some medium-sized branches (arrows) of the left gastric artery.

proximal to the tip may be used to occlude the origin of the catheterized artery, thus preventing reflux of the embolic material (Greenfield *et al.*, 1978).

Gelfoam pieces are used in bleeding from larger branches, as encountered in some Mallory–Weiss tears, some centrally located stress ulcers, and especially in chronic peptic ulcers. Three to ten Gelfoam fragments (mixed with contrast medium) are delivered into the catheterized artery, always under fluoroscopic control, to ensure that reflux does not occur. Depending on the number and size of the injected Gelfoam pieces, major branches or even the main superselectively catheterized artery itself, are occluded. In duodenal ulcers the gastroduodenal artery is often embolized. In ulcers of the descending duodenum, however, embolization of the gastroduodenal artery may fail to control haemorrhage because of collateral arterial supply. Here, superselective catheterization with occlusion of the bleeding branch artery itself, constitutes the most successful and safest approach (Fig. 10.13).

Special care must be taken when there are vascular anomalies, particularly an aberrant left hepatic artery originating from the left gastric (Fig. 10.14). In this situation, occlusion should be done only when the bleeding artery itself can be superselectively catheterized, allowing control of the bleeding without endangering hepatic arterial supply. If the

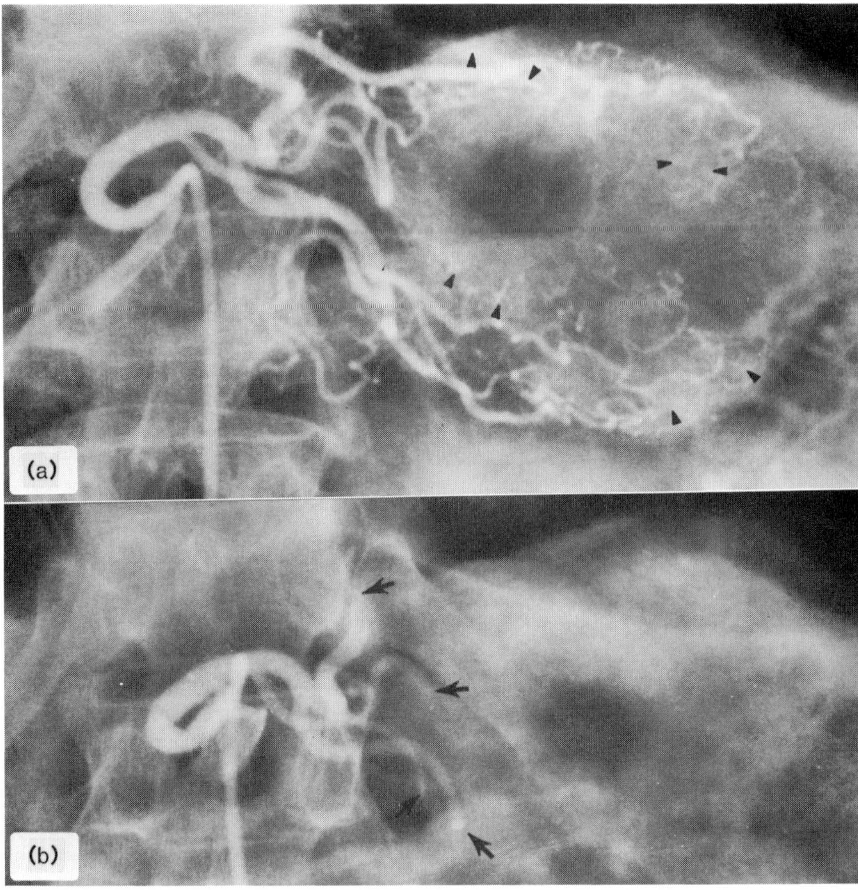

Fig. 10.12 Acute bleeding from erosive gastritis in the gastric fundus successfully controlled by selective embolization of Gelfoam powder. (a) Initial left gastric angiogram demonstrates multiple bleeding points (arrowheads) in the horizontally located gastric fundus. (b) Follow-up angiogram after injection of 4 ml of Gelfoam powder shows occlusion (arrows) of all medium-sized and some of the larger left gastric branches.

necessary specificity of catheter placement cannot be achieved, vasoconstrictive therapy is preferable (Fig. 10.15).

Success in vasoocclusive therapy is necessarily linked to catheterization success. In the hands of the experienced angiographer, primary branches of the coeliac and superior mesenteric arteries (hepatic, splenic, left gastric, pancreaticoduodenal, jejunal) can be entered in 90–95% and secondary branches in 80–85%. Once catheterized, use of the proper

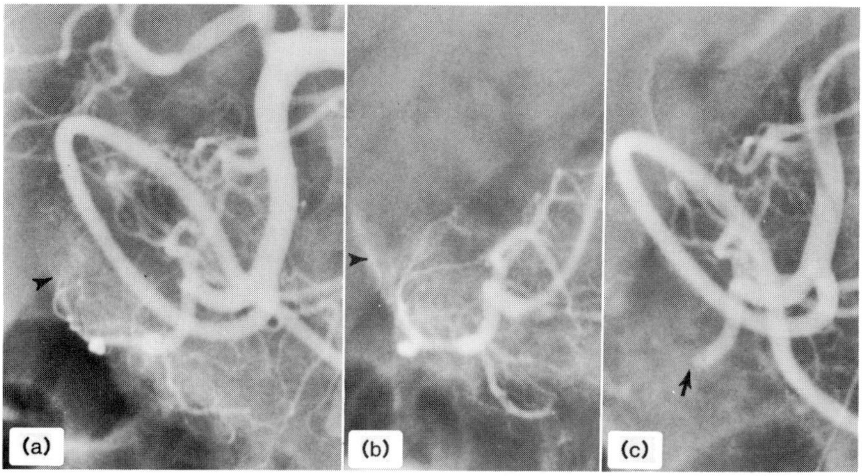

Fig. 10.13 Acute bleeding from a duodenal ulcer, demonstrated well at duodenoscopy, successfully controlled by occlusion of the bleeding duodenal artery by Gelfoam pieces. (a) Initial common hepatic angiogram shows only minimal bleeding in the duodenum (arrowhead). (b) Direct superselective angiogram of the bleeding duodenal artery demonstrates extravasation of contrast material (arrowhead). (c) Follow-up gastroduodenal angiogram after injection of three pieces of Gelfoam shows complete occlusion of the previously bleeding duodenal artery (arrow).

embolization material will result in successful occlusion in 95–100% of attempts. Particular caution should be exercised in patients with previous gastric resection, because of the diminished collateral vascular supply (Bradley and Goldman, 1976).

Embolization should not be performed in bleeding from arteries originating from those supplying other organs; for example, short gastric arteries arising from the splenic artery, sometimes involved in bleeding ulcers high on the greater curvature of the stomach. Here, too, vasoconstrictive infusions are preferable to embolization (Fig. 10.16). *Inability to catheterize the specific bleeding vessel or its main feeder contraindicates occlusive embolization whenever it poses the risk of uncontrolled infarction.*

Some angiographers have used vasoocclusive embolization to control bleeding from jejunal branches in anastomotic ulcers. We believe, however, that mesenteric arterial occlusion should be done only as a life-saving procedure in high surgical risk patients where vasoconstrictive infusion has failed. Superselective occlusion of the bleeding branch itself is imperative in the mesenteric circulation. Indications for vasoocclusion in the mesenteric bed are thus limited, since the required selectivity

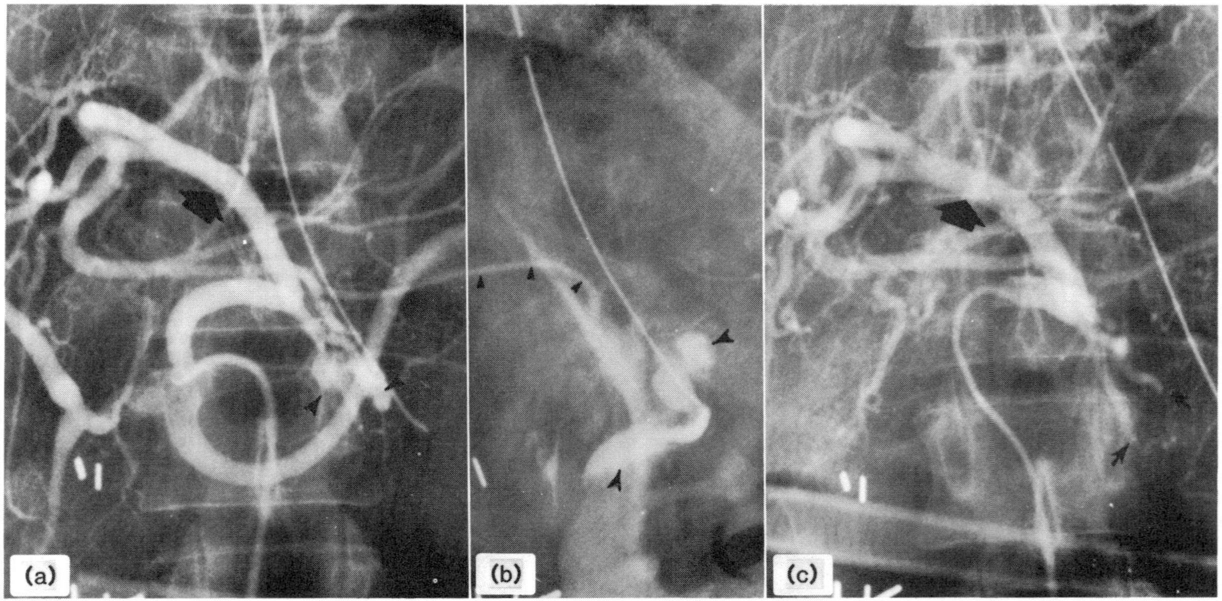

Fig. 10.14 Acute bleeding from a large ulcer on the lesser curvature of the stomach successfully controlled by selective embolizations of Gelfoam pieces into the bleeding branches. (a) Initial angiogram with the catheter tip at the left gastric artery origin shows extravasation of contrast medium (arrowheads) in the stomach. The left gastric artery gives origin to a large aberrant left hepatic artery (large arrow). (b) Superselective angiogram with catheter (small arrowheads) in the main bleeding branch reveals extensive extravasation of contrast medium into the stomach (arrowheads). (c) Follow-up left gastric angiogram after injection of two larger Gelfoam pieces demonstrates selective occlusion of the previously bleeding arteries (small arrows) with widely patent aberrant left hepatic artery (large arrow).

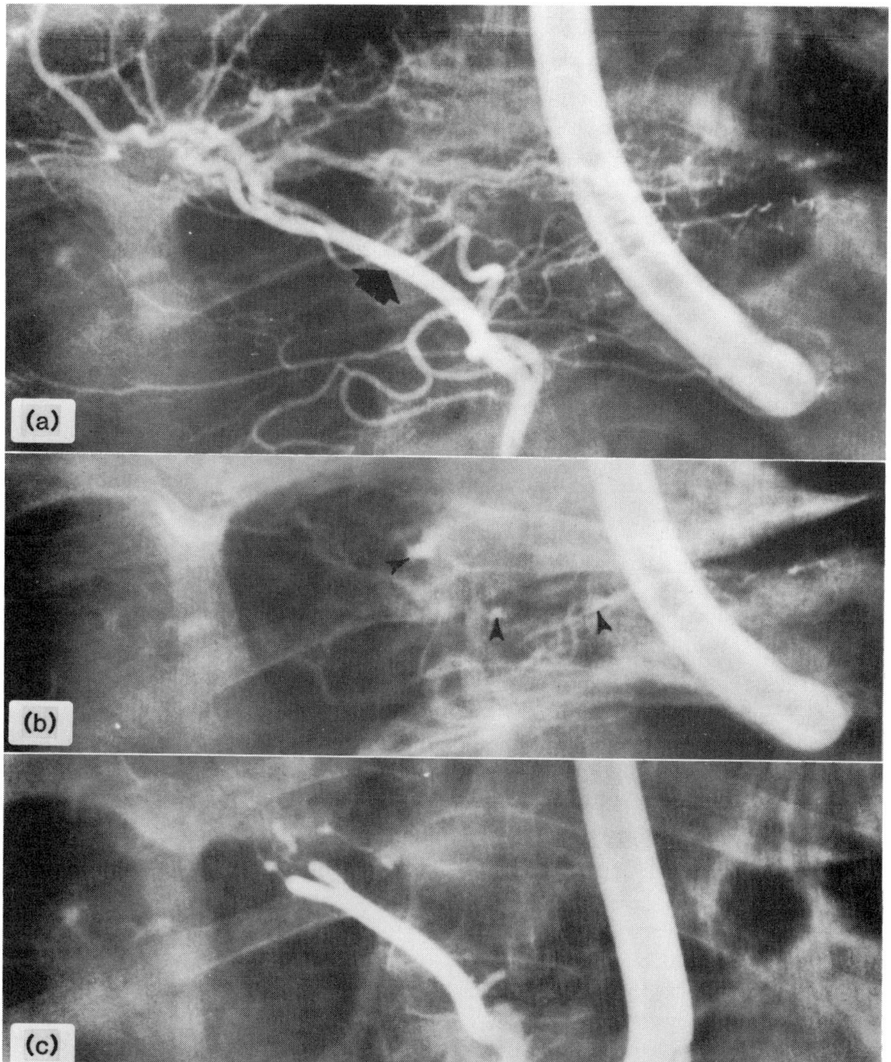

Fig. 10.15 Acute bleeding from multiple gastric stress ulcers successfully controlled by selective infusion of adrenaline into the left gastric artery. (a) Arterial phase of the initial left gastric angiogram demonstrates an aberrant hepatic artery originating from the left gastric (large arrow). (b) Later phase of the initial angiogram reveals several small extravasations of contrast medium in the stomach (arrowheads). (c) Angiogram after 30-minute selective infusion of adrenaline (12 mg/min) demonstrates extensive constriction of all branches of the infused left gastric artery, including the aberrant left hepatic, and no extravasation of contrast medium.

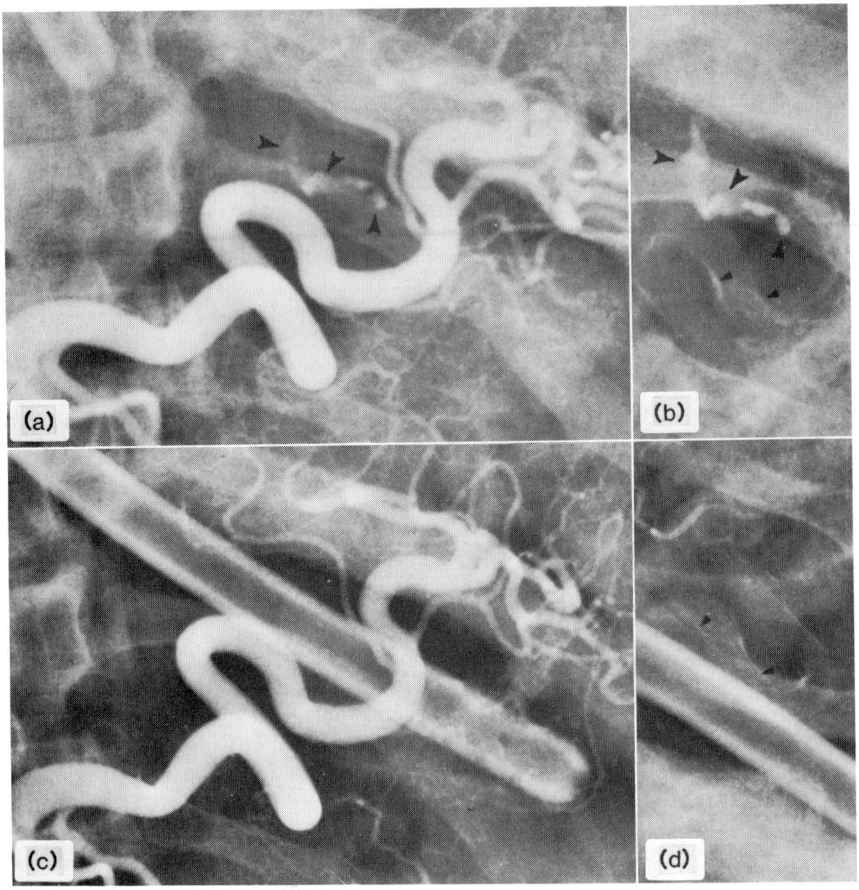

Fig. 10.16 Acute bleeding from an ulcer high on the greater curvature of the stomach. (a) Arterial phase of the initial splenic angiogram shows extravasation of contrast medium (arrowheads) on the greater curvature of the stomach. (b) Capillary phase of the initial angiogram shows persistence and increased amount of extravasation (larger arrowheads) and calcifications in the splenic artery (small arrowheads). (c) Arterial phase of the splenic angiogram performed 5 minutes after 30-minute infusion of adrenaline (19 mg/min) does not show any bleeding and reveals good perfusion of the spleen. (d) Capillary phase of the follow-up angiogram also does not demonstrate any extravasation. Calcifications in the splenic artery are again seen (small arrowheads).

cannot always be achieved. Where mesenteric arterial occlusion is to be done, a relatively fast lysing material, such as autologous or modified blood clot, is recommended. Permanently occluding materials can be considered in intractable bleeding due to a recurrent anastomotic malignancy where the heightened risk of ischaemia or infarction may be warranted.

To minimize the risks associated with transcatheter vascular occlusion, certain basic precautions should be observed. The bleeding site, its feeding vessel and regional vascular anatomy, must be delineated with precision. Occlusion should be produced only when catheterization of the specific bleeding vessel or, in certain cases, its feeder is possible. The proper occlusive material should be used and the occlusion accomplished under high definition fluoroscopic control. These simple guidelines can substantially decrease or eliminate complications. We have successfully done therapeutic transcatheter occlusions in over 50 patients with acute gastroduodenal arterial bleeding with no complications related to vascular occlusion. It must be emphasized that transcatheter occlusion can harm the patient, even endanger his life, if performed inappropriately by an inexperienced angiographer or without the necessary technical facilities and care.

APPENDIX 10.1

Catheters, drugs, and suppliers

Amicar (aminocaproic acid) – Lederle Laboratories, 201 University Avenue, Westwood, Massachusetts 02090.

Avitene (microfibrillar collagen haemostat) – Avicon, Inc., 6201 South Freeway, Fort Worth, Texas 76134.

Gelfoam (absorbable gelatin, sponge and powder) – The Upjohn Company, 7000 Portage Road, Kalamazoo, Michigan 49001.

Isobutyl-2-cyanoacrylate (tissue adhesive) – Ethicon, Inc., Somerville, NJ 08876.

Oxycel (oxidized cellulose) – Parke-Davis, Division of Warner–Lambert Co., 201 Tabor Road, Morris Plains, NJ 07950.

Renografin 76% (diatrizoate meglumine) – E. R. Squibb and Sons, Inc., P.O. Box 2013, New Brunswick, NJ 08903.

Torcon catheters – Cook, Incorporated, P.O. Box 489, Bloomington, Indiana 47401; or Wm. Cook Europe ApS, Poppelgaardsvej 14, DK 2860, Söborg, Denmark.

REFERENCES

Athanasoulis, C. A. (1976). Angiographic methods for the control of gastric hemorrhage. *Am. J. Dig. Dis.*, **21**, 174–81.

Athanasoulis, C. A. *et al.* (1974). Control of acute gastric mucosal hemorrhage. Intraarterial infusion of posterior pituitary extract. *New Engl. J. Med.*, **290**, 597–603.

Athanasoulis, C. A. *et al.* (1976). Angiography: its contribution to the emergency management of gastrointestinal hemorrhage. *Radiol. Clinics N. Am.*, **14**, 265–80.

Barr, J. W., Lakin, R. C. and Rösch, J. (1975). Vasopressin and hepatic artery: effect of selective celiac infusion of vasopressin on the hepatic artery flow. *Invest. Radiol.*, **10**, 200–5.

Baum, S. *et al.* (1965). The preoperative radiologic demonstration of intraabdominal bleeding from undetermined sites by percutaneous selective celiac and superior mesenteric arteriography. *Surgery*, **58**, 797–805.

Baum, S. *et al.* (1969), Selective arteriography in the diagnosis of hemorrhage in the gastrointestinal tract. *Radiol. Clinics N. Am.*, **7**, 131–45.

Bookstein, J. J. *et al.* (1974). Transcatheter hemostasis of gastrointestinal bleeding using modified autogenous clot. *Radiology*, **113**, 277–85.

Bradley, E. L. and Goldman, M. L. (1976). Gastric infarction after therapeutic embolization. *Surgery*, **79**, 421–4.

Carsen, G. M., Casarella, W. J. and Spiegel, R. M. (1978). Transcatheter embolization for treatment of Mallory–Weiss tears of the esophagogastric junction. *Radiology*, **128**, 309–13.

Dotter, C. T., Goldman, M. L. and Rösch, J. (1975). Instant selective arterial occlusion with isobutyl 2-cyanoacrylate. *Radiology*, **114**, 227–30.

Dotter, C. T. *et al.* (1972). Injectable flow-guided coaxial catheters for selective angiography and controlled vascular occlusion. *Radiology*, **104**, 421–3.

Eisenberg, H. and Steer, M. L. (1976). The nonoperative treatment of massive pyloroduodenal hemorrhage by retracted autologous clot embolization. *Surgery*, **79**, 414–20.

Frey, C. F., Reuter, S. R. and Bookstein, J. J. (1970). Localization of gastrointestinal hemorrhage by selective angiography. *Surgery*, **67**, 548–55.

Goldman, M. L. *et al.* (1976). Transcatheter therapeutic embolization in the management of massive upper gastrointestinal bleeding. *Radiology*, **120**, 513–21.

Grace, D. M. and Gold, R. E. (1978). Angiography in determining the cause and treatment of gastrointestinal bleeding. *Can. J. Surg.*, **21**, 171–4.

Granmayeh, M., Wallace, S. and Schwarten, D. (1979). Transcatheter occlusion of the gastroduodenal artery. *Radiology*, **131**, 59–64.

Greenfield, A. J. *et al.* (1978). Transcatheter embolization: prevention of embolic reflux using balloon catheters. *Am. J. Roentg.*, **131**, 651–5.

Hedberg, S. E. (1974). Endoscopy in gastrointestinal bleeding. A systemic approach to diagnosis. *Surg. Clinics N. Am.*, **54**, 549–59.

Janicki, P. and Alfidi, R. J. (1976). Selective visceral angiography in the diagnosis and treatment of gastroduodenal hemorrhage. *Surg. Clinics N. Am.*, **56**, 1365–73.

Kadir, S. and Athanasoulis, C. T. (1977). Angiographic management of gastrointestinal bleeding with vasopressin. *Fortschr. Geb. Röntgenstr. Nucklearmed.*, **127**, 111–9.

Katon, R. M. and Smith, F. S. (1973). Panendoscopy in the early diagnosis of acute upper gastrointestinal bleeding. *Gastroenterology*, **65**, 728–34.

Katzen, B. J. and McSweeney (1975). Therapeutic transluminal arterial embolization for bleeding in the upper part of the gastrointestinal tract. *Surg. Gynec. Obstet.*, **141**, 523–7.

Kaufman, S. L. *et al.* (1978). Transcatheter embolization with microfibrillar collagen in swine. *Invest. Radiol.*, **13**, 200–4.

Keller, F. S. and Rösch, J. (1979). Angiography in the diagnosis and therapy of acute upper gastrointestinal bleeding. *Schweiz. Med. Wschr.*, **109**, 586–91.

Merland, J. J. *et al.* (1978). Angiography and emergency embolisation of digestive haemorrhages. *J. Belge Radiol.*, **61**, 83–98.

Nusbaum, M. *et al.* (1972). Clinical experience with selective intra-arterial infusions of vasopressin in the control of gastrointestinal bleeding from arterial sources. *Am. J. Surg.,* **123**, 165–72.

Palmer, E. D. (1970). *Upper Gastrointestinal Hemorrhage.* Charles C. Thomas, Springfield.

Probst, P. *et al.* (1978). Which embolic material is best suited for which embolization procedure? *Fortschr. Geb. Röntgenstr. Nucklearmed.,* **129**, 447–54.

Rabin, A. *et al.* (1977). Hémorragies digestives et artériographie. Intérêt actuele et perspectives. *Ann. Radiol.,* **20**, 567–72.

Raja Rao, A. K. *et al.* (1978). The importance of the anomalous left gastric artery in the arteriography of gastric hemorrhage. *Br. J. Radiol.,* **51**, 260–1.

Reuter, S. T. and Bookstein, J. J. (1968). Angiographic localization of gastrointestinal bleeding. *Gastroenterology,* **54**, 876–83.

Reuter, S. T., Chang, V. P. and Bree, R. L. (1975). Selective arterial embolization of control of massive upper gastrointestinal bleeding. *Am. J. Roentg.,* **125**, 119–26.

Ring, E. J. *et al.* (1974). Angiography in the diagnosis and treatment of nonvariceal bleeding in patients with portal hypertension. *Surg. Gynec. Obstet.,* **139**, 205–19.

Rösch, J., Antonovic, R. and Dotter, C. T. (1976). Current angiographic approach to diagnosis and therapy of acute gastrointestinal bleeding. *Fortschr. Geb. Röntgenstr. Nucklearmed.,* **125**, 301–10.

Rösch, J., Dotter, C. T. and Antonovic, R. (1972*a*). Selective vasoconstrictor infusion in the management of arterio-capillary gastrointestinal hemorrhage. *Am. J. Roentg.,* **116**, 279–88.

Rösch, J., Dotter, C. T. and Brown, M. J. (1972*b*). Selective arterial embolization. A new method for control of acute gastrointestinal bleeding. *Radiology,* **102**, 303–6.

Rösch, J. *et al.* (1970). Selective arterial drug infusions in the treatment of acute gastrointestinal bleeding. *Gastroenterology,* **59**, 341–9.

Rosenbaum, A., Siegelman, S. S. and Sprayregen, S. (1975). The bleeding marginal ulcer: catheterization, diagnosis and therapy. *Am. J. Roentg.,* **125**, 812–5.

Twiford, T. W., Goldstein, H. M. and Zornoza, J. (1978). Transcatheter therapy of gastrointestinal arterial bleeding. *Am. J. Dig. Dis.,* **23**, 1046–55.

Wenz, W., Roth, J. F. and Brücknew, U. (1969). Die Angiographie bei akuter gastrointestinaler Blutung. *Fortschr. Geb. Röntgenstr. Nucklearmed.,* **110**, 616–29.

White, Jr., R. J., Giargiana, Jr., F. A. and Bell, W. (1974*a*). Bleeding duodenal ulcer control. Selective arterial embolization with autologous blood clot. *J. Am. Med. Ass.,* **229**, 546–8.

White, Jr., R. J. *et al.* (1974*b*). Pharmacologic control of hemorrhagic gastritis: clinical and experimental results. *Radiology,* **111**, 549–57.

White, Jr., R. J. *et al.* (1979). Therapeutic embolization with detachable silicone balloons. Early clinical experience. *J. Am. Med. Ass.,* **241**, 1257–60.

Wholey, M. H. (1977). The technology of balloon catheters in interventional angiography. *Radiology,* **125**, 671–6.

Wholey, M. H., Stockdale, R. and Tin Kan Hung (1970). A percutaneous balloon catheter for the immediate control of hemorrhage. *Radiology,* **95**, 65–71.

11 Gastric and duodenal polypectomy

E. SEIFERT

Until 1970, fibreoptic endoscopy of oesophagus, stomach and duodenum was only a diagnostic technique. The first time endoscopy was used for treating a gastric lesion was described in 1970 in a paper by Namiki *et al.* (1970) about local treatment of stomach ulcers. In the same year, Tsuneoka and Uchida (1970) reported a gastroscopic method to remove gastric polyps. They were using instruments made by the Machida Company in Japan, cutting the polyps mechanically. Improvements were possible by using high-frequency diathermy loops (Seifert and Elster, 1972, 1973, 1975; Classen and Fruehmorgen, 1976; Elster, 1976; Seifert, 1973, 1975a, 1977).

11.1 INDICATIONS FOR ENDOSCOPIC POLYPECTOMY

Many types of polyps occur in the upper gastrointestinal tract. The term 'polyp' is only a descriptive word incorporating a variety of histological structures. The size, number and location of polyps give little indication as to their type. Differentiation of epithelial polyps is possible by guided biopsy when they are uniform in their histological structure. A typical mesenchymal polyp can be recognized by the bridging folds and by being covered with normal mucosa. However, biopsy verification using forceps often fails because characteristic tissue cannot usually be obtained by biopsies of the overlying mucosa.

The exact classification of a gastrointestinal polyp, and the diagnosis of malignant change within a polypoid lesion, necessitates histological examination of the whole polyp. Polypectomy provides an effective form of treatment when polyps are the cause of haemorrhage or obstruction, and may be regarded as an effective form of cancer prevention. Generally, however, the major role of upper gastrointestinal polypectomy is diagnostic, i.e. to obtain sufficient material to enable an accurate histopathological diagnosis.

11.2 INSTRUMENTS

11.2.1 **Endoscopes**

It is advisable to use a fully flexible forward-viewing fibre-endoscope. Double-channel 'operating' endoscopes and endoscopes with a bigger biopsy channel have recently become available (see Chapter 1), but, in our opinion, they do not offer any advantage over normal instruments.

11.2.2 **Snares**

Today, many suitable high-frequency diathermy snares are on the market. In tubular organs like oesophagus and duodenum, oval-shaped snares are advantageous, but in the stomach, eccentric loops are more convenient to handle. It is useful to have different shapes and sizes of snares which can be adapted to the polyp size and to the width of the lumen (Fig. 11.1).

11.2.3 **Electrosurgical power units**

Several manufacturers of endoscopic equipment offer suitable electrosurgical power units for diathermy. A capability of 40 to 50 W, two amps, and 130 kHz has been reported satisfactory (Classen and Demling, 1971; Classen and Fruehmorgen, 1976; Seifert, 1973, 1975a, 1975b, 1977). We use a generator (Erbotom, Erbe Company, Tuebingen, West Germany) adjusted to produce 40–50 W at about 130 kHz.

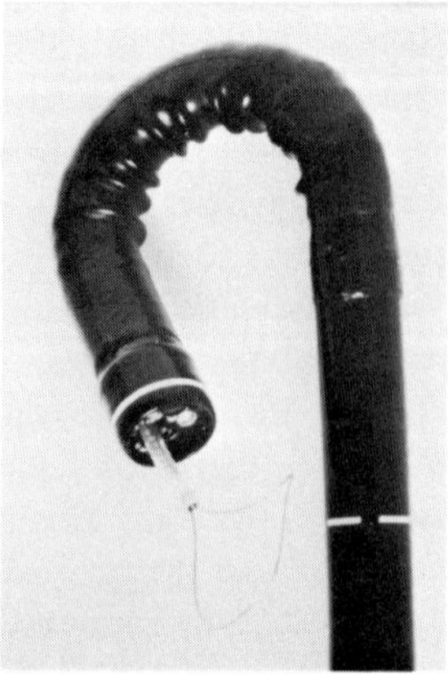

Fig. 11.1 Forward-viewing endoscope (Olympus GIF D3) with inserted open snare.

11.2.4 **Retrieval instruments**

The best method for retrieving a cut polyp is to hold it with special forceps. The best grasping forceps have three movable fingers, fixed to a strong piece of wire (Fig. 7.1(b)). Insertion is carried out in the closed position via the biopsy channel. After locating the object to be removed, the forceps are spread and the object is cautiously grasped with all three fingers.

Another successful method of grasping the polyp is to use a Dormia basket (such as those used after endoscopic papillotomy for removal of gallstones) (Fig. 7.1(e)). Grasping forceps and Dormia baskets are available from several manufacturers.

11.3 TECHNIQUE

Premedication of the patient is the same as for normal upper gastrointestinal endoscopy. We use 2 ml pethidine and 5 ml diazepam with 2 ml hyoscine *N*-butyl bromide. The procedure can be performed on outpatients.

The fibrescope is usually inserted with the patient in the left lateral position. After seeing the polyp, the snare, which has been passed through the operating channel of the instrument, is placed around the base of the polyp and cautiously tightened (Seifert and Elster, 1972; Seifert, 1975a) (Fig. 11.2(a), (b)). Polypectomy is performed by applying one or more pulses of 'coagulating' current. The polyp is retrieved by suction via the endoscope or by special forceps, or a Dormia basket. The polyps are then withdrawn together with the endoscope (Seifert, 1973, 1975a; Seifert and Elster, 1975). Retrieval is essential.

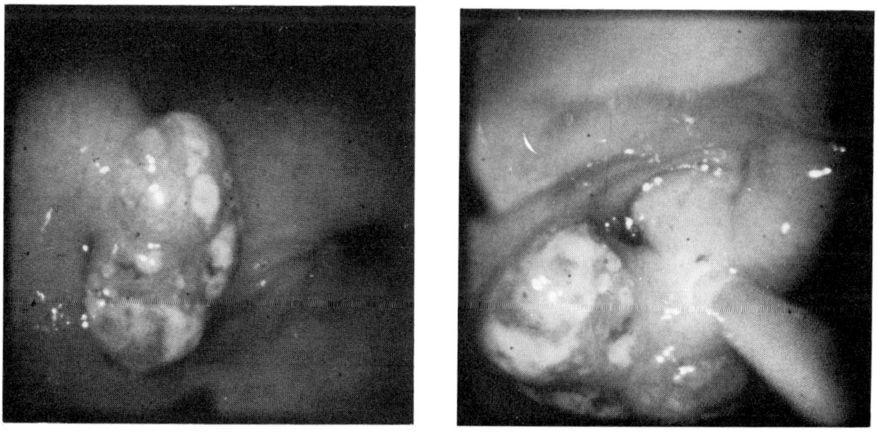

Fig. 11.2 (a) Epithelial gastric polyp, (b) snared polyp.

An ulcer will have been created at the site of the polypectomy, its size varying with the diameter of the base of the extirpated polyp (Table 11.1). Ulcers less than 5 mm in diameter heal in one week or less, leaving no scar. In 95% of cases, ulcers have healed within four weeks and in all by eight weeks (Table 11.2) (Ottenjann, Bartelheimer and Elster, 1971; Seifert, 1973, 1975a, 1975b). They do not need any treatment, since they are not real 'peptic defects' (Fig. 11.3(a), (b)).

11.4 COMPLICATIONS

These occur in less than one per cent of patients undergoing polypectomy (Seifert, 1973, 1975a, 1975b, 1977). In our cases, haemorrhage was observed in three of 800 polypectomy patients of whom two required surgical intervention. Postpolypectomy pain, which occurred in one patient, was ascribed to the ulcer which had developed at the site of extirpation.

Epithelial polyps with a base or stalk diameter of up to 3 cm may be

Table 11.1 Correlation between ulcer diameter, size and type of gastric polyps (no. = 44).

Polyp	*Ulcer diameter*	*<2 mm*	*3–5 mm*	*6–10 mm*	*11–15 mm*
Diameter	<10 mm no. = 98	●● ●●	●●●● ●●●● ●●●	●●● ●●	
	11–20 mm no. = 57	●	●●●● ●●● ●●●	●● ●● ●	●●
	21–30 mm no. = 21		●	●● ●●	●
Type (Yamada)	I no. = 19		●● ●●	●●●● ●●●●	● ●
	II no. = 41	●	●●●● ●●●● ●●●	●●● ●●	●
	III no. = 102	●● ●●	●●● ●●● ●	●	
	IV no. = 14				
	Total	5	22	14	3

Table 11.2 Findings at the original localization of gastric polyps one, four and eight weeks after electroresection (no. = 176).

	1 week	*4 weeks*	*8 weeks*
Normal	92	—	—
Scar	—	—	—
Protrusion with central depression	22	normal	—
Granulation tissue	9	normal	—
Ulcer	44	11 normal	
		25 scars	8 scars
		8 ulcers	
Polypoid remnant	9	4 normal	—
		3 scars	—
		2 polypoid remnant	2 scars

safely removed by endoscopic polypectomy. Mesenchymal tumours present special risks as they may penetrate the full depth of the wall of the viscus involved. Attempted resection may therefore cause a perforation. Endoscopic electrosurgery should be restricted to obtaining an adequate portion of tissue for diagnostic purposes. Such lesions are, in any case, usually recognized and correctly diagnosed by the endoscopist because of their appearance: the overlying mucosa is intact and has typical folds (Fig. 11.4).

11.5 GASTRIC POLYPS

It is now clear that gastric polyps of epithelial origin, or indeed any type of gastric polyp, cannot be accurately diagnosed when reliance is placed

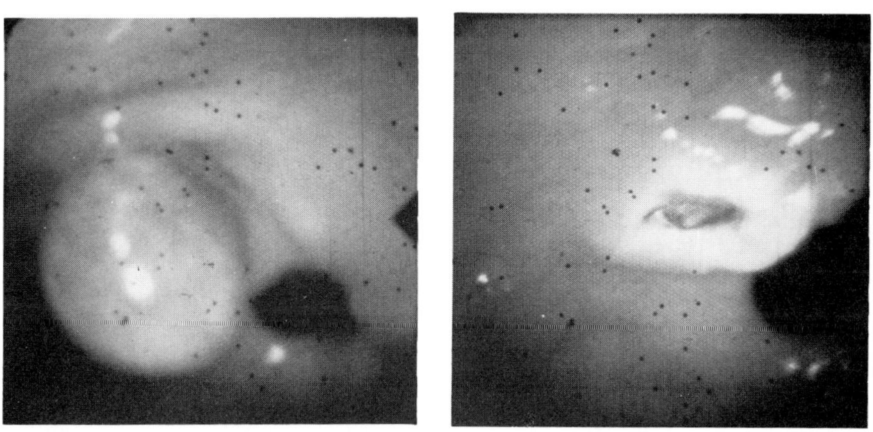

Fig. 11.3 (a) Epithelial gastric polyp in the prepyloric region. (b) Polypectomy site after electrosection.

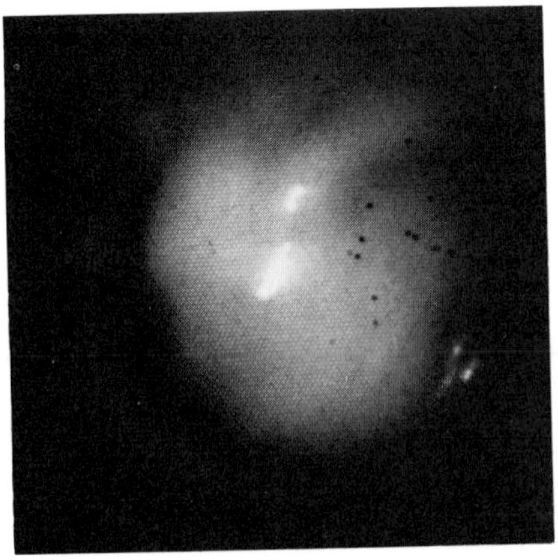

Fig. 11.4 Mesenchymal polyp with typical bridging folds.

on visual appearances and on the interpretation of endoscopic biopsy specimens (Seifert and Elster, 1972, 1973, 1975; Seifert, 1973, 1975a, 1975b; Seifert and Otto, 1973). When diagnoses based on biopsy material were compared with diagnoses derived from examination of whole polyps obtained by endoscopic polypectomy, there was no agreement in 53 out of 75 cases (70%) (Table 11.3). The cause of the difference in diagnoses is that epithelial polyps often contain a mixture of histological appearances, and that material forming the 'mother tissue' of mesenchymal tumours can almost never be obtained by biopsies of the overlying mucosa.

11.5.1 **Histological classification of gastric polyps**

Increasing experience has shown the need for a new classification of gastric polyps; such a classification was reported by Elster (1976) and is shown in Table 11.4.

(a) *Focal hyperplasia*
Focal hyperplasia of the foveolae (gastric gland orifices) and of the crest of the gastric rugae is not due to the formation of a polyp *sui generis* but is a reactive process (Seifert and Elster, 1972, 1973, 1975; Elster, 1976). The term hyperplastic polyp should be avoided when discussing gastric polyps, as false analogies with the classification and behaviour of colonic polyps may be drawn.

(b) *Hyperplasiogenic polyp (HPG-polyp)*
The histopathological appearances of the hyperplasiogenic polyp lie between those of focal hyperplasia and of a true adenomatous polyp.

Table 11.3 Discrepancies of histological findings of biopsy material and the tissue of the excised polyp (no. = 53).

Biopsy material	*n*	*Removed polyp*	
Focal hyperplasia	18	Hyperplastic-adenomatous	Hyperplasiogenic
	2	Hyperplastic-angiomatous	
	2	Hyperplastic-adenoangiomatous	
Adenoma	2	Hyperplastic-adenomatous	
	2	Adenomatous-cystic	
Foveolar pseudohyperplasia	7	Hyperplastic-adenomatous	
Superficial gastritis	1	Hyperplastic-adenomatous	
Adenoma	1	Hyperplastic	Focal hyperplasia
Foveolar pseudohyperplasia	1	Adenomatous	Adenoma
Superficial gastritis	3	Adenomatous	
	1	Xanthoma	
	2	Inflammatory pseudopolyp	
	1	Hyperplastic-neurogen	
	2	Brunneroma	
	4	Neurinoma	
	1	Pancreatic heterotopy	
Normal mucosa	1	Lipoma	
	1	Neurinoma	
	1	Neurofibroma	

Table 11.4 Classification of epithelial gastric polyps (from Elster, 1976).

Term	*Tissue of origin*	*Pathogenesis*	*Localization*
Focal hyperplasia	Foveolar epithelium	Hyperplasia	anywhere
Hyperplasiogenic polyp	Foveolar epithelium	Hyperplasia + glandular component	anywhere
Adenoma (highly differentiated)	Gastric glands (pyloric type)	Blastoma (neoplasia)	antrum – pylorus – cardia
Adenoma (moderately differentiated)	Neck cells	Blastoma (neoplasia)	predominantly cardia
Borderline lesion – protruded type (subtype IIa)	Neck cells	Hyperplasia with atypia – blastoma	anywhere
Early carcinoma type IIa + I	Neck cells	Blastoma (neoplasia)	anywhere

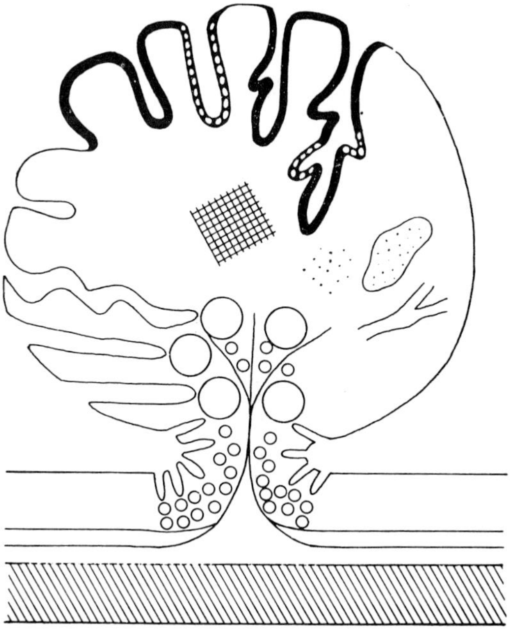

Fig. 11.5 Schema of morphology of hyperplasiogenic gastric polyp.

Hyperplasiogenic polyps comprise the majority of gastric polyps. The term is designed to stress that hyperplasia of glandular tissue is present, but that the fully developed appearance of the adenoma is lacking. This hyperplasiogenic polyp only occurs in the stomach (Fig. 11.5).

(c) *Adenoma*

True adenomas of the stomach are rare but when present are most likely to be found in the cardia and pyloric regions, i.e. near the mucosal transition zones (Seifert and Elster, 1972, 1973, 1975; Singer *et al.*, 1975; Elster, 1976).

(d) *Borderline lesions and early cancer*

Cellular atypia may be observed in the crypts of gastric glands and may assume the appearance of borderline lesions and even of early carcinoma of the stomach.

To this classification of gastric polyps of epithelial origin, based mainly on experience gained since endoscopic polypectomy became possible, must be added another relatively new histopathological concept, namely that of *corpus glandular cysts*, i.e. cyst formation in the glandular tissue, sometimes sufficient to cause single or multiple tumours or swelling with the endoscopic appearance of polyps (Fig. 11.6) but with typical, specific

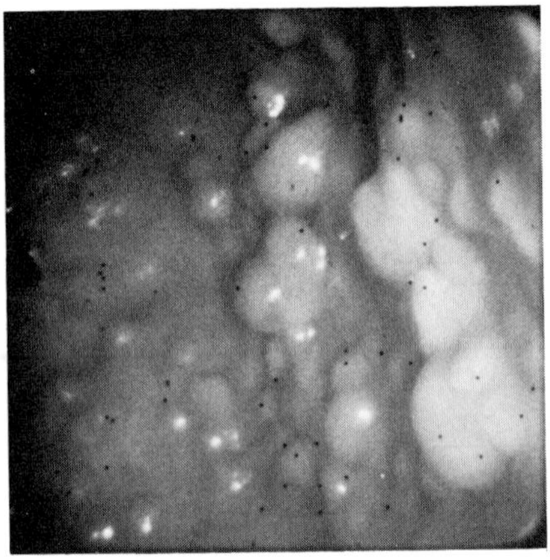

Fig. 11.6 Endoscopic appearance of multiple corpus glandular cysts.

and benign pathological appearances (Fig. 11.7) (Seifert and Elster, 1975; Elster, 1976; Elster *et al*., 1977). Our experiences with 706 gastric polyps removed by endoscopic polypectomy are shown in Table 11.5.

(e) *Gastric polyposis*

This is a condition in which there are 50 or more polyps present in the stomach. The pathological nature of these polyps may vary widely, but they are not of adenomatous type (Table 11.6). In polyposis, several polyps should be removed endoscopically for accurate diagnosis (Seifert and Elster, 1972, 1973, 1975), but, in general, polyposis is not an indication for surgery; the malignant potential depends on the type rather than the number of polyps present (Roesch, 1970; Seifert and Elster, 1972, 1973, 1975; Elster, 1976; Elster *et al*., 1977).

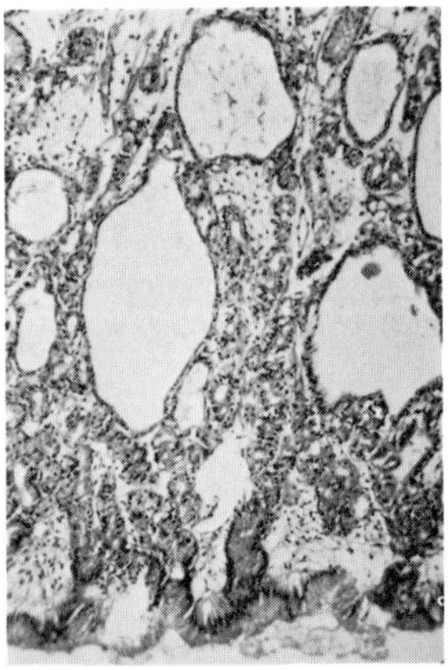

Fig. 11.7 Histological structures of corpus glandular cysts.

Table 11.5 Histological findings in 706 gastric polyps removed by endoscopic polypectomy (Single polyps: n = 358).

Histological findings	*n*		%	
1. Epithelial polyps	237			66.20
Focal hyperplasia		49	13.68	
Hyperplasiogenic polyps		158	44.13	
Adenoma		17	4.75	
Borderline lesion, protruded type		5	1.40	
Adenoma and borderline lesion		1	0.28	
Hyperplasiogenic polyp and borderline (BII-anastomosis)		1	0.28	
Early gastric cancer type I, IIa		4	1.12	
Polypoid cancer		2	0.56	
2. Carcinoids	5			1.40
3. Heterotopias	7			1.95
4. Mesenchymal tumours	20			5.59
5. Miscellaneous, not epithelial polypoid lesions	89			24.86
	358		100.00	

As there may be an association between gastric and colonic polyposis, patients with the former should be investigated for the latter (Seifert and Elster, 1973, 1975; Seifert and Otto, 1973).

Seifert (1977) has reported that a synchronous carcinoma was found in four of 80 patients with gastric polyposis. The polyps in each of these four were hyperplasiogenic in type. Follow-up examinations revealed no patients with premalignant or malignant conditions. Multiple corpus glandular cysts have no malignant potential and require no treatment.

Table 11.6 Histological findings in 706 polyps removed by endoscopic polypectomy (Polyposis: n = 27, removed polyps 348).

Histological findings	*cases* *n*	*polyps* *n*
Hyperplasiogenic polyps	12	140
Polyps in Peutz-Jeghers syndrome	3	53
Corpus glandular cysts	9	127
Mixed polyposis (hyperplasiogenic and multiple carcinoids)	2	24
Mixed polyposis (hyperplasiogenic and focal hyperplasia)	1	4
	27	348

Table 11.7 Follow-up examinations (after) polypectomy. Solitary and multiple polyps.

		Stomach			
		Recurrent polyps	*Polyps at other locations in the stomach*	*Non-discernible*	
	n	*n*	*n*	*n*	
After 1 year	223	11	11		22 = 9.9%
After 2 years	72		7		7 = 9.7%
After 3 years	38		4		4 = 10.5%
Within 3 years	333		22	25	58 = 17.4%
After 4 years	4		2		2
After 5 years	7				
	344	11 = 3.2%	24 = 7.0%	25 = 7.3%	60 = 17.5%

11.6 LONG-TERM RESULTS

We have collected the long-term results (Seifert, 1977) from seven endoscopic centres in Germany. Details of 344 patients over a period of five years were available (Table 11.7); 223 patients were re-examined one year after polypectomy, the remainder at periods up to five years post-polypectomy. In 3.2% of the cases the polyps recurred, and in 7% polyps grew at other gastric locations. In 7.3% there was no certainty whether a polyp had grown at the site of polypectomy or at a different location. Thus, we found recurrence in 17.5%. The follow-up examination revealed that recurrent polyps grew within one year, whereas the percentage of new polyps that developed at different gastric locations was about the same for the first to the third year. In the group of genuinely recurrent polyps the histology of the primary polyp and that of the recurrent ones was identical.

Table 11.8 Frequency of carcinomas in follow-up patients with benign primary gastric polyps subjected to follow-up examinations.

	n	*Ca*
Solitary or multiple polyps	277	6 = 2.1%
Polyposis	20	0
	297	6 = 2.0%

11.6.1 **Development of carcinoma after polypectomy** (Table 11.8)

Out of 277 patients who had undergone polypectomy for one or more benign gastric polyps during the previous one to three years, six (2.1%) developed carcinoma, all of the 'early' type. Each of these patients had had a hyperplasiogenic polyp (Seifert, 1977).

11.6.2 **Follow-up of patients with borderline lesions and early gastric cancer** (Table 11.9)

There were 14 subjects with early gastric cancer and 29 with borderline lesions, all treated by endoscopic electrosurgery alone. Only some of these patients were followed up. Two had a relapse within one year and three others developed a carcinoma (Seifert, 1977).

11.6.3 **Development of carcinoma in cases of gastric polyposis** (Table 11.10)

A histological examination of 80 patients with gastric polyposis (patients with more than 50 gastric polyps) revealed that 37 of them (46.3%) exhibited gastric glandular cysts. Because of their histological structure, gastric glandular cysts do not primarily contribute to the development of carcinomas. A re-examination of 22 polyposis patients (excluding gastric glandular cysts) showed that not a single carcinoma had developed. However, in four of 80 cases (5%), carcinomas grew simultaneously. In all of these cases the polyposis consisted of hyperplasiogenic polyps. These results indicate that gastric polyposis is not a precancerous stage. Neoplasia does not appear to be related to the number of polyps or their site, but rather to inherent biologic activity.

11.7 DUODENAL POLYPS

The most common type of duodenal polyp is the hyperplastic polyp, but brunneromas and lipomas are not uncommon. Tumours may also be caused by ectopic pancreatic tissue. From our own experience an adenoma in the duodenal bulb is a very rare condition. Most of the adenomas are located at the papillary region where they are more frequent than any other histological type of duodenal polyp. We have to be aware that focal carcinomas (adenoma with severe atypia) may arise in duodenal adenomas, as in colonic adenomas, and may become invasive cancer.

In the duodenal bulb, and in the upper part of the duodenum, polypectomy is performed by the method described for gastric polyps, and the resected tumours are removed. In the papillary region, however,

Table 11.9 Follow-up examinations (after) excision of protruded-type early cancer and borderline lesion.

Early cancer n = 14				*Borderline lesion n = 29*			
Period elapsed since polypectomy	*Recurrence*	*?*	*Died*	*Period elapsed since polypectomy*	*Recurrence*	*Carc.*	*Died*
2 months n = 2	1	1	0				
3 months n = 1	0	1	0				
1 year n = 5	0	3	1 after 13 months	1 year n = 18	2	3	0
2 years n = 2	0	0	0	2 years n = 1	0	0	0
3 years n = 2	0	0	0				
4 years n = 2	0	0	0				
? = 5 lost to follow-up				10 lost to follow-up			

Table 11.10 Gastric polyposis (n = 80)

37 (46.3%) of which were gastric glandular cysts	
Follow-up examination n = 22	Development of carcinoma: n = 0
Simultaneous carcinomas in 4 of 80 patients = 5%	

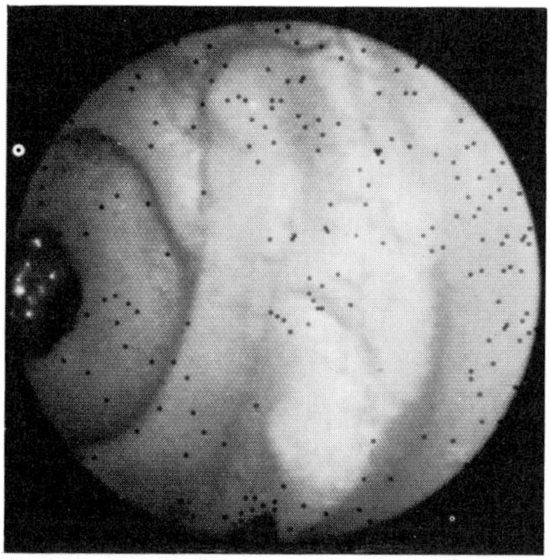

Fig. 11.8 Flat duodenal adenoma in the descending limb.

differentiation between benign adenomas and malignant tumours is essential for further treatment. From the macroscopic aspect it can never be decided whether a tumour at the papillary region is benign or not. Of 15 polypoid periampullary cancers, seven showed adenomatous structures on histology (Seifert, 1977). A precise diagnosis can never be accurately obtained by guided biopsy. Snare biopsy or, if possible, polypectomy is the method of choice. Because in most cases snaring the whole lesion is impossible (Oi, 1973; Blumgart and Kennedy, 1975; Read, 1977) the best method for verifying its nature is snare biopsy after endoscopic papillotomy (Hagenmueller *et al.*, 1977; Safrany *et al.*, 1977; Seifert, 1977). Normally after verification of a periampullary tumour, surgery is indicated. When the patient presents a high risk, and snare biopsy after endoscopic papillotomy does not show malignancy, endoscopic papillotomy and snaring the cut lesion may be good palliative treatment.

In our experience tubular adenomas of the duodenum are sometimes of the flat type, not indicating a polypoid lesion (Fig. 11.8).

REFERENCES

Blumgart, L. H. and Kennedy, A. (1975). Carcinoma of the ampulla of Vater and Duodenum. *Brit. J. Surg.*, **60**, 33.

Classen, M. and Demling, L. (1971). Operative Gastroskopie: Fiberendoskopische Polypenabtragung im Magen. *Dtsch. med. Wochenschrift*, **96**, 1466.

Classen, M. and Fruehmorgen, P. (1976). Therapeutische Endoskopie im Verdauungstrakt. *Internist,* **17**, 220.

Elster, K. (1976). Histologic classification of gastric polyps. In: *Topics in Pathology*, Vol. 63: *Pathology of the Gastro-intestinal Tract*, p. 77 (Morson, B. C., Ed.), Springer, Berlin, Heidelberg.

Elster, K. *et al.* (1977). Drüsenkörperzysten, eine polypoide Läsion der Magenschleimhaut. *Dtsch. med. Wochenschrift,* **102**, 183.

Hagenmueller, F. *et al.* (1977). Snare biopsy of the papilla of Vater. *Endoscopy,* **9**, 193.

Namiki, M. *et al.* (1970). Local injection treatment of gastric ulcer with fiberscope. *IInd World Congress of Gastrointestinal Endoscopy*, Rom, Kopenhagen.

Oi, I. (1973). Duodenoscopy in 14 cases of Papillary Cancer. In: *Endoscopy of the Small Intestine with Retrograde Pancreato-Cholangiography* (Demling, L. and Classen, M., eds), G. Thieme, Stuttgart.

Ottenjann, R. *et al.* (1971). Magenulkus nach endoskopischer Polypektomie. *Endoscopy,* **4**, 212.

Read, A. E. (1977). Periampullary cancer: clinical introduction. In: *Third Gastroenterological Symposium, Nice 1976, The Sphincter of Odii* (Delmont, J., Ed.), Karger, Basel.

Roesch, W. (1970). Polypen und Polyposis des Magen-Darm-Traktes. *Therapiewoche,* **20**, 1784.

Safrany, L. *et al.* (1977). Indications for surgical endoscopic procedures on the papilla of vater and biliary tract. *Endoscopy,* **9**, 184.

Seifert, E. (1973). Endoscopic polypectomy. *Gastroenterology Jap.,* **8**, 103.

Seifert, E. (1975*a*). Results in gastroscopic polypectomy. In: *Surgical Endoscopy* (Seifert, E., Ed.), Witzstrock, Baden-Baden, Bruessel.

Seifert, E. (1975*b*). New classification of gastric polyps, based on the experiences in polypectomy. In: *Surgical Endoscopy* (Seifert, E., Ed.), Witzstrock, Baden-Baden, Bruessel.

Seifert, E. (1977). Esophageal and gastric polypectomy – long-term results. In: *Operative Endoscopy* (Demling, L. and Koch, H., eds.), F. K. Schattauer, Stuttgart, New York.

Seifert, E. and Elster, K. (1972). Endoskopische Polypektomie am Magen; Indikation, Technik und Ergebnisse. *Dtsch. med. Wochenschrift,* **97**, 1199.

Seifert, E. and Elster, K. (1973). Wert der endoskopischen Polypektomie am Oesophagus und Magen. *Leber-Magen-Darm,* **3**, 155.

Seifert, E. and Elster, K. (1975). Gastric polypectomy. *Amer. J. Gastroent.,* **63**, 451.

Seifert, E. and Otto, P. (1973). Erfahrungsbericht über die endoskopische Polypektomie im oberen und unteren Verdauungstrakt. In: *Endoskopische Polypektomie im Gastrointestinaltrakt* (Demling, L. and Ottenjann, R., eds.), Vol. 51, G. Thieme, Stuttgart.

Seifert, E. *et al.* (1977). Duodenoscopic Guided Biopsy of the Biliary and Pancreatic Duct. *Endoscopy,* **9**, 154.

Singer, M. *et al.* (1975). Endoscopic polypectomy in the upper gastrointestinal tract. *Endoscopy,* **7**, 216.

Tsuneoka, K. and Uchida, T. (1970). Endoscopic polypectomy of the stomach. *IInd World Congress of Gastrointestinal Endoscopy*, Rom, Kopenhagen.

12 Duodenoscopic sphincterotomy and bile-duct stone retrieval

PETER B. COTTON

The diagnosis and management of biliary and pancreatic problems has been greatly facilitated by the development and increasingly widespread use of endoscopic cannulation of the papilla of Vater for retrograde cholangiography and pancreatography (ERCP) (Cotton, 1977). Endoscopic cholangiography has been particularly helpful in the diagnosis of patients with symptoms following biliary tract surgery; intravenous cholangiography is often not of diagnostic quality and both ultrasonography and percutaneous transhepatic cholangiography are at a disadvantage when the ducts are not dilated. By allowing greater confidence in excluding retained duct stones, endoscopic cholangiography has thrown the problem of 'postcholecystectomy pain' into clearer focus; endoscopic sphincter manometry has provided a new diagnostic dimension (Bar-Meir *et al.*, 1979).

The use of the duodenoscope to treat biliary tract disease is a recent development. Endoscopic diathermy sphincterotomy was first performed in man in 1973 (Kawai *et al.*, 1974; Classen and Demling, 1974). Thereafter the technique was mainly developed and championed in Europe. By 1978, Safrany was able to review a collected series of 3618 cases; with few individual variations, the success rate for performing sphincterotomy and removing stones from the common bile duct averaged around 90% with a complication rate of 7–10%, and a mortality around 1% (Safrany, 1978). Endoscopic sphincterotomy was quickly accepted as the best treatment for elderly and high-risk patients with common duct stones, in whom the hazards of orthodox surgical intervention are substantial; the reported mortality for common duct exploration in patients over the age of 60 years averages around 5% (Cotton, 1980), and the largest single series quotes a figure of 12.3% (Spohn *et al.*, 1973). The experts who have established the relative safety and value of the technique in high-risk patients are now exploring the use of endoscopic sphincterotomy in younger patients with common duct stones, in patients who still have a gallbladder *in situ*, and in those with biliary outflow obstruction due to benign stenosis or tumour.

12.1 TECHNIQUE

12.1.1 **Equipment**

Endoscopic sphincterotomy should be performed only by those endoscopists who have obtained sufficient experience with ERCP to have at least an 80% chance of achieving retrograde cholangiography; this usually means more than 200 examinations. The procedure should take place in the radiology department in a room with high quality fluoroscopy, and on an X-ray table which allows at least 45° head-up and head-down tilt. Co-operation with an experienced gastrointestinal radiologist is essential.

Sphincterotomy is performed using a side-viewing duodenoscope, of which many types are available. The latest instruments are electrically insulated, but the older types can also be used if an electrical safety wire is placed between the patient plate and any metal part of the instrument umbilical as it enters the light source. This provides a safety return for any leaking current.

The simple concept of the diathermy 'knife' was suggested by Classen and Demling in 1974. Knives can be obtained from the main instrument manufacturers, and consist of standard cannulation tubing with a wire extruding 2.5–3 cm near the tip (Fig. 12.1). It is convenient, but not essential, to have a radio-opaque marker at the tip. Most diathermy catheters allow the injection of contrast alongside the wire. The proximal end of the knife consists of an insulated handle with connections to the diathermy source. Many different sources have been used, and some are designed specifically for endoscopic work. Most experts use cutting current with occasional coagulation when some bleeding is seen. Electrical safety is of paramount importance; anyone starting endoscopic diathermy should make himself thoroughly familiar with the equipment.

Stone extraction baskets can be obtained from the major endoscope manufacturers. Long balloon tipped catheters (Edwards Company, Santa Ana, California) are useful in some circumstances, but are rather fragile.

12.1.2 **Patient preparation**

The patient should be admitted to hospital for the procedure. Because of the rare but serious complications, the hospital must be one capable of providing urgent blood transfusion and surgical facilities. It is wise for the endoscopist to discuss the procedure with a specialist surgical

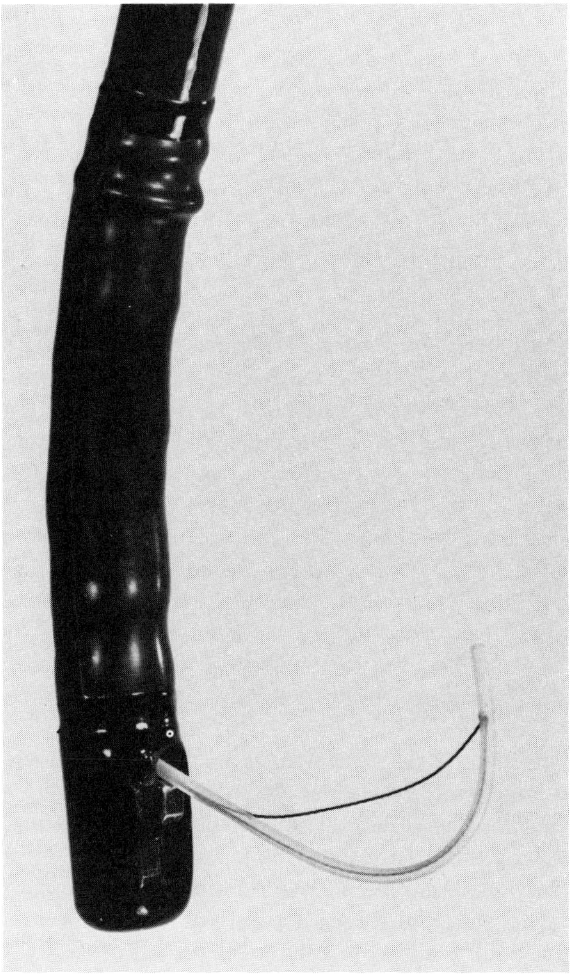

Fig. 12.1 Tip of fibreoptic duodenoscope and the diathermy knife in the bowed position.

colleague beforehand. Sphincterotomy should not be performed immediately before a weekend.

The patient's coagulation status is checked, and blood is taken for grouping. Written informed consent is obtained. The patient is fasted for at least eight hours, and an intravenous line is set up in the right arm. Experts now rarely use antibiotics (either in the contrast or parenterally). However, the beginner may spend more time over a procedure and may fail to provide adequate drainage. It may therefore be wise initially to use antibiotics (perhaps gentamicin and ampicillin), particularly if stasis exists after the procedure is completed.

12.1.3 **ERCP and sphincterotomy**

ERCP is first carried out in the standard manner under sedation. We use pethidine (Demerol) 25–100 mg and diazepam (Valium) 5–20 mg, given intravenously immediately before the procedure starts, and buscopan (hyoscine *N*-butyl bromide, 40 mg) on entering the duodenum. In countries where buscopan is not available, it is customary to use atropine (0.6 mg intramuscularly) followed by an intravenous injection of glucagon (in increments of 0.25 to 0.5 mg) to maintain duodenal ileus. Sedation requirements vary greatly between patients; care should be taken in the elderly, and in patients with respiratory insufficiency.

Retrograde cholangiography is performed with the standard catheter, using low density contrast materials (not more than 25%); denser contrast materials may obscure quite large stones. If the retrograde cholangiogram confirms the indication for sphincterotomy, the standard catheter is replaced by the diathermy wire, which should be inserted deeply through the papilla with the wire pointing upwards between about 11 and 12 o'clock. It is essential to ensure that the wire is in the bile duct, and not in the pancreatic duct; it is easy to be misled on fluoroscopy and wise to take spot radiographs before commencing diathermy. The best method is to pass the knife very deep into the common bile duct so that it can be seen in the common hepatic duct, possibly moving the stones around as it is 'jiggled'. Cutting the pancreatic duct may lead to severe complications.

When it is confirmed that the wire is in the correct duct, it should be withdrawn so that approximately half (10–15 mm) of the wire is visible outside the papilla (Fig. 12.2). The assistant then tightens the wire to produce a bowing effect, putting pressure on the roof of the lower bile duct. Diathermy is then applied in short bursts. Most experts use cutting or mixed current; the appropriate setting for the diathermy source must be established beforehand by reference to other users of the same equipment, or by experiment with a piece of meat. It is a mistake to start at too low a current setting, or to use purely coagulation current; the current and pressure will eventually have to be raised considerably to cut through the coagulated area, and usually results in a longer and uncontrolled incision with bleeding. The cut should be extended upwards in a controlled manner by lifting the knife with the cannula elevator of the endoscope, not by increasing the bowing of the wire. The cut is extended about 15 mm up to the covering transverse fold, and until the bile duct is entered freely; there is then a gush of bile into the duodenum (Fig. 12.3). The length is difficult to quantitate precisely, and must also be related to the size of the stones. Although some experts have made sphincterotomies up to 30 mm long, it is unusual, and probably dangerous, to exceed 20 mm. A small amount of bleeding is commonly

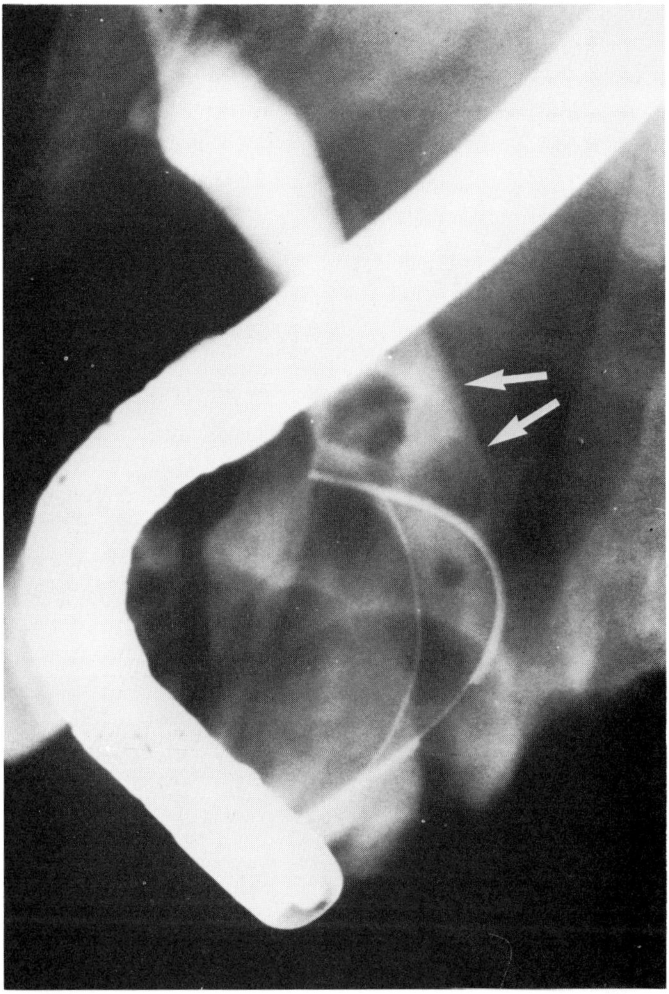

Fig. 12.2 Retrograde cholangiogram showing the knife in the lower bile duct, below two stones (arrowed).

seen during the sphincterotomy; severe bleeding is rare but obvious, as the view is lost within seconds.

12.1.4 **Precutting**

Occasionally it proves very difficult to place the diathermy wire deep into the bile duct. Some workers then recommend making a 'precut' which means attempting to cut the roof off the common channel. The idea is that this will facilitate access to the bile duct either immediately or

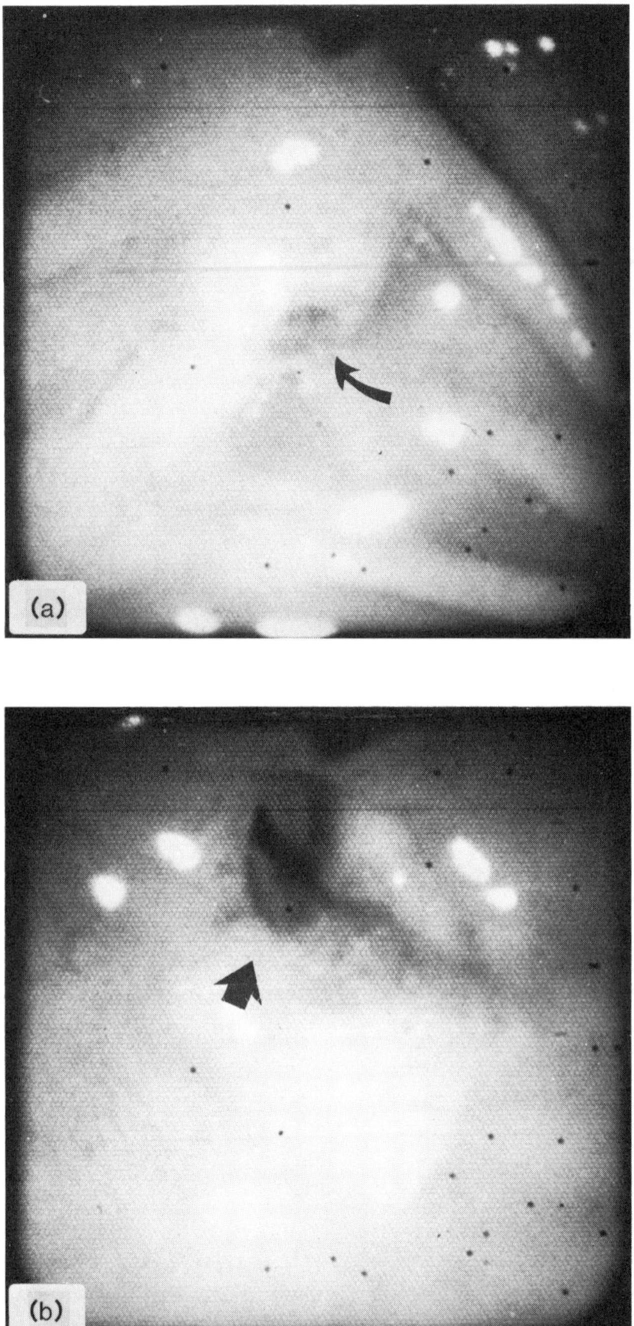

Fig. 12.3 Endoscopic views of the papilla of Vater before (a) and after (b) sphincterotomy (orifice arrowed).

after one or two weeks. Precutting should not be used by beginners; it is an uncontrolled process and may leave the patient worse off than before. Experts use this procedure in less than 5% of sphincterotomies.

12.1.5 **Postsphincterotomy care**

The severe complications of sphicterotomy (bleeding and perforation) are obvious within a few hours, and the other complications (pancreatitis and cholangitis) will be evident within the first two days. Most patients are kept nil by mouth for four hours; we then allow fluids for the remainder of that day, and normal food on the second day. During the first few hours it is useful to maintain a half hourly chart of pulse, blood pressure and temperature; this frequency can be reduced to four-hourly for the next day. It is wise to check the haemoglobin one to two days after sphincterotomy, and biochemical tests of liver function as appropriate.

The patient's length of hospital stay varies according to the method used for removing stones.

12.1.6 **Methods for removing duct stones**

There are many methods for clearing the common bile duct after sphincterotomy. If the patient has a T-tube in place, it is simple to flush distal stones into the duodenum with saline or contrast material at the time of sphincterotomy or on the following day. When stones are trapped above the upper limb of the T-tube, it is necessary to remove the tube (usually the next day) to allow the stones to descend.

It is convenient for the patient if the duct can be cleared of stones at the time of sphincterotomy – with various devices such as balloon tipped catheters, wire baskets or teflon loops. Teflon loops can be simply made, and have the advantage (over baskets) that stones cannot become trapped within them. Balloon catheters are atraumatic but rather fragile and expensive. They are ideal for small stones and biliary mud, and provide an excellent method for 'sweeping' the duct to be certain that all stones have been removed. The wire baskets (Fig. 12.4) provided by the instrument manufacturers and other agents are also rather fragile, at least those designed to pass through the standard duodenoscope, and tend to deform when force is applied to a large stone; but they are satisfactory for the removal of medium sized stones. Baskets should be passed in the closed position beyond the stone, and then opened completely, and withdrawn in the fully open position; attempts to close the basket around the stone are usually unsuccessful.

The simplest and most popular method for removing stones in patients

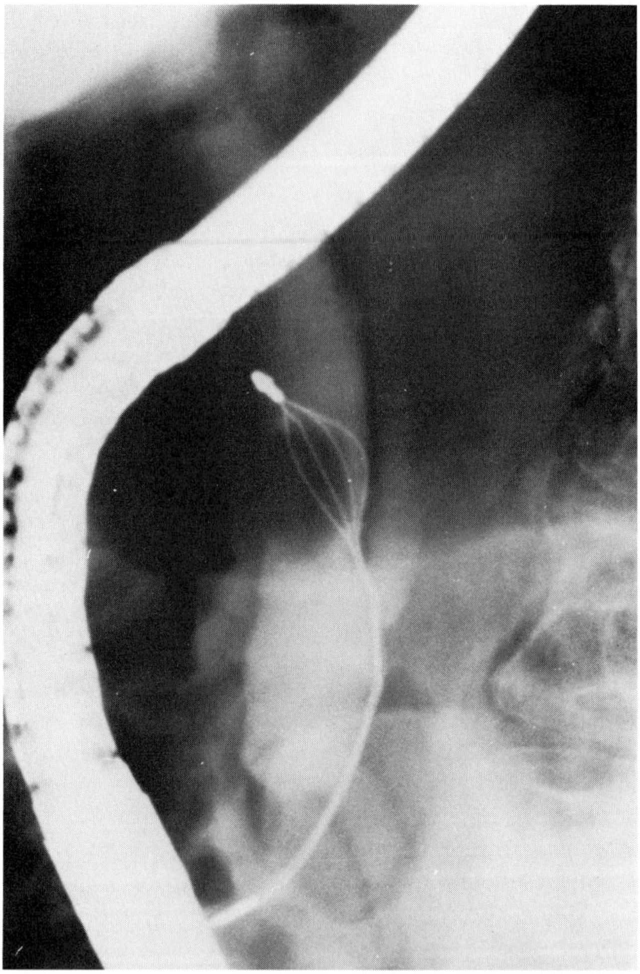

Fig. 12.4 Stone extraction with a wire basket.

without T-tubes is to allow them to pass spontaneously. Most stones less than 15 mm in diameter will pass within days or weeks of the standard sized sphincterotomy. If this expectant policy is pursued it is necessary to bring the patient back for a check ERCP, since intravenous cholangiography is usually inadequate in this context. A compromise solution is to leave a catheter in the bile duct after sphincterotomy, and bring it out through the patient's nose (Cotton *et al.*, 1979) (Fig. 12.5). This allows repeated transnasal cholangiography without discomfort to the patient, so that the passage of stones can be monitored over a few

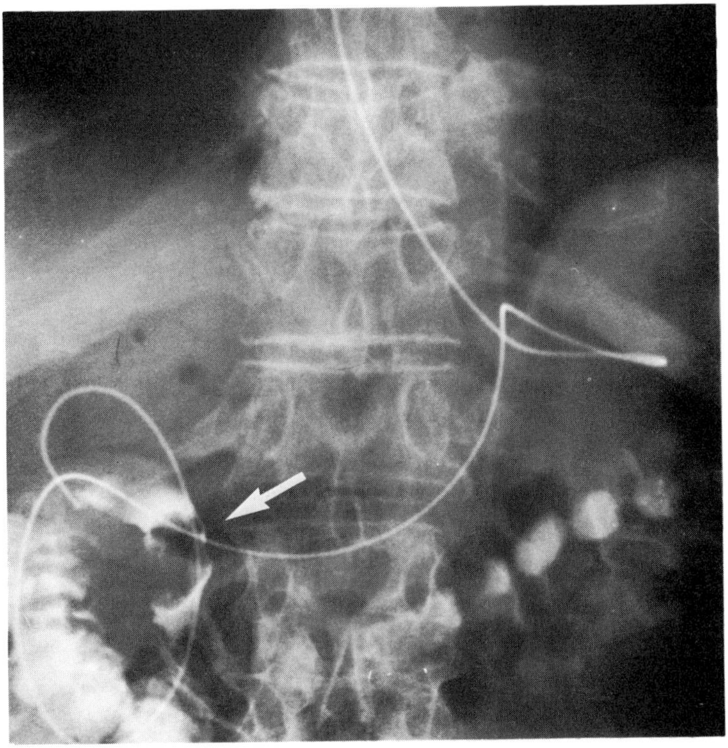

Fig. 12.5 Transnasal biliary catheter looped above a collection of stones in the lower bile duct (arrowed).

days after sphincterotomy; the tube also provides a route for infusion of saline to flush the duct. We use simple TWI8 teflon tubing (Polypenco Ltd., P.O. Box 56, Welwyn Garden City, Herts.) cut into 3 m lengths, with two large side holes cut at 1 and 2 cm from the tip; these holes should be large enough to weaken the catheter so that there is a natural tendency for it to loop in the bile duct as it is passed deeply. The duodenoscope is removed slowly as the catheter is further advanced through it, with fluoroscopy to check the position. A nasogastric tube is then passed, grasped in the pharynx and the tip pulled out through the mouth. The proximal end of the biliary tube is passed retrogradely through the nasogastric tube; traction on the nasogastric tube brings both out through the nose. The nasogastric tube is then discarded, and the biliary tube is allowed to drain into a bag. The amount of drainage varies considerably since most of the bile passes through the sphincterotomy itself into the duodenum.

12.1.7 **Usual procedure for stone removal**

If sphincterotomy has been simple and without significant bleeding, and if there are few stones, we usually attempt to remove them directly with balloon catheters or baskets. If attempts are certainly successful, the patient can be discharged the next day. If sphincterotomy is accompanied by bleeding, or if there are many stones, or if attempts to remove the stones are not completely successful, we use a transnasal biliary tube. A 'transnasal cholangiogram' is done on the following day. The radiologist can freely move the unsedated patient to take radiographs in different positions. If the stones have passed and the duct is clear, the radiologist removes the tube and the patient is discharged. If stones remain we normally perfuse the duct for a few days with saline (3–5 l/day) and repeat the transnasal cholangiogram. If stones are still present after duct perfusion, we repeat the endoscopy with a larger side-viewing instrument (gastroscope) which permits the use of larger and stronger baskets.

With this approach most of our patients leave hospital two to five days after sphincterotomy. The small group of patients who remain include those with the largest stones (see below).

12.2 CONTRAINDICATIONS AND TECHNICAL PROBLEMS

Sphincterotomy has the same contraindications as ERCP. It is unwise to examine patients who are potentially *infectious*, e.g. open tuberculosis or recent hepatitis, and rare patients with *oesophageal diverticula or strictures* cannot be treated. *Previous gastroduodenal surgery* may make access to the papilla difficult. A Billroth II partial gastrectomy provides a challenge which only the most expert can overcome (Safrany *et al.*, 1980). *Peripapillary diverticula* are common in patients with stones, but only rarely interfere technically with biliary cannulation. There does not appear to be any increased risk when performing sphincterotomy in the presence of a diverticulum, and many hundreds of such cases are now on record. *Previous surgery to the sphincter* zone may also make endoscopic sphincterotomy difficult; the duodenotomy may result in duodenal deformity and partial stenosis, reducing access to the area. Stenosis following surgical sphincterotomy or sphincteroplasty may extend for some distance up the duct, increasing the necessary length of endoscopic cut.

Coagulation defects considerably increase the risk of sphincterotomy, but also of the alternative surgical approaches. Sphincterotomy may be justified in such patients if every attempt is made to normalize coagulation at the time of the procedure by giving the relevant factors intravenously.

The lengths to which endoscopists should go in attempts to remove *large stones* must depend on previous experience and upon the alternatives for the individual patient. It may be justifiable to make many attempts to remove even very large stones in the oldest and illest patients; stones greater than 25 mm in diameter have been removed, but the chances of success diminish rapidly beyond this size, and there is a (very small) risk of gallstone ileus. Some of the largest ductal stones are 'primary' in nature, and can be partially fragmented within the duct using standard baskets and balloon catheters. There are several options if large stones cannot be easily extracted, or fail to pass spontaneously within a week or two of sphincterotomy. The incision can be enlarged, with a slightly increased risk of bleeding. Attempts can be made to reduce the size of the stones within the duct system by infusing chemicals through a transnasal catheter. Unfortunately, such perfusates pass rapidly into the duodenum, and most give rise to diarrhoea. We have discontinued the use of sodium cholate and mono-octanoin for this reason. Attempts have been made to 'crack' stones with electrical sparks and ultrasonic probes, but these methods are not yet safe enough for clinical use. It may be worth giving some patients oral agents such as chenodeoxycholic acid or rowachol.

12.3 IMMEDIATE RESULTS AND COMPLICATIONS

Most groups report more than 90% success rates for sphincterotomy and for stone extraction (Table 12.1). Series differ in the spectrum of patients treated, and in the precise methods used for stone extraction (Safrany *et al.*, 1979; Cotton, 1980; Liguory *et al.*, 1979).

Table 12.1 Results and complications of endoscopic sphincterotomy from three groups.

	Safrany et al., *1979*	*Liguory* et al., *1979*	*Author's series (unpublished)*
Total attempts	477	323	310
Successful sphincterotomy	94%	96%	96%
Bile duct cleared	94%	90%	92%
Complications			
cholangitis	8	6	7
haemorrhage	11	13	10
perforation	9	4	2
pancreatitis	5	4	1
impaction	2	0	2
cholecystitis	0	2	2
Total	35 (7.3%)	29 (9.4%)	22 (7%)
Urgent surgery	7 (1.5%)	6 (1.9%)	6 (1.9%)
Deaths	4 (0.9%)	3 (1%)	2 (0.6%)

Complications have occurred in 5.6% to 9.4% of procedures. *Haemorrhage* is the most common, and usually occurs immediately. Surgery for major bleeding can be formidably difficult, and a trial of conservative management is usually justifiable; angiographic embolization (see Chapter 10) would be logical, but results are not yet clear. Retroperitoneal *perforation* is usually recognized immediately by spillage of contrast outside the duct systems; in the largest collected series this was the commonest cause of death (Safrany, 1978). The precise indications for surgical intervention for this complication are not yet established. *Pancreatitis* may follow sphincterotomy when the pancreatic duct has been cut in error. However, pancreatitis has also occurred without interference with the pancreatic duct – possibly because of excessive coagulation in the area of the papilla. Episodes of pancreatitis have usually been mild and have responded to conservative management. *Cholangitis* may follow sphincterotomy if the procedure has been prolonged, with recurrent instrumentation, and if free drainage is not obtained. A transnasal drainage tube looped above any residual stones should reduce this hazard; however, it also seems reasonable to give antibiotics to such patients. Urgent surgery may be needed to provide drainage if cholangitis occurs in the presence of stasis. Experience is too small to make precise recommendations, but *spontaneous stone impaction* can be managed by repeat endoscopy with extension of the sphincterotomy and instrumental extraction. Rarely, a basket with a stone inside it may become impacted during endoscopy; it may work loose over a few days if the endoscope is removed. *Gallstone ileus* has been reported in at least three patients with stones greater than 25 mm diameter. Patients should be warned of this possibility, since it may occur after they leave hospital.

12.4 LONGER TERM RESULTS AND HAZARDS

Endoscopic sphincterotomy will remain controversial until long-term results are available. Most groups are now bringing back as many patients as possible for interview and repeat endoscopic studies at intervals. Postal questionnaires and enquiries of the family doctor should reveal any major problems occurring in those too frail or too distant to attend. Safrany (personal communication, 1979) collected follow-up information from several European centres. Of 1108 patients who had undergone sphincterotomy for stones after cholecystectomy, 70% were free of symptoms at one year, and 20% improved; 2% had experienced major biliary complications, and 0.5% had died as a result. Endoscopy was repeated on 438 similar patients. More problems were revealed, presumably partly because of selection bias; 5% had recurrent stones and 6% had developed papillary stenosis. Most of these complications were treated endoscopically. Clinical follow-up of 490 patients who had undergone sphincterotomy with the gallbladder in place revealed that 9% had subsequently undergone elective cholecystecomy; 6% had developed major biliary complications.

12.5 CURRENT INDICATIONS FOR ENDOSCOPIC SPHINCTEROTOMY

12.5.1 Patients with T-tube drains in place shortly after cholecystectomy

The technique described by Dr. Burhenne in Chapter 13 should be tried first if the T-tube is of adequate size and in the correct place. Sphincterotomy is used if these conditions are not fulfilled, or if the stones are too large to be extracted via the T-tube track, or if the patient has sufficient symptoms (despite T-tube drainage) that the necessary 4–6 weeks delay is not clinically acceptable.

12.5.2 Patients without T-tubes (or with unsuitable T-tubes) following cholecystectomy

Many patients present months or years after cholecystectomy with symptoms due to stones in the common bile duct. Treatment with currently available oral medications is not usually effective; the options are orthodox surgical intervention and endoscopic sphincterotomy. The choice will be influenced by local expertise, technical difficulties (size of the patient, previous surgery, etc.), the size of the stones, and by the fitness of the patient. Surgery is hazardous in elderly and ill patients, and in those with particularly complicated problems, including previous re-explorations. Endoscopic sphincterotomy is safer in high risk patients, and must be the preferred treatment in those with stones less than 20 mm diameter. It cannot, however, claim to be safer than surgery in young and fit patients; its convenience must be balanced against potential long-term hazards whose significance will only become apparent after longer follow-up studies.

12.5.3 Patients with a gallbladder in place

Sphincterotomy is logical in the presence of a gallbladder in any patient who is seriously ill due to complications of duct stones – such as severe cholangitis and septicaemia, and acute biliary pancreatitis (Safrany and Cotton, 1980). Sphincterotomy should result in adequate drainage and rapid clinical improvement. Cholecystectomy can be performed later with little risk; it may be postponed indefinitely in some elderly and frail patients, particularly those with shrunken gallbladders and large cystic ducts.

12.5.4 Papillary stenosis

The diagnosis of benign papillary stenosis is controversial. The endoscopic approach to the papilla has added a useful new dimension, including sphincter manometry (Bar-Meir *et al.*, 1979). Sphincterotomy provides a logical method of treatment, which is effective at least in the short term; follow-up studies are in progress.

12.5.5 Tumours of the papilla of Vater

Sphincterotomy can provide temporary relief of obstruction at the papilla caused by benign or malignant tumours. It may be used as palliation, or as a prelude to definitive surgery or the insertion of a tube prosthesis (Laurence and Cotton, 1980).

12.5.6 Sphincterotomy at the pancreatic duct orifice

Few groups have used endoscopic sphincterotomy to improve drainage of the pancreatic duct. It may be indicated to reduce pain in patients with malignant obstruction to the papilla, and in the rare patients with chronic pancreatitis and an isolated benign stricture at the orifice. Sphincterotomy has been used at the accessory papilla in patients with pancreatitis and pancreas divisum (Cotton, 1978).

12.5.7 Biliodigestive anastomoses

There are insufficient data to judge the efficacy and safety of using endoscopic sphincterotomy to enlarge stenosed biliodigestive anastomoses (such as choledochoduodenostomy and hepatodochojejunostomy); there are anecdotes of severe bleeding after endoscopic diathermy at choledochoduodenostomy stomas.

Some patients present with a biliary fistula above the papilla of Vater, caused by erosion of a duct stone or by previous surgical instrumentation. Sphincterotomy can be used to join the main papillary orifice with the fistula, or to enlarge the fistula upwards to release an impacted stone.

12.6 CONCLUSION

Endoscopic sphincterotomy has become accepted, at least in Europe, in a remarkably short period of time. It now provides an excellent method for treatment of common bile duct stones in elderly and high risk patients. As periods of follow-up lengthen, concern about long-term hazards diminish and the indications for sphincterotomy widen. It is crucially important that those performing this technique should remain conscious of its known and potential limitations, and should make every effort to review their own material on a regular basis. It will be particularly interesting (and relevant to the numbers of sphincterotomies subsequently performed) to follow the progress of those patients who still have a gallbladder in place.

Endoscopic methods for relieving benign and malignant biliary obstruction will be evolved and perfected over the next few years, and the role of sphincterotomy of the pancreatic orifice will be clarified.

REFERENCES

Bar-Meir, S. *et al.* (1979). Biliary and pancreatic duct pressures measured by ERCP manometry in patients with suspected papillary stenosis. *Dig. Dis. Sci.*, **24**, 209–13.

Classen, M. and Demling, L. (1974). Endoscopische Sphinckterotomie der papilla Vater. *D. Med. Wshcr.*, **99**, 496–7.

Cotton, P. B. (1977). Progress Report ERCP. *Gut*, **18**, 316–41.

Cotton, P. B. (1978). Duodenoscopic papillotomy at the minor papilla of Vater for recurrent dorsal pancreatitis. *Endosc. Dig.*, **3**, 27–28.

Cotton, P. B. (1979). Non-operative removal of bile duct stones: duodenoscopic sphincterotomy. In: *Developments in Digestive Diseases*, (ed. J. Edward Berk), Lea and Febiger, Philadelphia, pp. 127–39.

Cotton, P. B. (1980). Non-operative removal of bile duct stones by duodenoscopic sphincterotomy. *Br. J. Surg.*, **67**, 1–5.

Cotton, P. B., Mason, R. R., and Burney, P. J. (1979). Trans-nasal bile duct catheterisation after endoscopic sphincterotomy. *Gut*, **20**, 285–287.

Kawai, K. *et al.* (1974). Endoscopic sphincterotomy of the ampulla of Vater. *Gastrointest. Endosc.*, **20**, 148.

Laurence, B. H. and Cotton, P. B. (1980). Endoscopic placement of palliative drainage tubes in malignant biliary obstruction. *Br. Med. J.*, **1**, 522–6.

Liguory, C. *et al.* (1979). La sphinctertomie par voie endoscopique dans le traitement de la lithiase biliare. *Rev. Med.*, **22**, 1191–5.

Safrany, L. (1978). Endoscopic treatment of biliary tract diseases. *Lancet*, **2**, 983–5.

Safrany, L. and Cotton, P. B. (1980). Urgent duodenoscopic sphincterotomy for acute gallstone pancreatitis surgery. (in press).

Safrany, L. *et al.* (1979). Endoskopische Papillotomie. *Therapiewoche*, **29**, 4139–49.

Safrany, L. *et al.* (1980). Endoscopic sphincterotomy in patients with Billroth II gastrectomy. *Endoscopy*, **12**, 16–22.

Spohn, K., Fux, H. D., Mehnert, U. *et al.* (1973), Chlolecystectomie und Choledochotomie – Taktik und Techniken. *Lagenbecks Arch. Chir.*, **334**, 249–250.

13 Radiological retrieval of bile duct stones

H. JOACHIM BURHENNE

The tract of the T-tube placed in the common bile duct after cholecystectomy gives access to the biliary ducts in the postoperative period. A fibrous lining forms around the T-tube after it has been in place for about five weeks. This is the usual postoperative interval after which catheterization of the sinus tract is feasible.

This percutaneous approach lends itself to the retrieval of retained postoperative biliary duct stones, a surgical problem occurring in about 5% to 9% of patients undergoing common duct exploration (Longmire, 1979).

13.1 DIAGNOSIS OF RETAINED STONES

Retained stones in the biliary tract are identified on postoperative T-tube cholangiography. This radiological study is obtained seven to ten days after common duct exploration. It usually permits a better demonstration of retained stones than does operative cholangiography because fluoroscopy with radiographic spot filming is available at the time of postoperative T-tube cholangiography. Precise field collimation, spot filming in multiple projections, and proper contrast injection improve detail. Contrast dilution to about 25% iodine content is recommended for normal ducts up to 10 mm diameter, whereas further dilution to 12.5% iodine content is required for enlarged ducts. This permits radiographic penetration, whereas stones are often hidden in dense contrast material (Fig. 13.1).

Particular attention must be directed to the distal common duct at the duodenal entrance where spasm of the intramural portion of the common duct and its muscular closing mechanism may obscure retained material. A low hand injection pressure is required for good filling of the distal end of the common duct, for over-injection will result in spasm. When spot filming of the distal common duct has been completed, filling of the

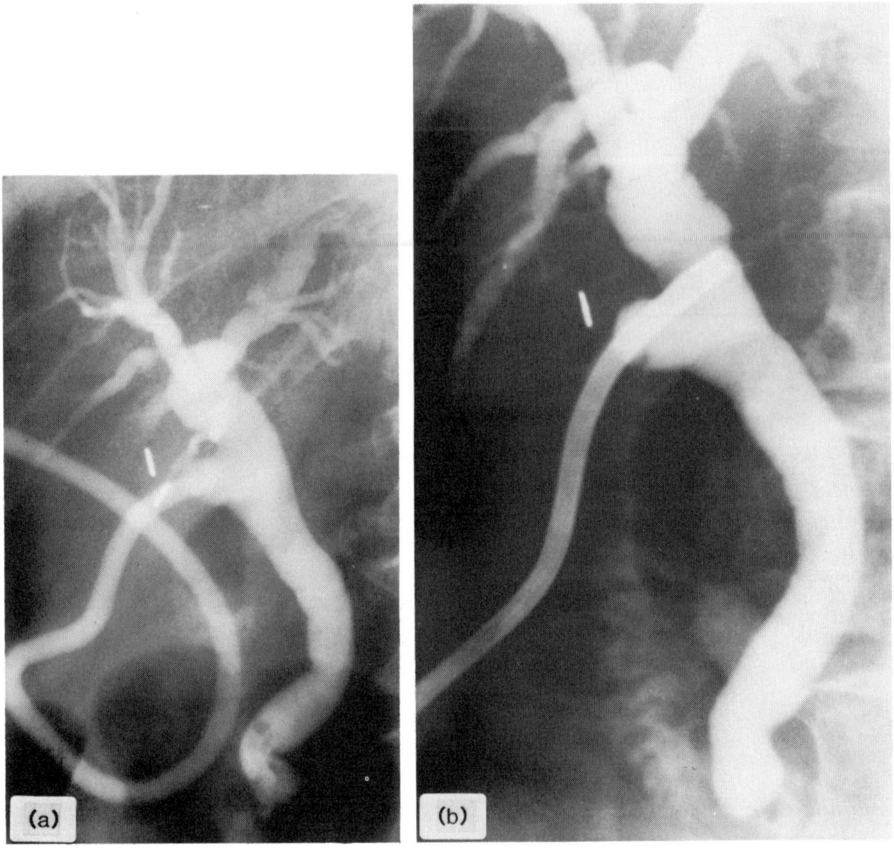

Fig. 13.1 (a) Dilute contrast with radiographic penetration identifies multiple, very small, retained distal common duct stones. (b) Poor radiographic penetration in the same patient is inadequate to ensure that all retained stones were removed. Note that one of the two surgical clips was inadvertently removed with the wire basket during stone retrieval.

intrahepatic radicals is required to identify any retained intrahepatic stones. The cystic duct remnant must also be filled.

Other postoperative abnormalities diagnosed on postoperative T-tube cholangiograms include malposition of T-tubes, strictures, neoplasms and other retained material such as blood clots and bile sludge (Figs. 13.2 and 13.3).

Care must be taken not to inject air during T-tube cholangiography. This is best accomplished by having the T-tube clamped for several hours and injection of contrast through a needle directly into the long arm of the T-tube.

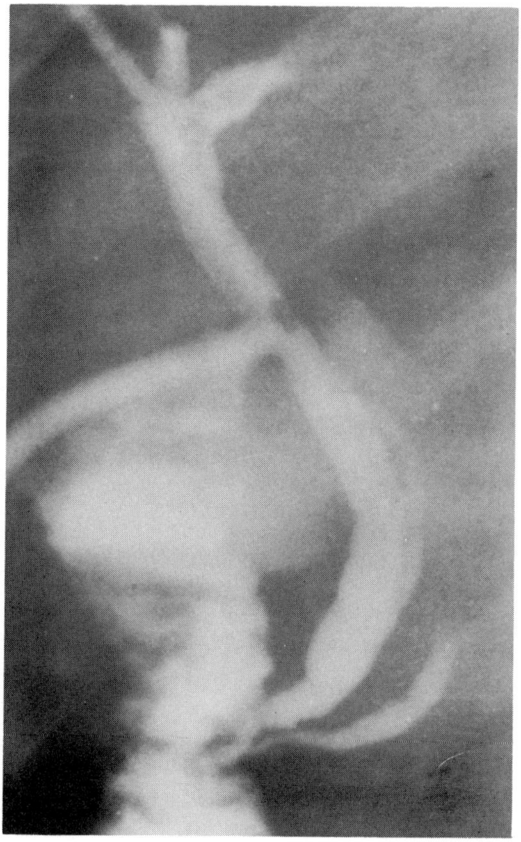

Fig. 13.2 Common hepatic duct defect may be misinterpreted as retained stone. It represents the cut-out in the T-tube at the junction of the long and short arms. Note that the T-tube was inserted into the common hepatic duct with a low insertion of a retained cystic duct stump. The operative report contains a statement that choledochotomy was performed.

13.2 EQUIPMENT

A special catheter has been designed for easy intrumentation of the sinus tract and the biliary ducts (Burhenne, 1973). Wires in the wall of the catheter permit guidance of the catheter tip from the outside. Catheters are available in 8, 10 and 13 French (F) diameters. The lumen of only the largest (13 F) steerable catheter allows passage of the Dormia stone extraction basket with its sheath. Smaller baskets from Cook and Meditech are available for the smaller steerable catheters, but the difficulty of instrumentation increases with decreasing size of the available sinus tract (Fig. 13.4).

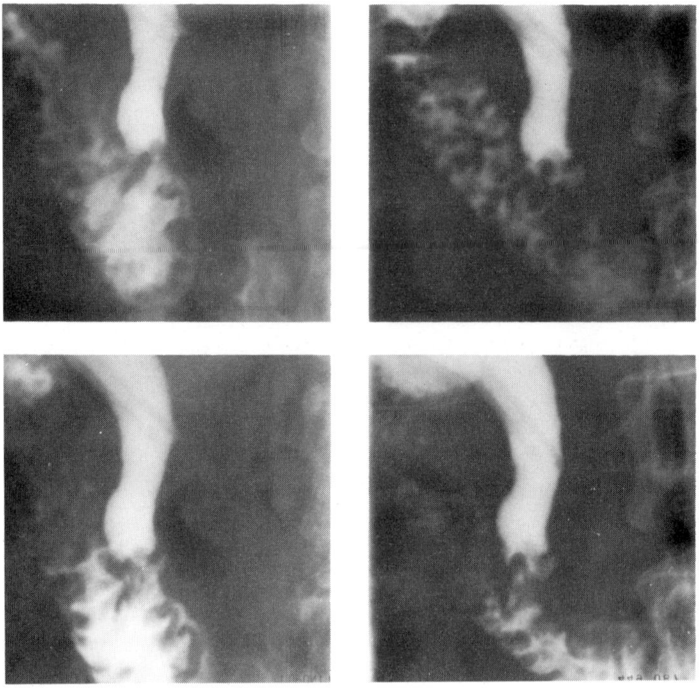

Fig. 13.3 Good filling of the distal common duct with multiple spot films demonstrating that the duct inserts into a small duodenal diverticulum. This is not a retained stone.

Dormia*, Medi-tech†, and Cook‡ stone baskets are used (Fig. 13.5). The first is available in only one size, the others in three sizes. Larger baskets are required for large stones and large common ducts. Ideally, the wires of the open basket should touch the walls of the bile duct resulting in easy stone engagement. Large baskets, therefore, are used even for retrieval of small stones if the bile duct system is dilated.

The wires at the proximal end of the steerable catheter are attached to a metal plate, and a steering handle surrounds the plate for single finger control. This handle also has side ports for contrast injection.

13.3 TECHNIQUE (Fig. 13.6)

Mondet (1962) pioneered the use of the postoperative T-tube tract for access to the bile ducts. He and Mazzariello (1970) used pliable forceps

*V. Mueller, Chicago, Ill., USA.
†Medi-Tech, Inc., Watertown, Mass., USA.
‡Cook, Inc., Bloomington, Ind., USA.

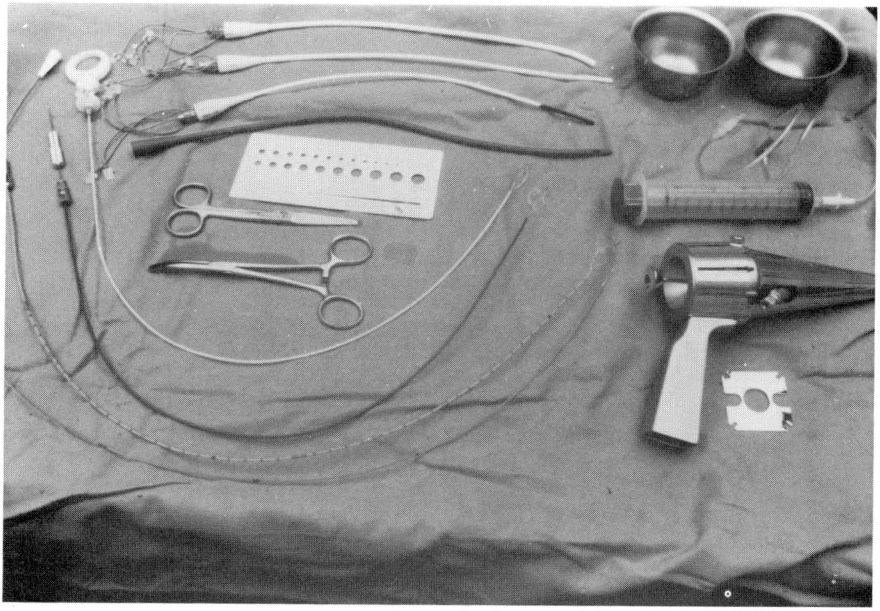

Fig. 13.4 Equipment for non-operative stone retrieval. Left row top to bottom: steerable catheters in 3 sizes, straight catheter, catheter measuring template, scissors, artery-forceps, 3 different baskets, Fogarty balloon catheter. Right row top to bottom: 4-in stainless steel bowls for mixing of contrast and saline, syringe for contrast injection with connecting tubing, pistol control handle and wobble plate for the steerable catheter.

for stone extraction. The first use of the Dormia ureteral stone basket was described by LaGrave (1969). This basket is still the most commonly used instrument for biliary stone retrieval. The combination of the stone basket with the steerable catheter has made non-operative stone extraction more practicable and less time-consuming. It also carries a lower complication rate.

The patient reports to the X-ray department about five weeks after operation. Almost all are treated as out-patients without premedication. Antibiotics are only used in patients with a history of previous pancreatitis, or if multiple intrahepatic stones require extraction.

The T-tube is extracted and the steerable catheter is passed through the sinus tract. Turns in the tract are demonstrated under fluoroscopic control during contrast injection. The steerable catheter can be manoeuvred around 90° turns in the sinus tract. An angle of more than 90° between the sinus tract and the common duct can also be negotiated.

After manipulation of the steerable catheter into the bile duct, the position of the retained stone is identified by cholangiography. The tip of

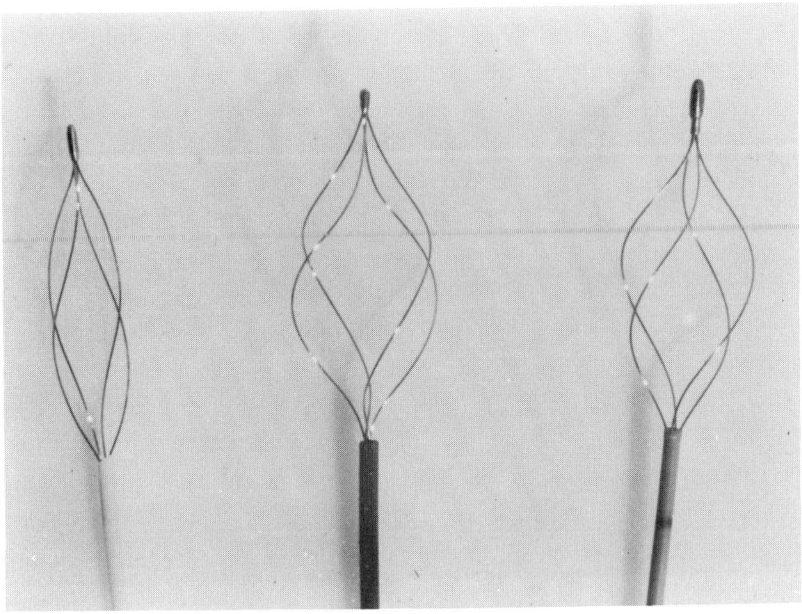

Fig. 13.5 Left to right: Medi-tech basket with white sheath, Cook basket with black sheath, Dormia basket with green sheath.

the catheter is then steered into that portion of the biliary tract containing the stone. It is positioned just beyond the stone if the duct diameter permits passage of the catheter alongside the stone. If the stone is blocking the duct, the steerable catheter is positioned with its tip just at the stone. The closed stone basket is then inserted through the steerable catheter and opened distal to the stone. Passage of the wire basket alongside the stone may be difficult, particularly if the duct is narrow and if the tip of the basket cannot be advanced parallel to the bile duct wall. Passage of the basket often requires making an obtuse angle between its tip and the duct wall. No perforations have occurred with this manoeuvre, but we do not advance the basket if it is at a right angle to the duct.

After opening the basket distal to the stone, it is slightly rotated during basket withdrawal. This usually results in stone engagement. We do not close the basket in the duct system after stone engagement. This used to be done, but it often resulted in stone fragmentation. Also, as the basket was closed, the stone often fell out. We now therefore use a continuous extraction movement as soon as the stone is seen within the basket.

Stones up to 6 millimeter diameter are usually extracted intact through the sinus tract of a No. 14 F T-tube. Larger stones require fragmentation.

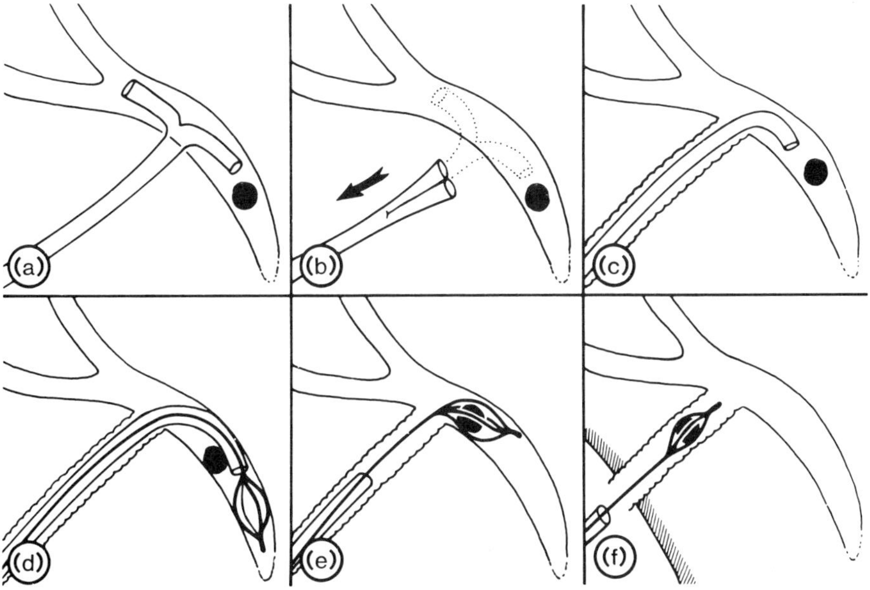

Fig. 13.6 Technical steps of stone extraction: (a) Identification of retained stone on T-tube cholangiography. (b) Extraction of T-tube. (c) Insertion of steerable catheter through the sinus tract. (d) Open basket in position distally to the retained stone. (e) Stone engagement in the wire basket. (f) Extraction of the stone through the sinus tract. (Reproduced with permission from *Am. J. Roentg.*, **117**, 388, 1973.)

13.4 PATIENTS

13.4.1 **Single sessions**

Our personal experience consists of 661 patients referred for retrieval of retained stones in the years 1972 to 1979. All patients undergo postoperative T-tube cholangiography for diagnosis.

Patients are only admitted as in-patients for extraction of difficult intrahepatic stones or if there is a history of previous postoperative pancreatitis. However, out-patients are asked to wait in the X-ray department for several hours after completion of the extraction procedure. This precaution was taken because some patients develop right upper quadrant pain following instrumentation of the distal common duct. This results from ampullary spasm and requires temporary external bile drainage.

The usual patient with a retained postoperative stone problem harbours a single common duct stone (Tables 13.1 and 13.2). An attempt is made to extract the stone and obtain a satisfactory closing cholangiogram in one sitting. This is often not possible. Blood clots or gas may

Table 13.1 Incidence of multiple stones.

Number of stones	*Incidence*
Single	72.5%
2–5	19.0%
6–10	8.0%
11–27	0.5%

Table 13.2 Location of stones.

Extrahepatic	529 (80%)
Intrahepatic	98 (15%)
Combined	34 (5%)
Total	661

accumulate in the duct system during stone removal. The patient is then asked to return several days later for a completion cholangiogram to ensure that all stones have been removed. A straight catheter is inserted through the sinus tract into the duct system during the interval (Fig. 13.7).

13.4.2 **Multiple sessions**

The removal of several retained stones may require multiple extraction sessions (Table 13.3). If a stone larger than the diameter of the sinus tract is extracted, this can result in injury to the wall of the sinus tract, or bleeding. It is then best to insert a straight catheter and have the patient return a week later for further stone extraction. We have learned that multiple sessions in patients with multiple stones are more likely to succeed in the extraction of the final stone. If one stone remains behind, the procedure is considered a failure. About 40% of all patients undergoing stone retrieval now attend for multiple sessions.

Table 13.3 Indications for multiple sessions.

1. Completion cholangiogram
2. Fragmentation
3. Multiple stones
4. Cystic duct stones
5. Intrahepatic stones
6. Tract manipulation
7. Impacted stones
8. Strictures
9. Penrose drains

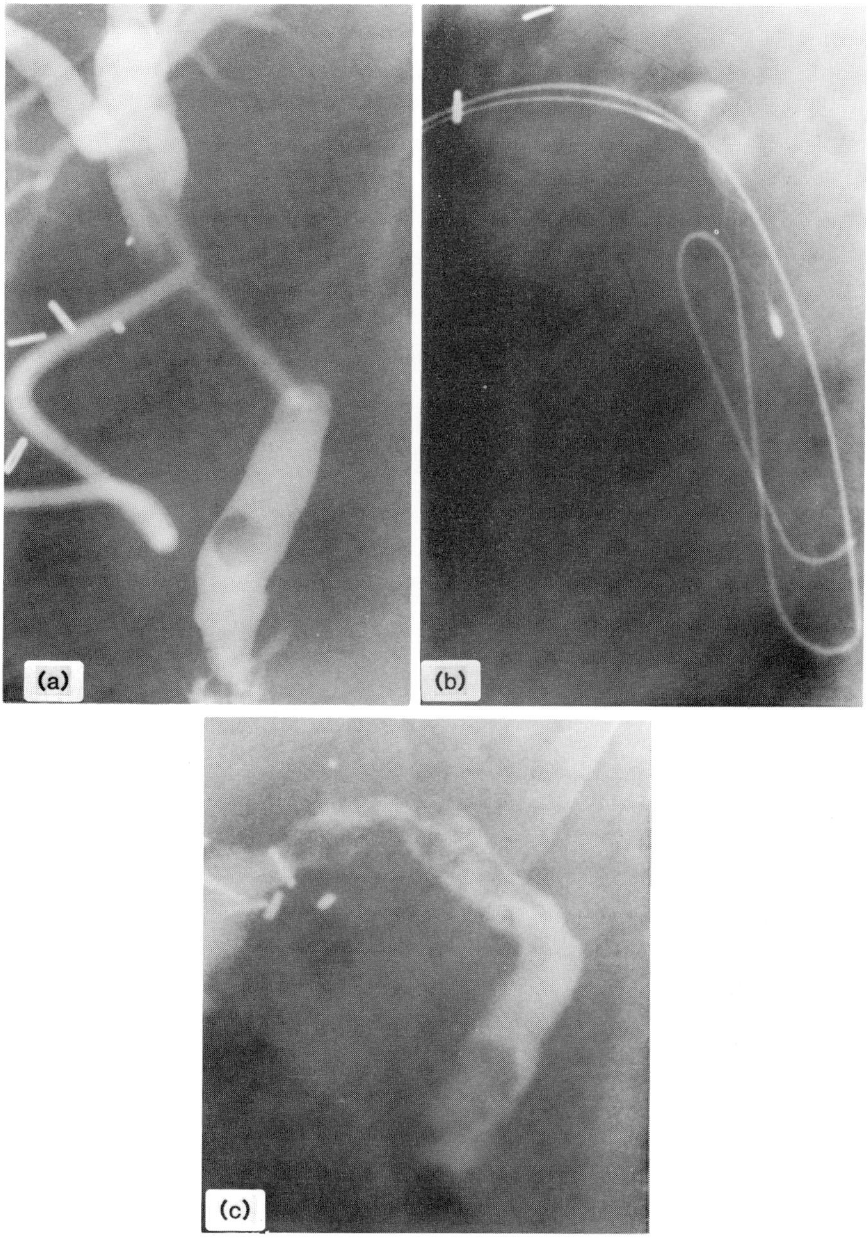

Fig. 13.7 (a) A distal retained common duct stone. (b) Wire basket in place distal to the retained stone. Note that a guide-wire was placed through the sinus tract and common duct into the duodenum for easier recatheterization of the sinus tract after extraction. (c) The retained stone has been fragmented, some fragments and several blood clots are present, requiring conclusion cholangiography at a subsequent session.

If a Penrose drain is in place adjacent to the sinus tract, we prefer to extract the drain and have the patient return at a later date. We have found that cross-connections exist between Penrose drains and T-tube tracts. This makes tract catheterization more difficult, and extravasation from the sinus tract may occur during the procedure.

Stone extraction is not attempted on the first day if small stones are present proximal to the short arm of the intraductal T-tube. The T-tube is simply extracted and a straight catheter is placed. This gives small stones a chance to pass spontaneously into the gut in the interval before the second visit.

It may be impossible to extract intrahepatic stones in second or third division radicals because of poor access with the wire basket. We prefer these patients to be ambulant for several additional weeks to give the hepatic stone a chance to move distally. Waiting in this way has contributed significantly to our high success rate.

Retained stones in cystic duct remnants are usually not accessible to the stone basket. If a low junction of common hepatic and cystic duct is present, surgical exploration and T-tube insertion has usually been performed into the common hepatic duct and the sharp angle from the common hepatic duct into the cystic duct remnant cannot be negotiated with the steerable catheter. Patients with stones retained in cystic duct remnants are positioned in a semi-erect or erect posture on the fluoroscopic table. This often results in downward movement of the retained stone so it can be extracted from the common duct. if this manoeuvre is unsuccessful, patients are asked to return several weeks later and the procedure is then started with the patient in a semi-erect position (Fig. 13.8).

13.4.3 **Small stones**

Small stones (up to 3 mm diameter) should pass from the common duct into the duodenum spontaneously if no ampullary narrowing is present. The T-tube can be clamped in almost all patients during the four week interval between T-tube cholangiography and stone extraction procedure. This increases the chance of passage of small stones or remaining fragments. Only rarely are distal common duct stones truly impacted, causing complete obstruction. We also clamp the indwelling straight tube between multiple sessions after fragmentation of large stones. This permits the passage of stone fragments.

Small stones are sometimes difficult to demonstrate during fluoroscopy on the television screen. Multiple spot films are then required for stone identification. Extraction with the open basket may then be a blind manoeuvre in the sense that the radiologist cannot see if the stone is being caught in the basket. Multiple passages with the basket may be

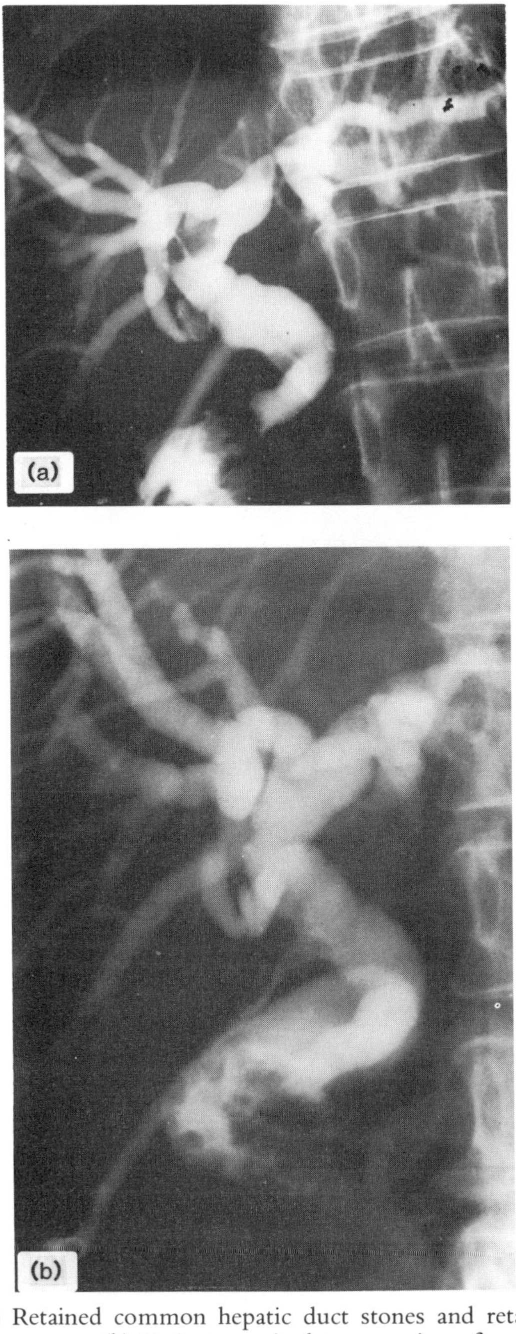

Fig. 13.8 (a) Retained common hepatic duct stones and retained stone in cystic duct remnant. (b) Patient required two sessions for removal of all retained stones. The cystic duct stone was extracted with the patient in a semi-erect position on the fluoroscopic table.

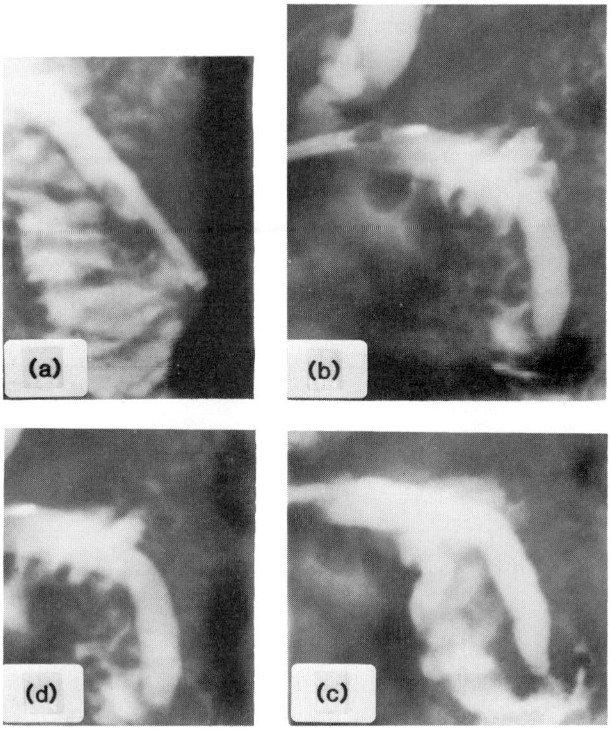

Fig. 13.9 Small distal retained common duct stone was engaged in the stone basket and extracted. The stone was difficult to visualize on the television monitor and multiple spot films throughout the procedure were required for visualization.

required to engage and extract small stones. We select the basket size so that the wires of the open basket touch the duct wall during extraction. This facilitates the engagement of small stones. A rotating motion on the wire stem of the basket further facilitates stone engagement (Fig. 13.9).

13.4.4 **Large stones**

Stones larger than the sinus tract, and stones with a diameter of more than 7 mm usually require fragmentation. The stone is engaged in the basket and brought to the junction of bile duct and sinus tract. Resistance is felt at this point, and traction is applied. A steady, slow increasing pull on the basket always results in fragmentation because the wire baskets are sufficiently thin and sharp to cut large stones. None of our 661 patients had retained large stones which were calcified. Large stones are primarily pigmented and relatively soft and can be crushed between finger-tips after extraction (Fig. 13.10).

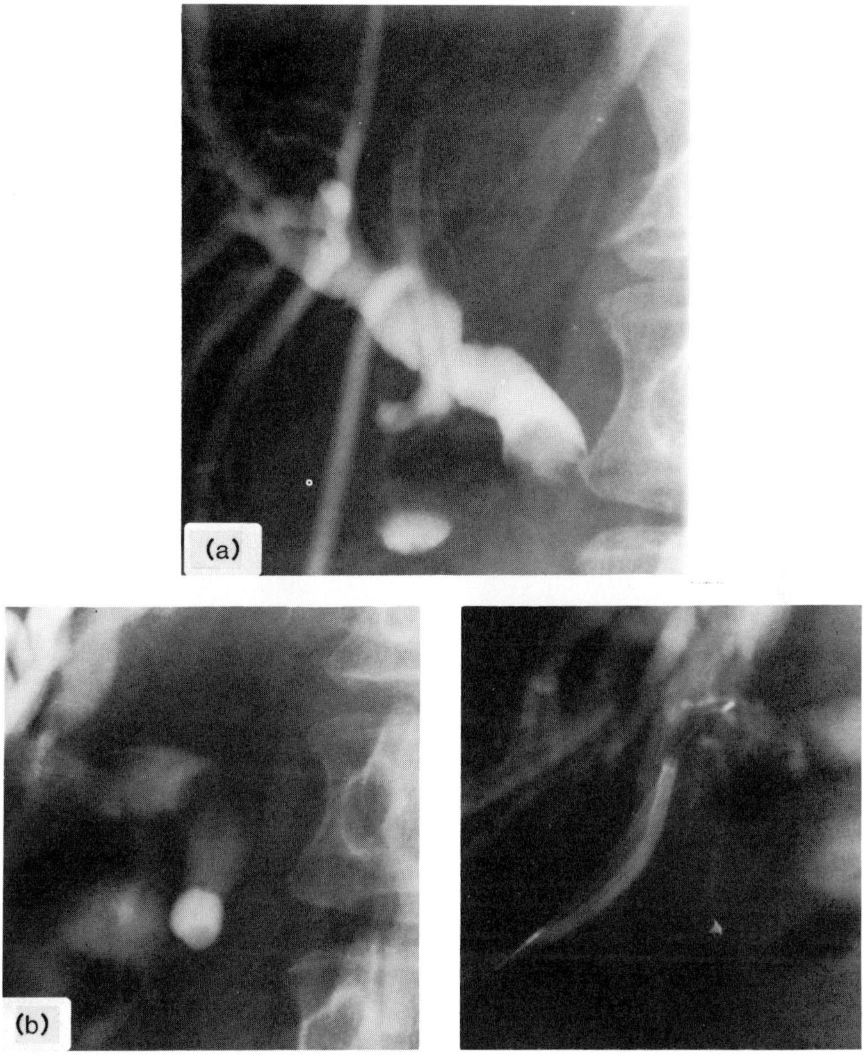

Fig. 13.10 (a) Partially impacted common duct stone. Note a leakage from the cystic duct stump. The proximal short arm of the T-tube is lying in the left hepatic radicle. (b) The large retained common duct stone was mobilized with use of Fogarty balloon. The balloon was inflated with contrast. Radiograph on the right shows the stone in the wire basket. The deformity of the wire basket is due to traction required for stone fragmentation.

Extravasation of contrast from the sinus tract due to injury of its fibrous wall may be seen after stone fragmentation in this fashion. We discontinue the procedure at that time and place a straight catheter for the interval to the next extraction session about one week later. It is necessarily time-consuming to remove all small pieces from the duct system after fragmentation of a large stone. Major fragments are extracted and small fragments are given a chance to pass spontaneously into the duodenum. As many as four sessions may be required if stone fragmentation involves several stones.

13.4.5 **Impacted stones**

Stones partially impacted in the distal common duct are more difficult to engage in the wire basket. We use a variety of manoeuvres to bring such a stone into a more proximal position in the duct before the basket can be opened distally to it. Suction through the steerable catheter may accomplish this change in stone location. A hand-held syringe is used for suction and the tip of the catheter is placed directly on the stone. Multiple attempts often succeed in moving the stone proximally. Other manoeuvres include rolling the stone proximally by bending the tip of the steerable catheter behind it. Contrast injected forcefully behind the stone sometimes results in the same movement. As a final manoeuvre, we use a Fogarty balloon catheter (Fig. 13.10(*b*)). The contrast filled balloon is positioned distal to the stone and gentle traction applied. The balloon is never inflated to a size greater than the bile duct diameter.

13.4.6 **Intrahepatic stones**

One or more stones may be retained in intrahepatic ducts after surgery. If a wire basket cannot be moved alongside the stone in the hepatic duct, or if the stone cannot be engaged by the basket, the stone has to be moved distally. This usually occurs after waiting for a longer interval than five weeks after surgery. Multiple return visits may be required. As a final resort, the Fogarty balloon catheter is employed. It is opened distal to the stone and gently pulled. No attempt at strong traction is made if the stone is seen to be wedged against the hepatic duct wall. The Fogarty balloon is carefully inflated with contrast under fluoroscopic vision to ensure that its inflated diameter is less than the diameter of the duct (Fig. 13.11).

We have removed as many as 27 intrahepatic stones in one patient in multiple sessions (Table 13.1).

13.5 COMPLICATIONS (Table 13.4)

A survey of 38 institutions was made to collect information on the complications of stone extraction (Burhenne, 1976). There was a 4.1% morbidity. This included postextraction fever, pancreatitis, sepsis, and extraductal bile collection. Contrast extravasations from injury to the

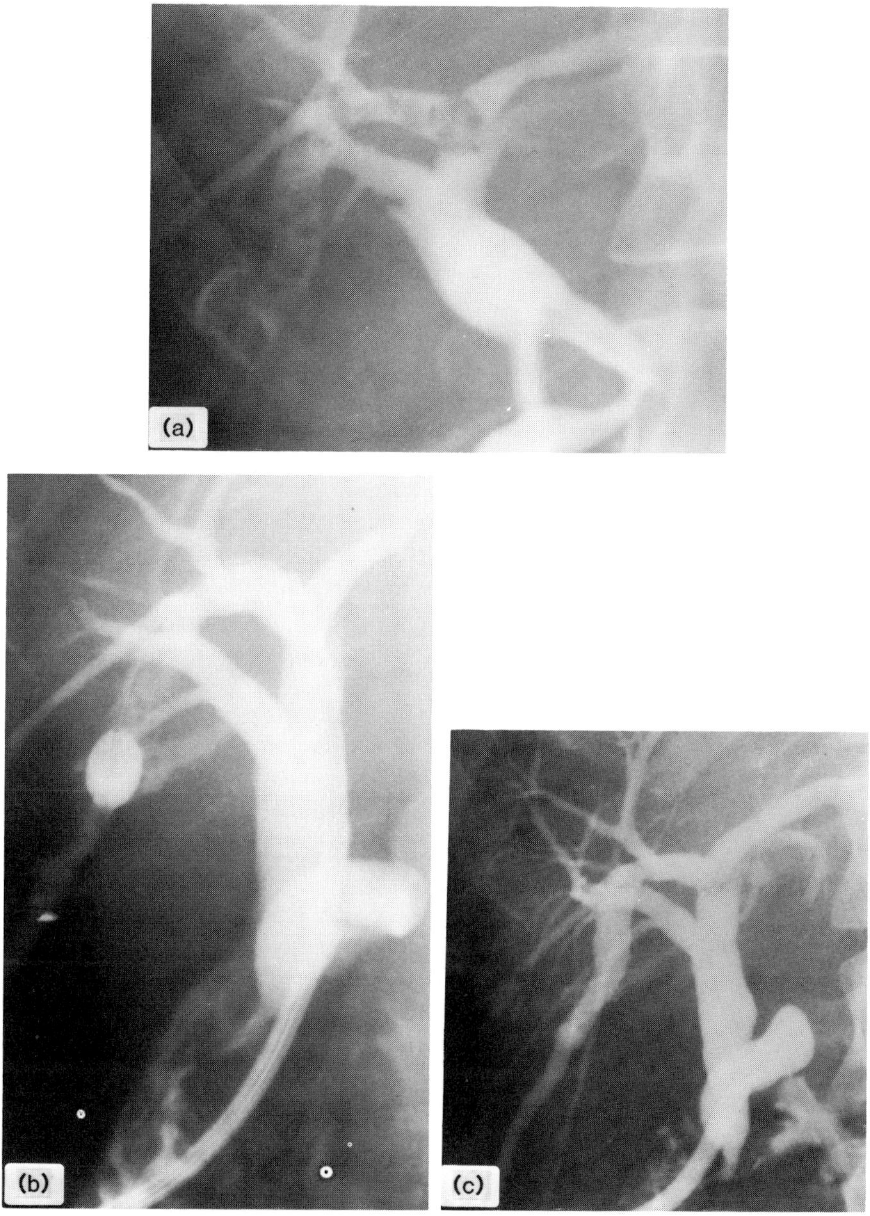

Fig. 13.11 (a) Multiple retained stones in second division hepatic radical. (b) Fogarty balloon in place during mobilization of retained intrahepatic stones. (c) All stones have been retrieved from the dorsocaudal branch of the left hepatic radicle.

Table 13.4 Complications.

1.	Sinus tract leak	7
2.	Peritoneal spill	2
3.	Bile collections	2
4.	Fever	11
5.	Sepsis	2
6.	Pancreatitis	2
7.	Vasovagal reaction	1
		27

sinus tract wall were usually confined. Free extravasation into the peritoneal cavity was seen in two patients. All signs and symptoms in patients with complications subsided within 48 hours. Patients with pancreatitis and sepsis were placed on antibiotics.

(Routine premedication with antibiotics is not used for our stone extraction procedures, but patients with a history of previous pancreatitis, and patients with multiple intrahepatic stones are placed on antibiotics before extraction is attempted.)

No mortality occurred in our group of 661 patients, though one death from acute pancreatitis following stone extraction has been reported in the literature (Polack *et al.*, 1977). [This group had experience of three extraction procedures before they attempted to remove a distal impacted common duct stone in a patient with a history of previous pancreatitis. The patient was transferred from one radiological room to another with instruments in place. Spot films were obtained in the second room where it was found that the stone had passed into the duodenum.]

13.6 SUCCESS AND FAILURE

All stones were removed in 95% of our 661 patients, obviating reoperation. Failures were experienced in 5% of patient (Tables 13.5 and 13.6) (Fig. 13.12).

Our success rate has been duplicated by other investigators (Garrow,

Table 13.5 Failures.

1.	Inability to catheterize	5
2.	Inability to recatheterize	7
3.	Cystic duct remnant stones	4
4.	Inability to engage hepatic stones	15
5.	Impacted distal stones	2
		33

Table 13.6 Failure by location.

Extrahepatic	18 (3.5%)
Intrahepatic and combined	15 (11%)
Total	33 (5%)

1977). A radiologist usually requires experience of about 20 stone retrievals before his success rate rises above 80%. However, the procedure can readily be learned.

Failure of stone extraction occurs usually in patients with intrahepatic stones, as such impacted stones may not permit instruments to pass alongside. Other failures include distally impacted stones, and stones retained in cystic duct stumps. It is sometimes impossible to enter the sinus tract of the T-tube, particularly in patients with T-tubes brought out through a midline incision. Failure may also result from injury to the sinus tract during removal of the first stone, and inability to re-enter the sinus tract for extraction of further stones. It is the extraction of the last remaining stone which determines success or failure.

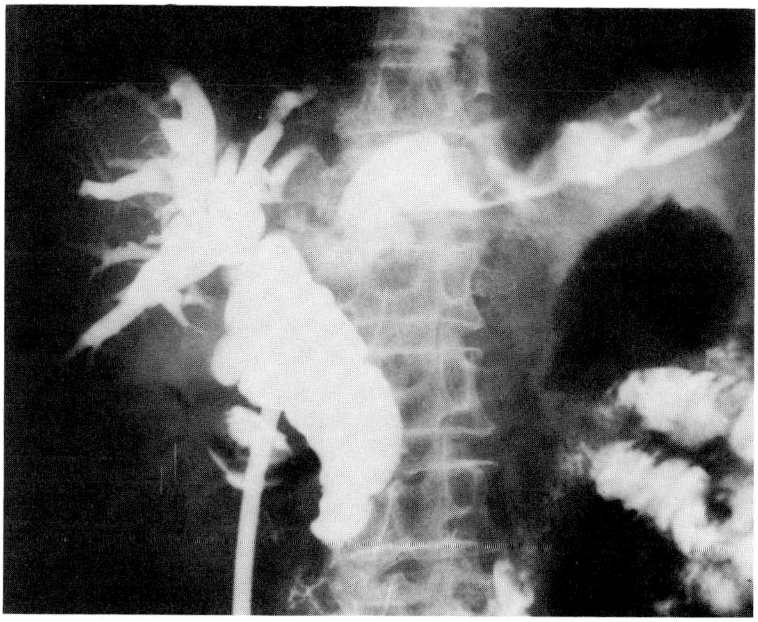

Fig. 13.12 Large retained stone in enlarged left hepatic radicle with narrowing at the porta hepatis. We were unable to extract this retained stone.

13.7 SURGICAL IMPLICATIONS

Successful non-operative retrieval of retained bile duct stones eliminates a problem for the surgeon, so his operative technique should be designed to facilitate postoperative stone removal.

A sufficiently large T-tube should be used routinely. The long arm of the T-tube should never be smaller than a No. 14 French. The short arms of the T-tube can usually be adjusted and bivalved to fit to a small bile duct. A T-tube with a large calibre long arm, originally described by Burhenne (1975), has now been made available by Moss *et al.* (1976).*

The long end of the T-tube should be brought out through a lateral anterior stab wound in the abdominal wall. Placement through abdominal midline incisions often makes extraction procedures impossible.

Routine operative cholangiography and operative choledochoscopy are more reliable techniques for detection of common duct stones than reliance on probing with surgical instruments. The passage of probes, dilators, or catheters through the distal end of the common duct into the duodenum is particularly unreliable for the demonstration of distal common duct stones. Our experience has shown that steerable catheters and baskets almost always pass easily alongside distal common duct stones into the duodenum.

13.8 OTHER POSTOPERATIVE RETRIEVAL METHODS

The use of the T-tube tract for passage of an endoscope has been described, with basket instrumentation for stone retrieval. This method is more expensive, less successful and requires hospitalization because sinus tract dilatation is required in most patients (Yamakawa *et al.*, 1976). However, X-ray exposure is reduced and it is easy to distinguish between stones, air bubbles and blood.

Attempts at stone dissolution show a poor success rate in the use of retained common duct stones. It is also expensive, requires hospitalization and is often associated with complications (Way, 1973).

Retained common duct stones after surgery may be extracted by endoscopic retrograde cannulation of the bile duct followed by sphincterotomy and basket extraction (see Chapter 12). This method, however, is difficult to learn and shows a low success rate for large and intrahepatic stones (Classen, Koch and Demling, 1975).

Non-operative percutaneous retrieval under fluoroscopic control carries the highest success rate and is associated with fewest complications. If a T-tube is in place, it is the therapeutic technique of choice for the retrieval of retained stones (Classen and Ossenberg, 1977).

*Davol, Inc., Cranston, R.I.

REFERENCES

Burhenne, H. J. (1973). Nonoperative retained biliary tract stone extraction: a new roentgenologic technique. *Am. J. Roentg.*, **117**, 388–99.

Burhenne, H. J. (1975). Nonoperative instrumentation of the postoperative biliary tract. In: *Surgery of the Liver, Pancreas and Biliary Tract.* (eds. J. S. Najarian and J. P. Delaney) Symposia Specialists, Miami, Florida. pp. 177–207.

Burhenne, H. J. (1976). Complications of nonoperative extraction of retained common duct stones. *Am. J. Surg.*, **131**, 260–2.

Classen, M., Koch, H. and Demling, L. (1975). Papillotomy and treatment of gallstones by means of endoscopy. In: *Surgical Endoscopy.* (ed. E. Seifert) Witzstrock: Baden-Baden, pp. 187–284.

Classen, M. and Ossenberg, F. W. (1977). Progress report: non-surgical removal of common bile duct stones. *Gut*, **18**, 760–9.

Garrow, D. G. (1977). The removal of retained biliary tract stones: report of 105 cases. *Br. J. Radiol.*, **50**, 777–82.

LaGrave, G. *et al.* (1969). Lithiase biliaire residuelle. Extraction a la sonde de Dormia par le drain de Kehr. *Mem. Acad. Chir.*, **95**, 430.

Longmire, Jr., W. P. (1979) The Treatment of Retained Gallstones: The Western Journal of Medicine, Vol. **130**, 422–37.

Mazzariello, R. (1970). Removal of residual biliary tract calculi without reoperation. *Surgery*, **67**, 566–73.

Mondet, A. (1962). Técnica de la extracción incuenta de los cálculos en la litiasis residual del colédoco. *Bol. Trab. Soc. Circug. Buenos Aires*, **46**, 278–90.

Moss, J. P., Whalen, J. G. and Fry, D. E. (1976). Unsuccessful Postoperative Extraction of Retained Common Duct Stones. *Am. J. Surgery*, **135**, 785–9.

Polack, E. P., Fainsinger, M. H. and Bonnano, S. V. (1977). A death following complications of roentgenologic nonoperative manipulation of common bile duct calculi. *Radiology*, **123**, 585–6.

Way, L. W. (1973). Retained common duct stones. *Surg. Clinics N. Am.*, **53**, 1139–47.

Yamakawa, T. *et al.* (1976). An improved choledochofiberscope and non-surgical removal of retained biliary calculi under direct visual control. *Gastrointest. Endosc.*, **22**, 160–4.

14 Jejunal biopsy by endoscopy

BRIAN J. PROUT

In the management of patients with intestinal malabsorption, histological examination of the jejunal mucosa is essential. We are particularly concerned in this chapter with the role of small intestinal disease and how the clinical gastroenterologist can narrow the differential diagnosis by the use of endoscopy.

A sample of small intestine can be examined histologically, biochemically and by immunofluorescence. There may be a recognizable histological abnormality in the mucosa, with or without a demonstrable biochemical disorder, or the structure of the mucosa may be normal in the presence of a biochemical disorder. The list of diseases and conditions in which abnormalities of the jejunal mucosa may occur has lengthened with the practice of the technique. Small intestinal biopsies may be obtained by the following methods, but in this chapter we shall emphasize those techniques using fibreoptic endoscopy.

14.1 'BLIND' SUCTION BIOPSY

The Crosby capsule was described by Crosby and Kugler in 1957. This capsule, or some modification of it, is at present the most widely used method of obtaining a jejunal biopsy. The Crosby capsule does however give a good sized biopsy as its main advantage. This advantage can be fully utilized in the combined endoscopic biopsy technique to be described in detail later.

The main cause of delay in this 'blind' method of obtaining a jejunal biopsy is the time taken for the capsule to enter the pylorus and pass on through the duodenum, which in some patients can be several hours. Most experienced gastroenterologists have also had experience of the capsule turning back into the stomach or the tubing tying itself into a knot.

To guide the capsule through the pylorus Wicks and Glain (1972) suggested a guide-wire to insert down the tubing and then manipulate the capsule through the pylorus under fluoroscopic control. In the method of Evans *et al.* (1970) the stiffening effect of an outer polythene sleeve around the biopsy tubing facilitates manual manipulation of the capsule through the pylorus. In these methods of manipulation the patient is exposed to X-radiation while the pylorus is located, and during corrective manipulations when the capsule is turning retrogradely.

Other types of suction biopsy instruments are available, including the Rubin tube, Shiner tube, Quinton tube, Oregon tube, and the Cooke–Chaudhury capsule.

14.2 DIRECT VISION BIOPSY WITH A SMALL INTESTINAL FIBRESCOPE

Mucosal biopsies may be obtained by ordinary biopsy forceps used with a standard forward-viewing gastroduodenoscope. Although it has been reported that these biopsies are comparable to those obtained by capsules from the jejunum (Scott and Jenkins, 1980), they are necessarily ***duodenal*** and not jejunal, and the biopsy size is small. Even if histological interpretation can be made, the material is unsuitable for disaccharide assay.

Manufacturers of fibreoptic endoscopes are now producing enteroscopes for viewing the interior of the small intestine. It has been pointed out that this instrument might be used only in a few centres (Classen *et al.*, 1972; Salmon *et al.*, 1973) and certainly the instrument has limited applications.

The author has been somewhat disappointed by the small size of the biopsies obtainable with these instruments in comparison with those obtained by the Crosby capsule. The 'grasp' biopsy forcep is limited in size by the necessarily small biopsy channel in the present fibreoptic enteroscopes. The method does, however, have the advantage of direct vision of the site of biopsy and the whole of the small intestine, and any lesion seen can be biopsied. The enteroscope can also be used with a Rubin-type suction biopsy capsule so that larger multiple biopsies can be taken under direct vision, but this is an expensive method of performing a jejunal biopsy and applicable only in special circumstances (Salmon, 1979). The technique of small intestinal endoscopy through an enteroscope is similar to that for routine endoscopy of the upper oesophagus, stomach and duodenum. Although the view is improved by a longer pre-examination fast, in practice overnight fasting is sufficient.

14.3 COMBINED UPPER GASTROINTESTINAL ENDOSCOPY WITH CROSBY OR WATSON CAPSULE JEJUNAL BIOPSY

The advantage of this technique is that both instruments – a Crosby (or Watson) biopsy capsule and a forward-viewing gastrointestinal fibrescope – form part of the standard equipment of a gastroenterological unit. The author uses an Olympus GIF D2 and D3 but the method could be used with other forward-viewing fibrescopes. The method was reported first by the author in 1974 (Prout, 1974) and has been adopted in other centres (Holdstock, 1978).

The main reasons for the development of this technique were to speed the process of obtaining a jejunal biopsy and to avoid involving an X-ray department.

The technique has the following advantages:

(a) A biopsy can be obtained more quickly.
(b) It can be performed without fluoroscopy.
(c) Patients who have been biopsied by the 'blind' method and later by the combined fibrescope and capsule method, prefer the latter.
(d) Upper gastrointestinal endoscopy can be performed simultaneously.
(e) The biopsy obtained from a Watson or Crosby capsule is of good size.
(f) Problems such as the capsule not returning through the pylorus do not occur as the fibrescope is holding the pylorus open.

The disadvantages of the technique are:

(a) It requires experience in fibreoptic endoscopy.
(b) Repeated biopsies cannot be taken unless the fibrescope and capsule are withdrawn and the capsule reloaded.

To ensure good results, in addition to having a well-maintained fibrescope the following technical points concerning the capsule should be observed:

1. Clean the capsule thoroughly.
2. Keep the knife edge sharpened; but not its outer edge, otherwise the knife does not approximate the inner wall of the capsule.
3. Use radio-opaque tubing with the capsule (see Appendix) and cover the capsule with a rubber jacket (Salem *et al.*, 1965).
4. Use a Teflon-coated guide-wire, dimension T 160 (0.92 mm). The special coating gives the guide-wire a smooth and even surface (Appendix).
5. When fitting the radio-opaque tubing to the capsule be sure that the flange is not so small that the tubing is pulled out of the capsule. Alternatively, too large a flange, not seated properly into the vertex of the instrument, will interfere with cocking the instrument.
6. Ensure the spring is in good condition and well hooked into its groove.
7. Check that the capsule fires reliably and that the pin is not bent.
8. If more than one biopsy is required, then the capsule can be modified

with two aspiration holes (Dawson and Sladen, 1979) which may be useful in patients with suspected patchy lesions (Manuel *et al.*, 1979).

14.3.1 **Method**

The prothrombin time is measured and vitamin K given if necessary; until the prothrombin time is normal, biopsy is inadvisable. The patient is fasted overnight. The examination is carried out in the endoscopy area or X-ray room. It is to be emphasized, however, that it is possible, and indeed usual, in this technique to obtain biopsies without the use of X-ray screening. The patient is placed in the left lateral position and sedated with intravenous diazepam, until satisfactory relaxation is achieved. The stiffening wire is now threaded into the biopsy capsule tubing, and together the tubing and wire are threaded up through the

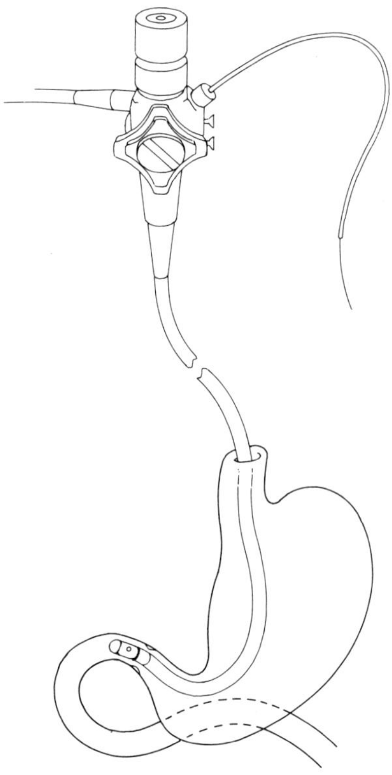

Fig. 14.1 The diagram shows the Crosby capsule sitting against the distal end of the fibrescope and being passed through the pylorus. At the proximal end of the fibrescope, protruding from the biopsy channel, is the radio-opaque tubing attached to the capsule with the stiffening wire *in situ*.

distal end of the endoscope, until the capsule is sitting against the distal end of the endoscope. The capsule is held firmly in this position by slight tension being exerted on the proximal end of the capsule tubing, where it is protruding from the biopsy channel near the eye-piece (Fig. 14.1). The endoscope and capsule are then passed into the pharynx and on into the oesophagus as one fixed unit. If necessary the capsule can be pushed from the end of the fibrescope and the oesophageal mucosa viewed. It is, however, usual to proceed directly into the body of the stomach and to view the pylorus, again by freeing the capsule from the end of the fibrescope. The combined unit can then be passed into the duodenum, after the stomach has been inspected (Figs. 14.1 and 14.2). The fibrescope is advanced as far into the second part of the duodenum as possible (Fig. 14.3) and from here the capsule is passed ahead of the distal end of the fibrescope, by pushing at the proximal end of the capsule tubing. The wire gives the required additional rigidity. Occasionally it may be

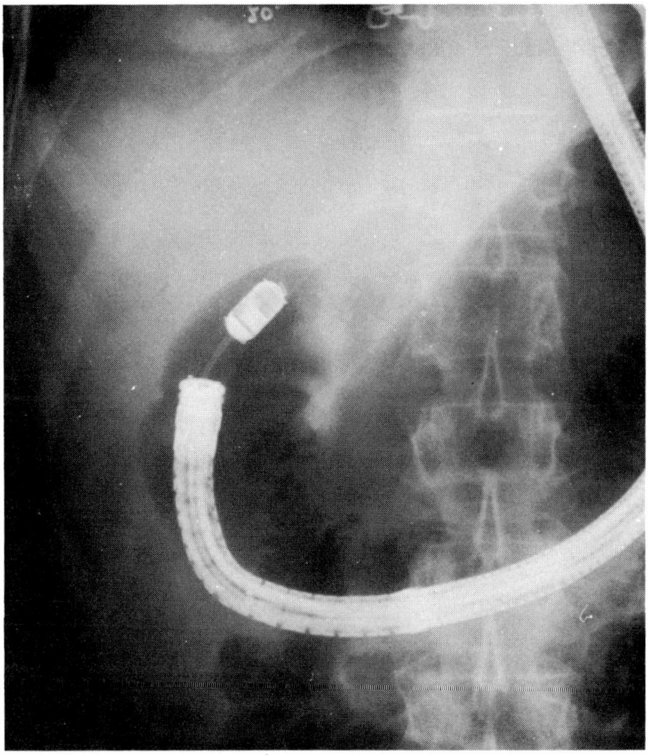

Fig. 14.2 The X-ray shows the distal end of the fibrescope with the capsule and its radio-opaque tubing separated from the fibrescope tip and being passed into the duodenum (from Prout, 1974).

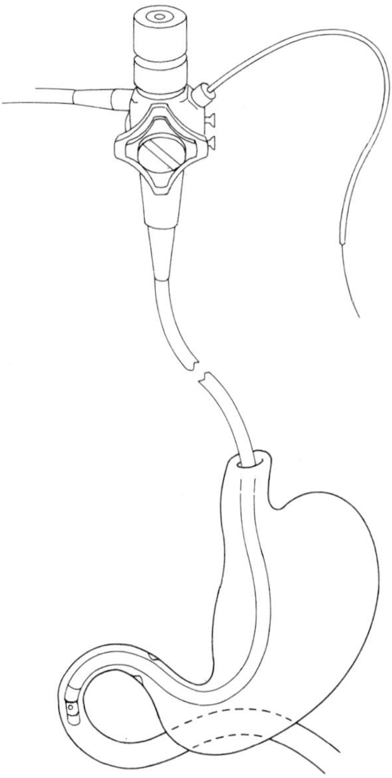

Fig. 14.3 The fibrescope and capsule are passed together into the second part of the duodenum.

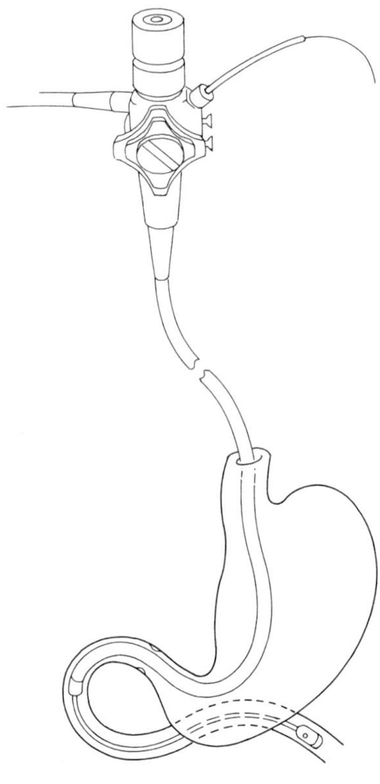

Fig. 14.4 The final stage of the procedure. The capsule, tubing and wire have been pushed into the biopsy channel to advance the capsule from the fibrescope tip to the duodeno-jejunal flexure.

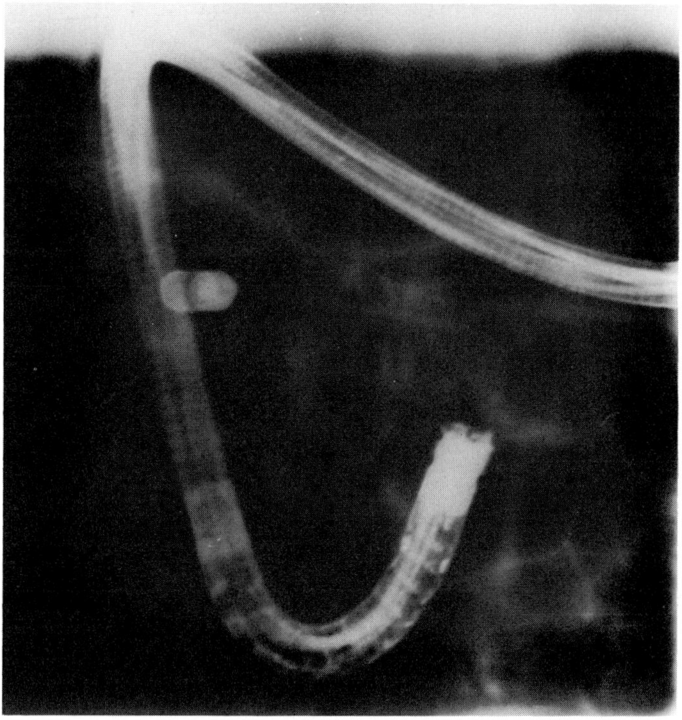

Fig. 14.5 The X-ray shows an example of the successful passage of the fibrescope tip into the third part of the duodenum and the advancement of the biopsy capsule towards the duodenojejunal flexure.

difficult to advance the tubing, and if so one should attempt to straighten out the fibrescope to minimize the curves that the tubing is having to circumvent. With practice it is possible gently to manoeuvre the fibrescope and capsule independently of each other to achieve forward progression of the capsule. It is not usually necessary to lubricate the moveable parts, but occasionally a drop or two of silicone lubricant down the biopsy channel is helpful. The capsule is thus manipulated to a position estimated to be at or beyond the duodenojejunal junction (Fig. 14.4).

In some patients the fibrescope can be pushed into the third part of the duodenum and the capsule advanced to the jejunum (Figs. 14.5 and 14.6). In Fig. 14.7 the ease with which the fibrescope and biopsy capsule can be separately manoeuvred is demonstrated radiologically. When the capsule is in the correct position it is helpful to flush the tubing with saline after removing the guide-wire. If any food particles have been seen, flushing is essential, or a biopsy may not be obtained.

To fire the capsule, one should use a 20 ml syringe at the proximal end of the tubing. If the syringe plunger is pulled quickly, then a thin superficial specimen is obtained from the mucosa, which is desirable in small frail patients, especially if malabsorption is severe. This will minimize the risks of haemorrhage or perforation (although the author has not experienced this hazard). To obtain a larger and deeper specimen, give a slow pull on the syringe plunger. When the capsule has fired, it is withdrawn until it is once again seated against the distal end of the fibrescope. The whole unit is then withdrawn slowly and steadily from the patient. The stomach can be viewed again at this point by separating the capsule from the end of the fibrescope (Fig. 14.8).

The routine procedure for care of the patient, with particular relevance to removal of any mouthpieces or indwelling needles, is followed (Prout and Schiller, 1976). The patient is moved to the ward, and observed overnight to detect the potential hazards of haemorrhage or perforation.

14.3.2 **Preparation of the specimen**

To obtain the best results this stage of the procedure is vital. Preliminary discussion with the pathologist will have been carried out particularly if an obscure condition is suspected. As soon as the capsule is withdrawn from the patient the biopsy specimen should be gently removed from the capsule. The clinician taking the biopsy should remove the specimen with care to avoid damage and place it mucosal surface upwards on a square of absorbent paper. Often the biopsy specimen rolls up and if after inspection with a hand lens it is still difficult to determine which is the mucosal surface, for example in total villous atrophy, then the convex surface is usually the mucosal surface. The contraction of the *muscularis mucosae* is the cause of the rolling up of the specimen and it usually causes the specimen to curl in this particular direction. When mounted, the specimen is placed into a previously labelled pot containing 10% buffered formaldehyde or formol calcium.

In patients with suspected disaccharidase deficiency the specimen should be divided, and the portion sent to the biochemists should be unfixed. If histochemistry is required the specimen should be fixed cold, transferred to gum sucrose, and cut with the cryostat. The specimen can

Fig. 14.6 This X-ray shows the fibrescope tip in the third part of the duodenum with the capsule in the proximal jejunum.

Fig. 14.7 The X-ray shows the ease with which the two pieces of apparatus may be separately manoeuvred. The fibrescope has been withdrawn over the tubing of the Crosby capsule leaving the capsule in position. The stomach and duodenum were inspected and then the two pieces of apparatus were removed together (from Prout, 1974).

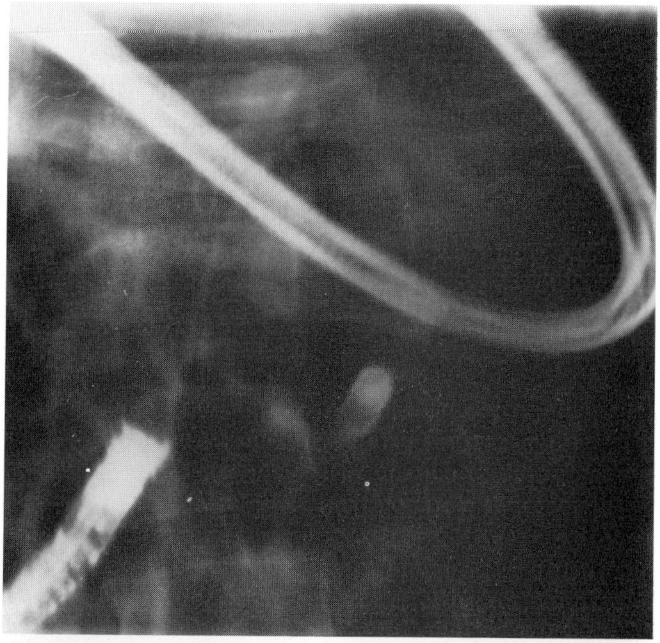

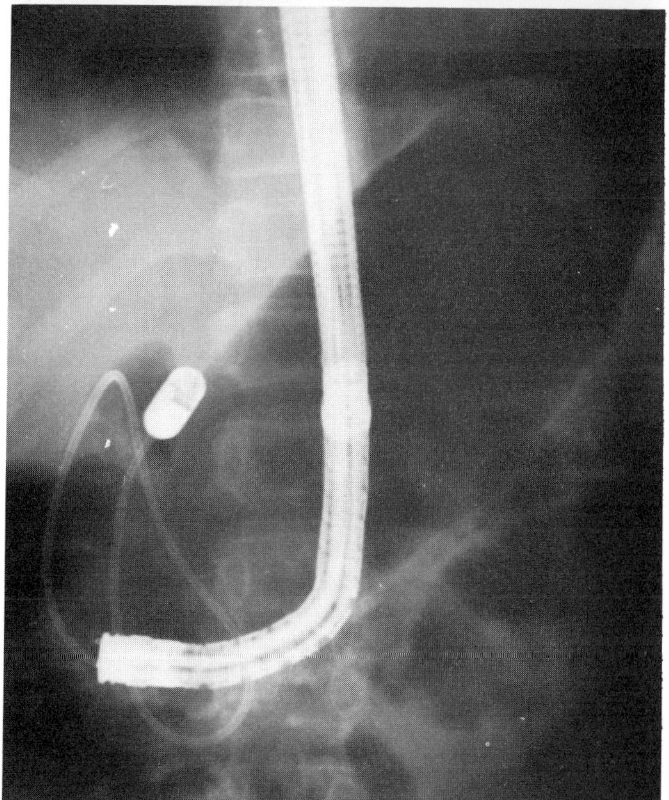

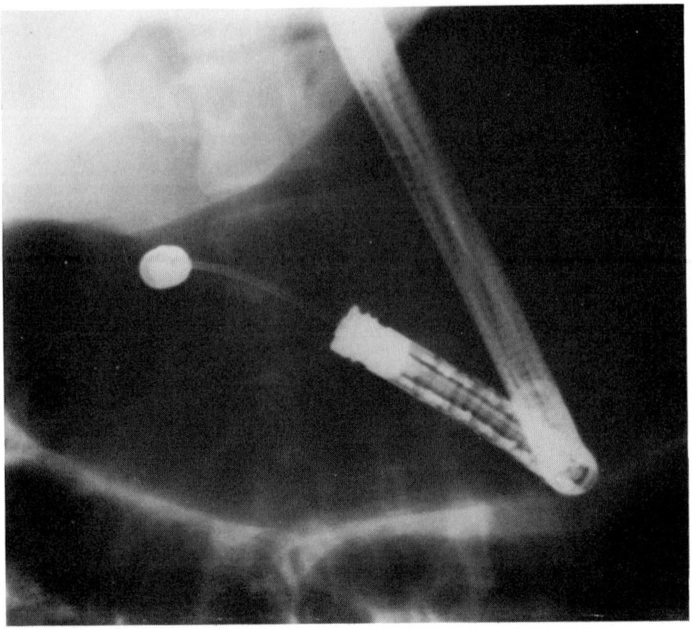

Fig. 14.8 This X-ray shows the stomach outlined by air. The capsule, seen end on, has been separated from the fibrescope tip, in order to inspect the gastric mucosa.

also be examined histochemically after a longer delay by routine paraffin wax embedding.

Close liaison with the pathologist is always advisable and becomes even more important if one is contemplating electronmicroscopy, although this method of examination is probably only of value in suspected Whipple's disease or congenital β-lipoprotein deficiency (Trier and Rubin, 1965; Trier, 1968).

APPENDIX 14.1

1. Radio-opaque polythylene tubing A/S Surgimed, Surgical Medical and Electronic Products. SMØ Rumnedre, 2760 Malov, Denmark. Red special soft, dimension 1.9 to 1.1 to 0.4 mm.
2. Guide-wires and tubing from Coloplast Ltd., St. Ives, Huntingdon, PE17 4LN. Telephone: (St. Ives) 0480-62600.

REFERENCES

Classen, M. *et al.* (1972). Enteroskopie fiberendoskopie son jejunum und ileum. *Dt. Med. Wschr.*, **11**, 409–11.

Crosby, W. H. and Kugler, H. W. (1957). Intraluminal biopsy of the small intestina; the intestinal biopsy capsule. *Am. J. Dig. Dis.*, **2**, 236–41.

Dawson, I. and Sladen, G. (1979). Procedures in medicine. *Medicine*, **14**, 705–6.

Evans, N. *et al.* (1970). New techniques for speeding small intestinal biopsy. *Gut*, **11**, 88–89.

Holdstock, G. (1978). Jejunal biopsy without the need for screening. *Lancet,* **1**, 1236–7.

Manuel, P. D., Walker-Smith, J. A. and France, N. E. (1979). Patchy enteropathy in childhood. *Gut*, **20**, 211–5.

Prout, B. J. (1974). A rapid method of obtaining a jejunal biopsy using a Crosby Capsule and gastro-intestinal fibrescope. *Gut*, **15**, 571–2.

Prout, B. J. and Schiller, K. F. R. (1976). *Modern Topics in Gastro-intestinal Endoscopy*, William Heinemann Medical Books, London, Chapter 4.

Salem, S. N., Salt, R. H. and Truelove, S. C. (1965). Crosby small intestinal capsule with radio-opaque tube and latex sheath. *Gut*, **6**, 99–100.

Salmon, P. R. (1979). Endoscopy. *Medicine*, **14**, 719–21.

Salmon, P. R. *et al.* (1973). Examination of the duodenum and jejunum employing a new fibreoptic enteroscope. *Gut*, **14**, 823.

Scott, B. B. and Jenkins, D. (1980). Are endoscopes small-intestinal forceps biopsies suitable for histological interpretation? *Gut*, **21**, 9446.

Trier, J. S. (1968) *Handbook of Physiology*, Sect. 6. Vol. 3. American Physiological Soc., Washington DC, Chapter 63.

Trier, J. S. and Rubin, C. E. (1965). Electron microscopy of the small intestine – a report. *Gastroenterology*, **49**, 574–603.

Wicks, T. and Glain, D. (1972). A guide wire for rapid jejunal biopsies with the Crosby capsule. *Gut*, **13**, 571.

15 Tube placement under radiological guidance

MARCIA K. BILBAO

This chapter describes the principles of antegrade intestinal intubation, with radiological guidance, for diagnosis, feeding and intestinal decompression, and some methods of prevention and treatment of tube complications. No attempt will be made to assign priorities for tube innovations. Those interested in the history of intubation are referred to Dr. Ingelfinger's delightful essay (Ingelfinger, 1978). The use of radiology enables the operator to see both tube and route during insertion. Special methods of catheter guidance, adapted from angiography, and the ability to exchange one catheter for another, make it possible to design a tube for its ease of placement or for its functional efficiency without attempting to combine these attributes in a single tube.

The blind passage of a tube is the simplest method even if not the most effective, and suffices in many instances. Where more sophisticated methods are needed, the advantages of fluoroscopically controlled gastrointestinal intubation are that it is faster, safer, and surer than passing a tube blindly, and usually less traumatic and expensive than passing it endoscopically. Additionally, contrast material used during placement may allow a concomitant diagnostic study in cases of obstruction, and the demonstration of effectiveness when feeding tubes have been inserted.

The disadvantages are the added time, expense, and trouble in transporting the patient to the X-ray department and using the radiological resources. Additionally there is radiation exposure, although this is nearly all fluoroscopic, with few radiographs, and therefore less than that of a standard gastrointestinal series.

15 1 INDICATIONS

Radiological guidance gives clear evidence of safe, appropriate postioning of feeding or decompression tubes. Fluoroscopically-aided placement is indicated when blind passage has failed or is likely to be difficult or dangerous, for example in patients with strictures, tumours, fistulaes, injuries, or surgical anastomoses, and in patients with swallowing difficulty, depressed gag reflexes, or abnormal peristalsis. Radiologically guided intubation is also faster. Duodenal intubation in five minutes and jejunal intubation in 10 to 30 minutes is usually possible with radiological aid (Bilbao and Dotter, 1975; Edlich *et al.*, 1968; Shipps *et al.*, 1979).

Relative contraindications to fluoroscopically-controlled intubation are related to radiation exposure (especially in pregnant or young patients) and to the choice of contrast agents. Air is simplest but least effective. Barium is the safest, most effective agent except in instances of suspected perforation or large bowel obstruction, or in positioning a tube for small intestinal biopsy where it may interfere with histological examination. Iodinated contrast agents, because of their high osmolarity (six times that of saline), are less safe. In infants they may cause hypovolaemic shock, as well as diarrhoea and vomiting (Harris *et al.*, 1964). Furthermore, because of dilution, they are less effective diagnostically (Nelson, 1965).

There are circumstances where any method of intubation may be hazardous carrying the risk of haemorrhage (bleeding diathesis, varices, anomalous mediastinal vessels) or perforation (recent surgical anastomoses, ulceration, tumours). If intubation is done in all in these instances fluoroscopic methods are safer than blind passage.

15.2 PRINCIPLES

Fluoroscopically-aided tube passage is easy: the fluoroscopist 'sees' the route and controls the tube, moving the tube past obstacles, and shaping tube and route into conformity. Afterward he may exchange the tube for another which is more functional, comfortable, sturdier or cheaper. The tube is advanced partly by peristalsis and by gravity, but mainly by pushing, which requires that it be at least temporarily stiff enough. Stiffening is accomplished either coaxially by inner wire guides or outer tubes, or by outrigged coupling to a pilot tube. These same techniques are used for tube exchanges. Coaxial layers are made movable and removable by straightening bends, and by lubrication. Passing obstacles involves decongesting, lubricating (and anaesthetizing), smoothing and distending corrugated mucosal surfaces, and then 'dancing' the tube across them by revolving it and shaking it (or shaking the surface).

The tube is bent by gravity, by palpation, or by the use of steerable tube-tips or preshaped or steerable wire guides. The shape of the route may be altered, using gravity to shift the viscera by positioning the patient and tilting the table, by palpation with either the fluoroscopist's or patient's hands, and by the patient's posturing – breathing, arching, stretching, flexing, leaning, 'undulating and fluttering' (like panting), and so forth. The patient may help more if he watches himself on the fluoroscopic monitor. Each sequential bend in the tract can be straightened in front of advancing tube.

15.3 TUBES

There is no perfect tube. Features which make it comfortable – small size, limpness, elasticity – also make it uncontrollable; features which make it easy to place, like stiffness and large size, also make it uncomfortable and more traumatic. Three general types of intestinal tubes are of interest to radiologists. *Diagnostic tubes* used for rapid short term nasoenteric intubation are simple, versatile, easily placed, large-bore, and inexpensive. *Feeding tubes* for long term comfort and safety are soft, rubbery, and as small as possible while still allowing a liquid feed to be forced through them. *Decompression tubes* are to be propelled by the gastrointestinal (GI) tract, large-bored enough for aspiration of intestinal content, yet soft enough for the patient to tolerate without undue discomfort and without ulcerating his mucosa.

15.3.1 **Constitution**

Materials used in GI tubes include *natural rubber*, which is soft, flexible, and not irritating, but too elastic for use with a guide-wire and prone to get coated with and clogged by detritus. Also, it hardens and weakens when exposed to gut contents. *Polyvinylchloride* is soft, flexible, can be made radio-opaque, and can be used with a wire guide. Polyvinylchloride is excellent for short term applications and for small feeding tubes, even though the plasticizer, which makes it soft, leaches out, irritates mucosal surfaces, and causes the tube to harden gradually after the first two weeks (Duke and Vane, 1968; Cowper, 1968; Editorial, *Lancet*, 1975). *Polyurethane* is soft, flexible, inert, good for feeding tubes and can be used to a limited extent with guide wires. *Silicone rubber* is extremely soft, durable, inert, comfortable, does not collect detritus nor tend to plug, and does not harden. It is difficult to use with a wire guide, but it is excellent for long term feeding tubes if it can be placed.

15.3.2 **Size**

The length of the tube and guide is crucial, since every inch increases the friction. The lumen size affects performance, since flow through tubes varies with the fourth power of the diameter; thus reducing tube diameter to a half reduces the tube flow to a sixteenth. Flow through a hole varies with the square of the diameter (MacIntosh *et al.*, 1963). Hole position is important. An end-hole is needed for coaxial exchange over a guide-wire and should be fabricated as needed.

For some purposes, like investigating strictures, side holes in tubes for diagnostic studies are disadvantageous because they deliver contrast agent too far from the site to be examined, thereby obscuring the route. Feeding tubes should have holes located near the end to avoid delivery proximal to the target. Decompression tubes should have holes over a considerable length to decompress more than one segment of the GI tract at a time.

Friction is the major impediment in GI intubation. There is friction between tube and guide, tube and GI tract, tube and coaxial tube, and tube and the fluid it carries. Friction increases directly with tube length, with every additional curve and with sharpness of curvature. Therefore, it is important to shorten the tube and make the curves fewer and gentler, especially while trying to move coaxial elements. One way is to move both guide and tube together around bends and advance the guide within the tube only when it is straight. Another way is to straighten the tube by external palpation on the abdomen while the guide is advanced. Kinks or surface irregularities in either tube or guide increase friction. A guide considerably smaller than the tube reduces contact. Friction is greatest with the most elastic materials such as rubber and silicone rubber, less, but still considerable with polyvinylchloride. Everything should be thoroughly lubricated to create a surface which floats instead of binds. Silicone fluid (medical grade) in a spray can with propellant is particularly useful (Fig. 15.1). It can be sprayed directly on the tube and guide, and also into the tube; it can be sprayed on gauze and wiped on the guides. It may be put into a syringe and injected down the tube. Residual dissolved propellant boils out and carries the silicone forcefully to the tube's end. Using a 'Y' adaptor, this can be done while the tube is in the patient, even with a spring guide in place. Silicone is inert, widely used in the food industry, and harmless in the gut. Silicone on the outside of the tube makes it less traumatic during passage, less irritating, and less likely to get crusted with adherent blood and mucous. To emphasize: 'dripping wet' lubrication of tubes and guides is a crucial element in successful intubation.

15.3.3 Selection of tube and guidance method

Usually the radiologist is asked to help after simpler methods have failed. Before trying to pass a tube it is best to consult the referring clinician and see the patient. What job is the tube to do? What has been tried so far? What can be deduced about the reasons for failure? What tube is already in the patient? (If the same tube is wanted, have a new one on hand.) Will the physician allow a different tube to be used if you are unable to pass the one the patient has? What compromises is he willing to make? (For example, a polyvinyl tube or a Cantor single-lumen

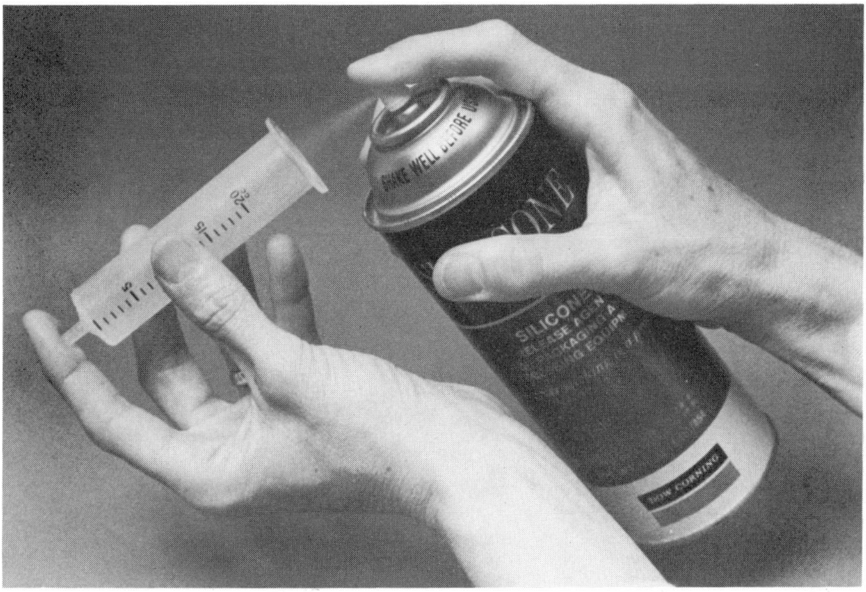

Fig. 15.1 Silicone lubricant can be sprayed into a syringe and injected into a nasoduodenal tube to reduce friction between tube and guide. The residual dissolved propellant carries the silicone forcefully down the tube even with a wire guide in the tube.

mercury-weighted tube placed in the distal duodenum or jejunum for decompression is better than a Miller Abbott tube that cannot be manoeuvred out of the stomach; a straight, small polyvinyl feeding tube placed across an anastomosis is better than a silastic tube coiled above it.) Where possible, tube systems which separate placement features from functional features have advantages in versatility and cost. It is useful to have on hand a supply of tubing, guides and fittings, as well as tools for their *ad hoc* fabrication (see Appendix).

Having decided what jobs the tube must do, how fast, for how long, in what order of priority, and what difficulties in placement are likely, the equipment and method is selected with regard to material, internal and external diameters, and position and size of holes, and length. (To estimate nasojejunal length measure nose to ear plus ear to xyphoid plus 25 cm.) Preliminary bench trials – marking lengths, lubricating and testing the frictional resistance to tube and guide movement – are invaluable.

(a) *Nasoduodenal diagnostic tubes*

For diagnostic and general short-term purposes the Bilbao–Dotter duodenal tube (Fig. 15.2) made of radio-opaque polyvinylchoride has

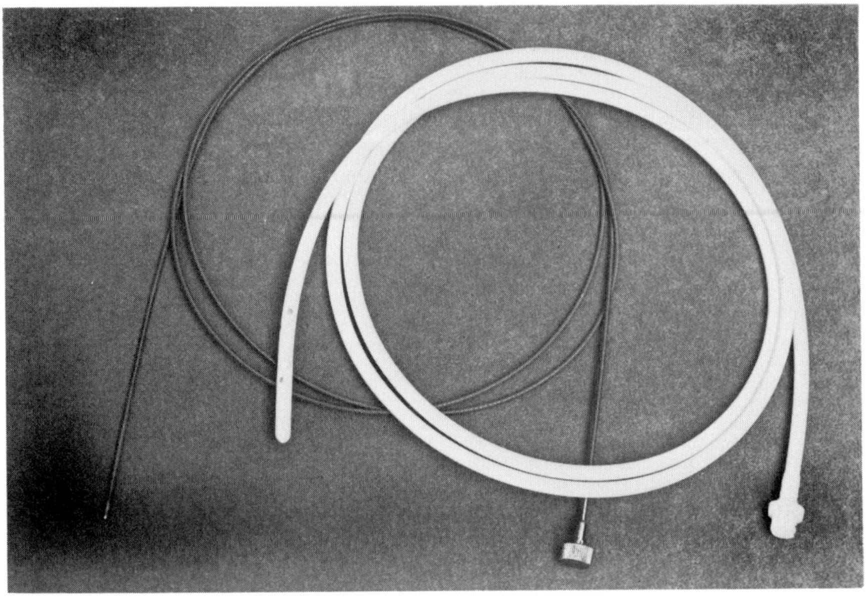

Fig. 15.2 Bilbao–Dotter duodenal tube with torque control wire guide.

been useful. It has a wide lumen and relatively thin wall (14 F, 5 mm OD and 4 mm ID) making it soft and flexible but able to accept wire stiffening guides 0.065 and 0.095 in (1.65 and 2.4 mm) diameter. These are teflon coated for reduced friction. The wire guides are double wound like speedometer cables so that a curve in the tip can be directed by turning a knob on the outer end (Gianturco, 1967).

The stiffening and controllability afforded by the guide make it easy to intubate the duodenum in less than 5 min. This tube is used for hypotonic duodenography (Bilbao *et al.*, 1967; Bilbao *et al.*, 1968) and for small bowel examination (Sellink, 1971). It is useful as a pilot tube beside which to pass a smaller feeding tube (*c.f.*) It has been adapted to accept, coaxially, adult and paediatric biopsy cannulas (Bilbao *et al.*, 1975). For this the tube is placed using the wire guide, enteric aspirations or other tests are done, and then the biopsy cannula is introduced coaxially. A double balloon modification has also been made for reflux study of enterobiliary anastomoses (Bilbao and Dotter, 1975).

A versatile, but more fragile and expensive, family of tubes is the Medi-tech system (Fig. 15.3). A control handle attached to four wires in the tube wall makes the tip easy to control. Medi-tech controllable catheters are made of radio-opaque polyvinylchloride in 5 to 13 F size and 30 to 270 cm long. Different varieties are used in the vascular system,

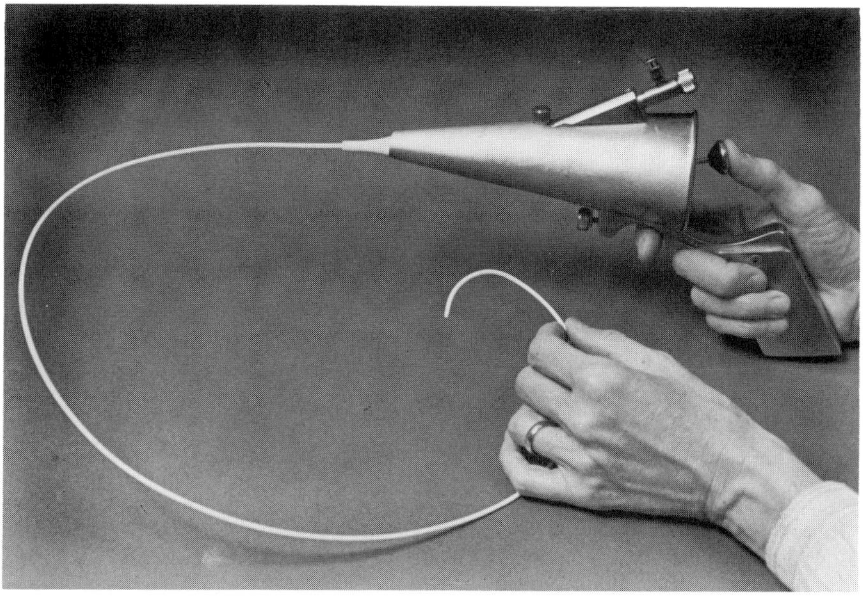

Fig. 15.3 Medi-tech steerable catheter and control handle. 'Y' adaptor on the handle allows the apparatus to be used with wire guide and contrast injection simultaneously. The single end hole allows catheter exchange over wire guide and the 'jet lumen-seeking' method of negotiating a narrowed lumen.

biliary, bronchial, genitourinary, and GI tracts, along with accessory baskets, biopsy instruments, forceps, and brushes. The GI catheters include an adaptation for intestinal biopsy (Linscheer and Abele, 1976) and another for intestinal decompression. GI tubes accept wire guides 0.025–0.052 in (0.6 mm–1.3 mm) diameter. The Medi-tech system has a 'Y' adaptor in the handle allowing contrast agent injection while a guide is in place. The catheter has a single end hole, useful for exchanging tubes over guide wires, and helpful in threading strictured or difficult routes (Ho and Lipinski, 1978; Dodds *et al.*, 1976; Wendth *et al.*, 1973) by demonstrating the lumen with injected contrast material.

Medi-tech GI catheters are sometimes not stiff enough to be effective but can be stiffened coaxially with a larger outer tube. At times it is difficult to manage the control handle and catheter simultaneously; these are minor disadvantages compared with its versatility and usefulness.

(b) *Intestinal decompression tubes*

Radiological placement methods can reduce the time required to pass a decompression tube from hours or days to minutes. There are several

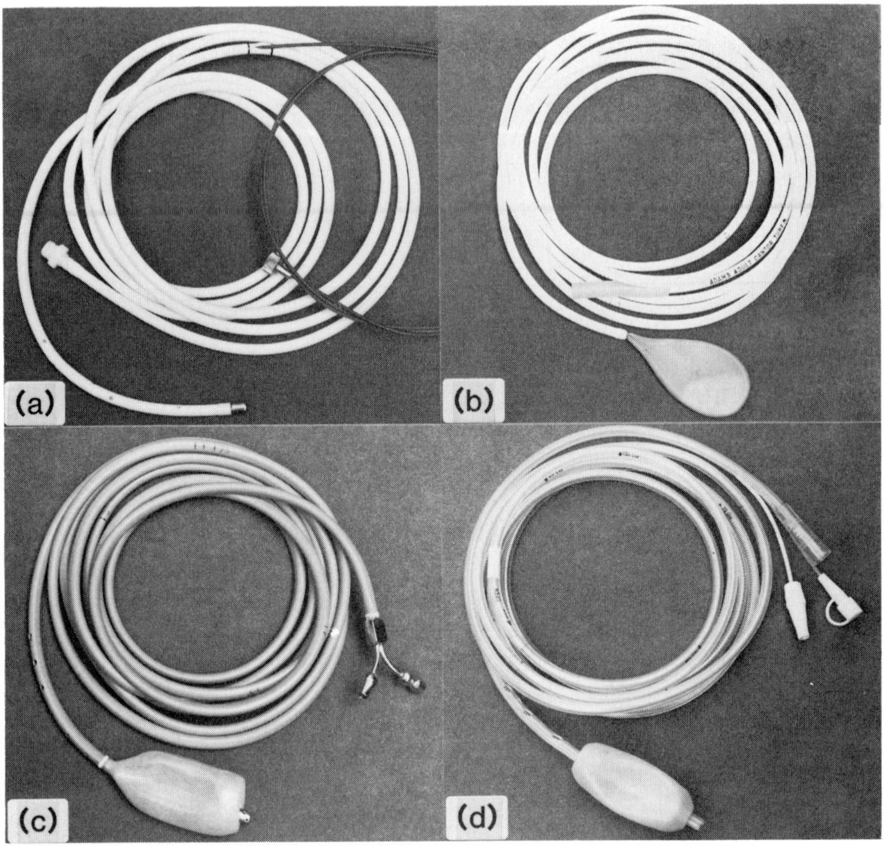

Fig. 15.4 Decompression tubes. (a) Shipps 14 F polyvinylchloride single lumen tube and guide. (b) Cantor 16 F polyvinylchloride single lumen mercury weighted ballon tube. (c) Miller–Abbott 16 F double lumen natural rubber mercury weighted inflatable balloon tube. (d) Medi-tech triple lumen mercury weighted inflatable balloon with sump conduit.

types of decompression tubes. The *Shipps tube* (Fig. 15.4(*a*)) is a long intestinal tube similar to the Bilbao–Dotter tube. It is made of radio-opaque polyvinylchloride 14 F, 90 in long with a slit 60 in from the tip for inserting a wire guide. There are three teflon-coated wire guides, double wound for torque control, each designed specifically for negotiating a troublesome part of the GI route. Using this intubation system and 10 min fluoroscopic time, Shipps and his associates succeeded in reaching the jejunum in 39% and the duodenum in 76% of 400 cases (Shipps *et al.*, 1979).

Single lumen tubes like the 16 F *Cantor* (Fig. 15.4(*b*), *Harris or Kaslow tubes* are made of radio-opaque polyvinylchloride. They have a closed balloon for a mercury bolus and a lumen large enough for a curved-tip torque control wire guide introduced through a side slit (Gianturco, 1967; Gelfand, 1978) or through the entire tube (Sargent and Meyers, 1969). A new tube should be used and the mercury bolus should be limited to 1.5 ml, lest its weight interfere with guided placement. With these long tubes friction is a prime consideration. The well lubricated tube must be forcibly 'milked' off the wire guide into the duodenum lest the guide be trapped in the tube by additional friction from bending around the duodenal flexures. Using guided placement of a Cantor tube in 25 patients, Sargent succeeded in intubating the duodenum in all 25 and the jejunum in 11 (44%).

Double lumen tubes like the *Miller Abbott Tube* (Fig. 15.4(*c*)) have the advantage of a balloon which can pass through the pylorus with a mercury bolus and then be inflated with air for rapid propulsion through the small intestine. However, it is not possible to stiffen them with a wire guide. The balloon is placed against the pylorus until peristalsis takes it through, a process taking hours or days but which is eventually successful in most patients (Smith, 1945; Deitel, 1967).

The *Medi-tech decompression tube* (Fig. 15.4(*d*)) is an elegant version of one reported by Edlich in 1967. It is made of 16 F polyvinylchloride and has both end and side holes. It has a fine coiled spring throughout the forward end to reduce friction, a sump conduit for decompression and (optional) a doughnut-shaped terminal balloon with a conduit for inflation. It is guided by a Medi-tech steerable catheter 7 F which is inserted through a slit in the rear. With his earlier tube Edlich succeeded in intubating the jejunum in less than 30 min in 96% of 30 cases with intestinal obstruction (Edlich *et al.*, 1968).

Which tube is best? All these decompression tubes are large, uncomfortable and begin to stiffen after about a week as the toxic plasticizer leaches out. In a normal dog's jejunum Murata *et al.* (1967) found that the Cantor polyvinylchloride tube with mercury bolus progressed faster than others tested. In my experience, any tube that can be persuaded to pass the pylorus is acceptable; any tube that can be placed promptly in the jejunum is a fast tube; all tubes, once in the jejunum, proceed promptly to an obstruction.

Decompression tubes also have diagnostic value. Barium injected though the tube may show the site and often the nature of small intestinal obstruction; it can differentiate unequivocally between mechanical obstruction and paralytic ileus. Immediately afterwards the barium can be removed by suction (Sargent and Meyers, 1969; Nelson and Christoferidis, 1968).

(c) *Feeding tubes*
Feeding tubes (Fig. 15.5) are made of *polyurethane*, *silicone rubber*, or *polyvinylchloride*. The first two have a mercury bolus for passage by gravity. They have so much inherent friction that wire guides are not useful, being difficult to retrieve once the tube is passed. I prefer polyvinylchloride tubes because they can be used with a wire guide. There are a number of methods for stiffening these sticky tubes, all intended to overcome friction. A gelatine guide is available to stiffen silicone rubber tubes. After use it is dissolved away by cold (not hot) water. Since frictional resistance increases with length, one way to make a stiffener retrievable is to insert it only a short distance inside the tube. A slit part way along the tube for guide insertion is one way (Fig. 15.6(*a*)). Using the rearmost side hole to insert it is another (Fig. 15.6(*b*)). Once the tube is in position, the wire guide is removed. One commercially available silicone rubber feeding tube is stiffened with an outer polyvinyl sheath (Fig. 15.6(*c*)); once in place the feeding tube is extruded from the outer tube by a jet of water (flow-guided principle) (Griggs and Hoppe, 1979). There are several other ways to deliver feeding tubes (Fig. 15.7). Polyvinyl tubes can be passed coaxially along preplaced wire guides. Silicone rubber and polyurethane tubes can be tip-connected using a gelatin capsule to a pilot tube. By cutting the ends off the capsules one can make a temporary ring-like coupler. The end hole of the pilot tube, being free, can be passed over a guide or used for lumen-seeking as described above. The capsule melts in a few minutes allowing removal of the pilot tube. Once placed, the tube should be tested for patency by injecting barium.

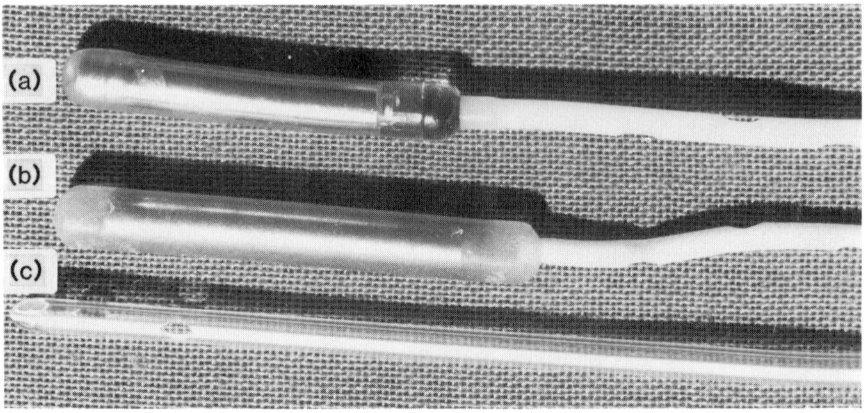

Fig. 15.5 Feeding tubes. (a) Polyurethane (Dobbhoff 8 F). (b) Silicone rubber (Keofeed 6 F). (c) Polyvinylchloride (Argyle 8 F).

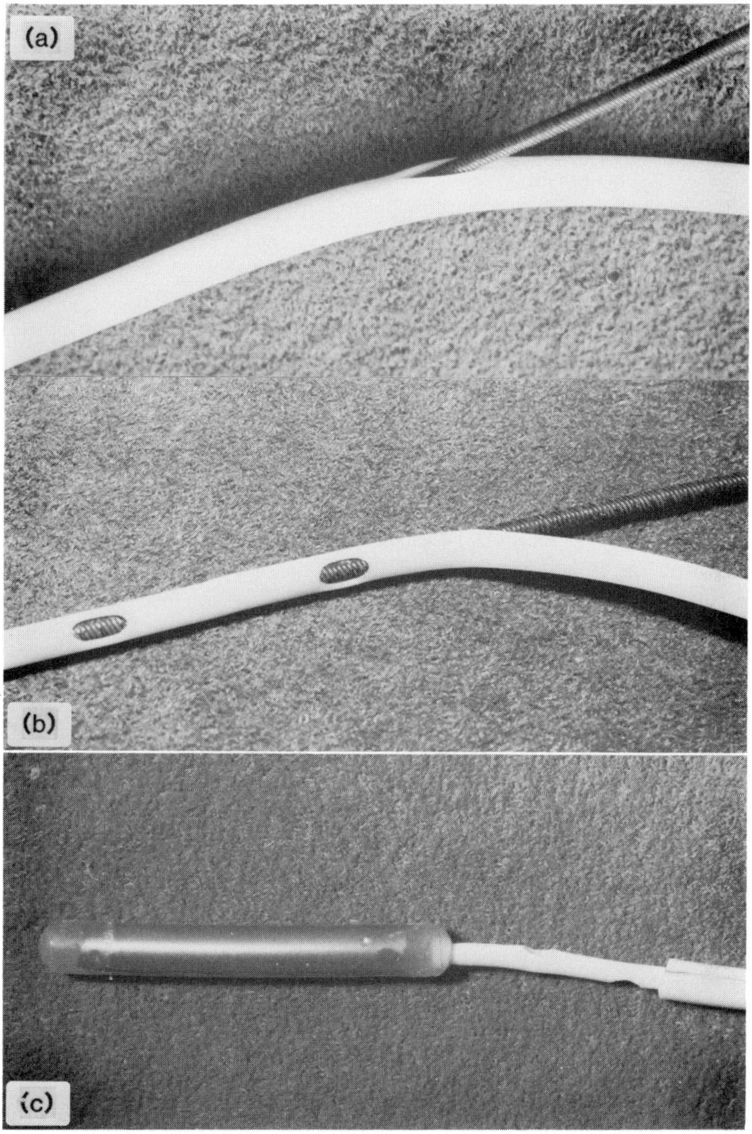

Fig. 15.6 Ways to stiffen a rubbery tube (frictional resistance increases directly with length). (a) Teflon-coated wire guide inserted through a slit 3 ft from the end of a Cantor polyvinyl tube. (b) Teflon-coated wire guide inserted in the rearmost side hole and advanced about 3 in to the tip of a polyurethane feeding tube. (c) Polyvinyl 10 F outer sheath stiffens this mercury weighted 5 F silicone rubber feeding tube. Once in place the inner catheter is extruded from the outer sheath by a jet of water (flow-guided principle).

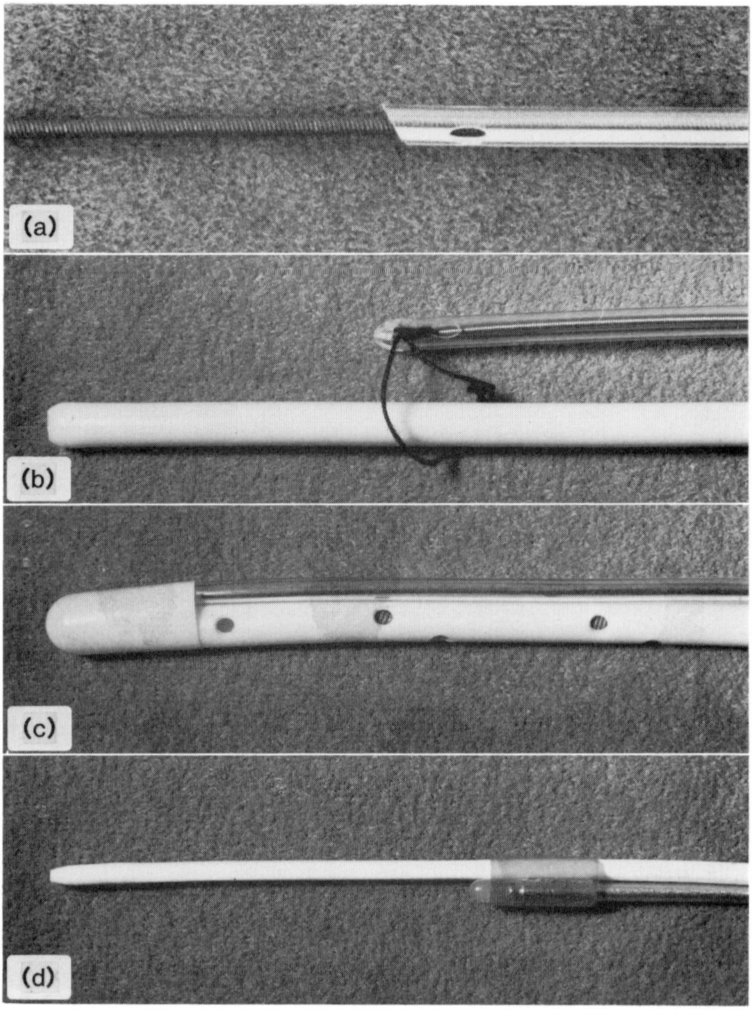

Fig. 15.7 Ways to deliver a limp tube. (a) Coaxially, over a preplaced wire guide. The tip has been cut off a polyvinylchloride feeding tube. (b) Outrigged 'piggyback' style, tethered with a suture to a preplaced Bilbao–Dotter tube. The vinyl feeding tube has been stiffened with a wire guide. (c) A polyvinylchloride feeding tube has been outrigged, jammed in half a gelatin capsule with a wire guide stiffened Bilbao–Dotter pilot tube. (d) Silicone rubber feeding tube collared by an amputated gelatin capsule to the pilot, a steerable Medi-tech catheter. The front of the steerable catheter has been left free to move.

15.4 METHODS

Premedication may make the stomach hypotonic and is best omitted except in infants where chloral hydrate is helpful. The patient normally lies supine. If the tube has a mercury weight, a 45° head-up tilt allows gravity to aid advancement.

The nasal fossa passes straight posteriorly from the nostril toward the ear. The passage is opened and gently intubated by using a nasal decongestant spray and then filling it completely with a local anaesthetic agent in water-soluble lubricating jelly. Enough should be used to anaesthetize the pharynx also. While the patient widely opens his eyes (and thereby the inside of his nose), the tip of his nose is elevated and the tube passed backwards along the nasal floor with a gentle oscillating or rotational movement of the tube. During all ensuing tube advancements one should always push gently backwards and downwards, not up into the turbinates.

The nasopharynx is straightened by extending the head. Although there is usually no problem intubating while the patient swallows a few sips of water, difficulties passing the pharynx may be resolved by fluoroscoping the patient in lateral view. It is then easy to advance the tube tip posteriorly past the epiglottis even in a patient who cannot swallow. In frontal view the tube will be seen to curve laterally around the larynx; any tube directly in the midline should be suspected of being misplaced in the trachea.

The oesophagus is more or less straight and a good place to hold the tube during insertion of a wire guide. The tendency for the guide to exit through a hole is thus minimized (Gelfand, 1978). Before the wire is inserted, a little barium is injected into the stomach.

The gastroesophageal junction passes obliquely posterolaterally; it directs the tube into the fundus lying in the left paravertebral gutter where the tube often coils. This is avoided by first turning the patient right side down or right prone oblique, allowing the stomach to fall toward the right, straightening the oesophagogastric junction, and directing the tube and guide toward the greater curvature. Manoeuvring the tube through the *pars media* which passes ventrally over the spine is also aided by placing the patient right side down, injecting some barium and air to separate the walls and show the route, and inserting the stiffening wire. Rotating the tube, pushing cephalad on the greater curvature, turning the patient prone, even knee–chest or semi–upright, all help to allow the stiffened tube to fall ventrally and to the right across the spine into the antrum lying in the right paravertebral gutter. The tube now must pass cephalad and posteriorly to the pylorus. This can be aided by putting the patient supine, head down, and pushing cephalad along the greater curvature, and then turning the patient to the left supine oblique position. By now barium should be showing the pylorus which can be seen and straightened as the stomach slumps to the left. The tube is now lined up with the pylorus and pushed up and to the right on the greater curvature, shaking the stomach gently as it advances. Difficulties at the pylorus are usually related to poor radiological demonstration, malalignment, or being impacted on a mucosal fold. The pylorus is most easily passed if it can be seen with contrast agent (a single 'end-hole' jet of contrast agent is ideal for this). Even when closed, it is not an impassable barrier. Emptying the stomach helps (Gianturco, 1967; Shipps *et al.*, 1979) as does lining up the thrust of the tube with the presumed orifice. Often the tube tends to push adjacent to rather than against the pylorus. The patient's efforts at breathing, shaking, and manoeuvring his own stomach can help here. The *superior duodenal flexure* is straightened in the left supine oblique position. It is helpful to push on the patient's back behind his duodenal bulb while he alternately protrudes and retracts ('undulates') his abdomen as the tube is advanced. The *inferior duodenal flexure* is straightened in the left lateral position. The tube must then cross the spine again, passing anterior, left and cephalad to the duodenojejunal flexure. At the *duodenojejunal flexure* the route is a hairpin-shaped bend passing anteriorly and caudally. The weight of an obese abdomen, abdominal muscles, pressure of the table top in the prone position and pressure from adjacent viscera all tend to keep the flexure acute. It is helpful to show the route with contrast agent, keep a little forward pressure on the tube, and try a number of manoeuvres to straighten the flexure long enough to allow the tube to pass. One can try to have the patient 'belly roll' ('suck up, push forward, bear down'), or adopt the knee–chest position or its equivalent with pillows, palpate and shake his abdomen, and so on. Having him watch the fluoroscope helps.

15.5 COMPLICATIONS

Some tube complications can be prevented by radiological guidance; among them the misplaced feeding tube or the blindly advanced, knotted decompression tube. No 'blind' way to ascertain correct stomach tube placement is fool-proof. Listening over the stomach for injected air did not detect a misplaced small feeding tube in the right main bronchus of an asymptomatic patient (Rombeau, 1979). Aspirating 'stomach' contents and listening for injected air did not detect decompression tubes passed inadvertently through basal skull fractures into the brain (Bouzarth, 1978; Gustavson *et al.*, 1978; Fremstad and Martin, 1976; Greogory *et al.*, 1978). Less spectacular, but more common, is the slightly misplaced feeding tube with some of the side holes above the cardia (making aspiration a potential hazard).

Other tube complications can be treated with radiological guidance. Obstructed feeding tubes can sometimes be cleared with wire guides. If this fails, they can be replaced using the 'piggyback' catheter exchange system already described. Long tubes tied into knots in the stomach can sometimes be untied by judicious manoeuvring under fluoroscopy. The manoeuvres used depend on individual circumstances, but useful principles include making the tube radio-opaque enough to be clearly visible fluoroscopically, reducing friction with silicone, and using wire guides or piggyback stiffeners to aid control of the tube. Catheter fragments in the jejunum can be snared via a guideable long intestinal tube (Bilbao *et al.*, 1971). Since 1971 improved equipment has become available, such as the Medi-tech catheter, stone retrieval baskets and snares developed for vascular catheters. A tube complication readily treated under radiological guidance is gaseous distention of the balloon of a single lumen long intestinal tube (Fricke and Niewodowski, 1976; Rozanski and Klenfeld, 1975). This complication may occur after prolonged intubation of ten days or more and may cause intestinal obstruction. The balloon can be easily and safely decompressed percutaneously using a Chiba 22 gauge 'skinny' needle (Coleman *et al.*, 1977).

15.6 RESULTS OF INTUBATION AT THE UNIVERSITY OF OREGON

Our own experience with feeding tube placement has been mainly where 'blind' placement has already failed in a patient with an abnormal gastrointestinal tract. In such cases we have used polyvinyl catheters 8 or 10 F size. In some, a Bilbao–Dotter tube with wire guide was placed first, following which the polyvinyl catheter, stiffened with a wire guide and with two or three loops of silk thread tied to it, was passed alongside the Bilbao–Dotter tube. In others a Medi-tech 10 or 13 F catheter with wire guide and single end hole was used to find and negotiate the lumen after which a double length wire guide was placed. The Medi-tech catheter was removed and a polyvinyl catheter was exchanged over the wire guide and left in place. We have done one case successfully using a polyvinyl feeding tube stiffened with a Cook deflector wire guide and several others with a simple wire guide stiffener. Using these methods in 29 consecutive patients aged 1 to 95 years old with various anatomical barriers we succeeded in intubating all but one (97%). The failure was in a patient later found to have a totally obstructed gastrojejunostomy.

Of 117 consecutive intubations for diagnosis, feeding or decompression we had only four failures, all of which were successful on a second attempt except for the totally obstructed patient mentioned above. Two of our three failures were attempted intestinal biopsies in children under three years old, and one was a Miller–Abbott tube placement. There were no failures with the Bilbao–Dotter tube. The overall success was 97%.

APPENDIX 15.1

INTUBATION EQUIPMENT AND SUPPLIERS

Medications

Item	*Purpose*	*Supplier*
1/4% Adrenaline	shrink nasal mucosa	Winthrop Laboratories 90 Park Ave., NY, NY 10016
2% Viscous lignocaine	topical anaesthetic agent	Astra Pharmaceutical, Inc. Worchester, Mass. 01606
Silicone spray	tube and guide lubricant	Dow Corning Corp. Midland, Mich. 48640
Stop-cock grease	guide lubricant	Dow Corning Corp. Midland, Mich. 48640
Elemental mercury	decompression tube balloon	
Barium Renografin 60, Gastrografin	GI demonstration	
Tincture of benzoin	taping tube	
Alcohol	clean tubing and patient before taping	
Chloral hydrate	premedication	
Empty gelatin capsules, assorted	temporary tube attachment	pharmacy

Tubes and tubing

	*Material and size			Side ports and tip			
Item	Mat.	Fr.	Length	No.	Tip	Purpose	Supplier
Nasal topical anaesthesia tube	PV	14	15 cm	0	metal end hole	nasopharyngeal anaesthesia	Homemade
Bilbao–Dotter	PV	14	125 cm	6	closed end	hypotonic duodenography	Cook, Inc. P.O. Box 439 Bloomington, Ind. 47401
Bilbao–Dotter	PV	14	125 cm	6	open end		Cook, Inc.
Oregon intestinal biopsy set	PV	14	125 cm	12	open end	suction biopsy	Cook, Inc.
Bilbao–Dotter Sellink modification	PV	14	160 cm		closed end	decompression tube	Cook, Inc.
Bilbao–Dotter	PV	12	160 cm		closed end	small bowel enema	Cook, Inc.
Shipps decompression tube	PV	14	90 in		closed end	decompression	Cook, Inc.
Bilbao–Dotter	PV	14	125 cm	0	closed end	*ad hoc* fabrication	Cook, Inc.
Bilbao–Dotter	PV	14	125 cm	0	open end	*ad hoc* fabrication	Cook, Inc.
Dobbhoff feeding tube	PU	8	43 in		mercury bolus		Biosearch Med. Products Raritan, N.J. 08869
Keofeed feeding tube	SR	6 to 18	36 in		mercury bolus		Hedeco (Health Dev. Corp.) Mt. View, Ca. 94043
Medpro feeding tube	SR	10, 7	36 in		closed end		Medpro Ltd. Sunprairie, Wisc. 53390
Argyle feeding tube	PV	5, 8, 10	36 in		closed end		Sherwood Medical Ind. St. Louis, Mo. 63103
Cantor decompression tube	PV	16, 12	8, 6 ft		balloon	decompression	Clay Adams of Beckton, Dickinson, Parcippany, N.J.

Tubes and tubing *(continued)*

	**Material and size*			*Side ports and tip*			
Item	*Mat.*	*Fr.*	*Length*	*No.*	*Tip*	*Purpose*	*Supplier*
Medi-tech intestinal decompression tube	PV	18, +8	8 ft + 150 cm		balloon	steerable catheter placement decompression	Medi-tech Cooper Scientific Corp. Waterton, Mass. 02172
Medi-tech steerable catheters	PV	13, 10, 8, 7	30–170 cm		directable	multipurpose	Medi-tech
Medi-tech biopsy set		10	150 cm		biopsy capsule		Medi-tech
Assorted silicone rubber tubing							Dow Corning Corp. Midland, Mich. 48640

*PV = Polyvinylchloride; PU = Polyurethane; SR = Silicone Rubber.

Wire guides

	Diam.	Length	Purpose	Supplier
	(in)	(cm)		
Angiography wire guides	0.035	145	stiffening tubing	Cook, Inc.
(teflon coated heavy straight	0.038	260	catheter exchange	P.O. Box 439
fixed core)	0.045	300	catheter exchange	Bloomington, Ind. 47401
	0.052	300	catheter exchange	
GI wire guides	0.065	125	duodenal intubation	
(teflon coated torque cables)	0.095	125	duodenal intubation	
Long torque cables	0.065	345	jejunal intubation	
	0.095	345	jejunal intubation	
Hubless torque cables	0.065	345	catheter exchange	Cook, Inc.
	0.095	345	catheter exchange	Cook, Inc.
Shipps wire guide set	0.065	125	jejunal intubation	Cook, Inc.
Gelatin guide				Hedeco
Defector wire guide				Cook, Inc.

Connectors, catheter accessories

Plastic Luer Lok adaptor	female Luer Lok to Tuohy-Borst adaptor (3–7 F catheter)	*ad hoc* fabrication	Cook, Inc.
		scavanged front and rear plastic and metal	
Side arm fitting	female side Luer Lok to male Luer Lok	closes flow around wire guide for injecting	Cook, Inc.
Multipurpose tubing adaptor	female to tapered hose end 10–30 F 20–40 F	*ad hoc* fabrication	Cook, Inc.
3-Way plastic stop-cocks			

Miscellaneous items

Rubber condoms	balloon fabrication
Hole punch, flaring tool 1.14 mm 0.45	*ad hoc* fabrication
Iris scissors	converting to open end catheters for coaxial passage over guide
Straight scissors	
Suture set	piggyback loop method
Assorted suture silk	piggyback loop method
Paper tape	sealing slit in tube
Scalpel, No. 11 blades	*ad hoc* fabrication
Syringes 5 to 60 cc	
Gauze 4 × 4, no cotton filling	traction on slippery tubes
Glass, straws	
Hypodermic needle, 21 gauge	mercury into Cantor tube
Elastic bandage 6 in wide, adhesive backed	immobilizing infants
Brat board	immobilizing infants

Fluoroscopy equipment

Fluoroscope	
Tilting table	
Foot board	
Shoulder braces	
Lead gloves	
Lead shield on table top	protect operator's hands during pharyngeal intubation under fluoroscopy

REFERENCES

Bilbao, M. K. and Dotter, C. T. (1975). Reflux cholangiography in sphincteroplasty or enterobiliary anastomosis. *Radiology*, **115**, 585–8.

Bilbao, M. K. *et al.* (1975). Small bowel biopsy by coaxial catheter. *Radiology*, **116**, 199–201.

Bilbao, M. K. *et al.* (1967). Hypotomic duodenography. *Radiology*, **89**, 438–43.

Bilbao, M. K., Krippaehne, W. W. and Dotter, C. T. (1971). Catheter retrieval of a foreign body from the gastrointestinal tract. *Am. J. Roentg. Radiat. Ther. Nucl. Med.*, **111**, 473–5.

Bilbao, M. K. *et al.* (1968). Hypotonic duodenography in the diagnosis of pancreatic disease. *Sem. Roentg.*, **3**, 280–7.

Bouzarth, W. F. (1978). Intracranial nasogastric tube insertion. (Editorial) *J. Trauma*, **18**, 818–9.

Coleman, S. L. *et al.* (1977). Nonoperative retrieval of an impacted long intestinal tube. *Am. J. Dig. Dis.*, **22**, 462–4.

Cowper, S. G. (1968). What's in PVC? (Letter to editor), the *Lancet*, **2**, 221.

Deitel, M. (1967). Successful use of the Miller-Abbott tube. *Can. J. Surg.*, **10**, 245–57.

Dodds, W. J. *et al.* (1976). Use of steerable catheter for intubating patients with Sencher's diverticulum. *Am. J. Dig. Dis.*, **21**, 47–48.

Duke, H. N. and Vane, J. R. (1968). An adverse effect of polyvinylchloride tubing used in extracorporeal circulation. *Lancet*, **2**, 21–23.

Editorial (1975). PVC, plasticizers and the pediatrician. *Lancet*, **2**, 1172.

Edlich, R. F. *et al.* (1968). New long intestinal tube for rapid nonoperative intubation. *Arch Surg.*, **95**, 443–50.

Fremstad, J. D. and Martin, S. H. (1976). Lethal complication from insertion of nasogastric tube after severe basilar skull fracture. *J. Trauma*, **18**, 820–2.

Fricke, F. J. and Niewodowski, M. A. (1976). Hazardous gaseous distension of intestinal balloons. *J. Am. Med. Ass.*, **235**, 2611–3.

Gelfand, D. W. (1978). An easy method for passing an intestinal intubation tube under fluoroscopic guidance. *Radiology*, **129**, 532.

Gianturco, C. (1967). Rapid fluoroscopic duodenal intubation. *Radiology*, **88**, 1165–6.

Griggs, B. A. and Hoppe, M. C. (1979). Nasogastric tube feeding, *Am. J. Nurs.*, **3**, 481–5.

Gregory, J. A., Turner, P. T. and Reynolds, A. F. (1978). A complication of nasogastric intubation: intracranial penetration. *J. Trauma*, **18**, 823–4.

Gustavson, S. *et al.* (1978). The accidental introduction of a nasogastric tube into the brain. *Acta Chir. Scand.*, **144**, 55–56.

Harris, P. D., Newhauser, E. B. D. and Gerth, R. (1964). The osmotic effect of water-soluble contrast media on circulating plasma volume. *Am. J. Roentg. Radiat. Ther. Nucl. Med.*, **91**, 694.

Ho, C. S. and Lipinski, J. K. (1978). Selective intubation of the afferent loop. *Am. J. Roentg. Radiat. Ther. Nucl. Med.*, **130**, 481–4.

Ingelfinger, F. J. (1978). Tubes. *Gastroenterology*, **74**, 310–18.

Linscheer, W. G. and Abele, J. E. (1976). A New directable small bowel biopsy device. *Gastroenterology*, **71**, 575–6.

MacIntosh, R., Muskin, W. W. and Epstein, H. G. (1963). *Physics for the Anesthesiologist*. 3rd edn., F. A. Davis Co., Philadelphia, pp. 157–237.

Murata, A. *et al.* (1967). The rate of progression of long intestinal tubes in a dog with a jejunal fistula. *Am. J. Dig. Dis.*, **12**, 1091–4.

Nelson, S. W. (1965). Facts versus folklore. *Am. J. Surg.*, **109**, 543.

Nelson, S. W. and Christoferidis, A. J. (1968). The use of barium sulfate suspensions in the diagnosis of acute diseases of the small intestine. *Am. J. Roentg. Radiat. Ther. Nucl. Med.*, **104**, 505–21.

Rombeau, J. L. (1979). (personal communication), University of Pennsylvania.

Rozanski, J. and Kleinfeld, M. (1975). A complication of prolonged intestinal intubation: gaseous distention of the terminal balloon. *Dig. Dis.*, **20**, 1067–70.

Sargent, E. N. and Meyers, H. I. (1969). Wire guide and technique for Cantor tube insertion; rapid small bowel intubation. *Am. J. Roentg. Radiat. Ther. Nucl. Med.*, **107**, 150–5.

Sellink, J. L. (1971). *Examination of the Small Intestine by Means of Duodenal Intubation*. H. E. Stenfert Kroese, N. V. Leiden.

Shipps, F. C. *et al.* (1979). Fluoroscopic placement of intestinal tubes. *Radiology*, **132**, 226–7.

Smith, B. C. (1945). Experiences with the Miller Abbott tube. *Ann. Surg.*, **122**, 253–9.

Wendth, A. J. *et al.* (1973). Hypotonic duodenography: a modified technique using the selector catheter system. *Radiology*, **108**, 274.

16 Tube placement by endoscopy

ROBIN TEAGUE

The development of fibreoptic endoscopy of the upper and lower gastrointestinal tract has provided the means for direct visual monitoring of tube placement. This has meant that areas of the intestine, which were difficult or impossible to intubate by conventional means, may now be explored. When a tube needs to be placed in the upper alimentary tract, the choice of techniques will be determined by several considerations, including the skills available at the time. An endoscopist may understandably choose to place a tube in the stomach or duodenum via a fibreoptic endoscope; if he were not available, radiology might serve equally well (Chapter 15). The comments made in Chapter 1 relating to tube materials, lubricants and guide wires are opposite when considering endoscopic tube placement.

Basically, there are three methods of endoscopic tube placement. The tube may be passed down the biopsy channel of the endoscope with the endoscope resting at, or near, the desired position. Secondly, it may be passed before endoscopy and then manipulated into its final position with forceps inserted down the biopsy channel of the endoscope. Thirdly, the tube may be held outside the endoscope and passed with it to the desired site. Double-channel instruments allow combinations of the three techniques to be used. Endoscopic tube placement is most commonly employed in the upper gastrointestinal tract, but some methods are particularly useful in the colon. Patient preparation for endoscopic tube placement is the same as is used for routine endoscopy.

16.1 TECHNIQUES FOR TUBE PLACEMENT

16.1.1 Insertion through the biopsy channel of the endoscope

This technique is extremely useful for the placement of small calibre feeding tubes (Table 16.1) into the duodenum or upper jejunum. The endoscope is passed until the distal tip lies at or near the required position. A tube is chosen which is preferably at least 0.3 mm smaller in

Table 16.1 Nasogastric feeding tubes. Narrow calibre feeding tubes (2.64 mm or less).

Type	*External diameter (mm)*	*Material*
Aldon feeding tubes	1.98 2.64	PVC (non-radio-opaque) PVC (non-radio-opaque)
East Grinstead feeding tube (fitted with male Luer)	1.8	PVC (radio-opaque)
Dobbhoff enteric feeding tube	2.64	Polyurethane (radio-opaque)
Wallace feeding tubes	1.65 2.64	PVC (non-radio-opaque)

external diameter than the biopsy channel of the endoscope (Table 16.1 and Table 16.2). The tube is generously lubricated with a silicone oil and is inserted down the biopsy channel until it can be seen through the endoscope. It is then placed in position under direct vision and the endoscope is withdrawn. At the same time as the endoscope is withdrawn from the patient the tube is fed into the biopsy channel so that its distal tip remains in position. It is obviously essential that the tube to be used is at least twice as long as the endoscope so that the endoscope can be completely withdrawn over the tube. It is also necessary to relax as much as possible any angulation of the endoscope and to maintain it as straight as possible.

During this procedure it may be helpful to position the distal opening of the tube against the mucosa whilst suction is applied at the proximal end with a pump or syringe. By this means the tubing can be made to adhere tightly to the mucosa and is less likely to be dislodged by

Table 16.2 Size of biopsy channel of gastroscopes.

Manufacturer	*Model*	*Size of channel (mm)*
ACMI	T × 8 T × 7 T × 82 (two-channel)	2.97 2.31 3.63 and 2.64
Fujinon	FGQBF	2.8
Olympus	GIF P2 JF B3 GIF B2 GIF K GIF D3 GIF Q TGF 2D (two channel)	2.1 2.1 2.9 2.9 2.9 2.8 2.8 and 3.7

withdrawal of the endoscope. This technique is therefore applicable when any size of tubing is used and when other methods of tube placement are employed. It is, however, limited to tubes having only one opening at the distal tip, and some double lumen tubes.

After withdrawal of the endoscope, tube position is verified radiologically. If the tube used is radio-opaque this can be performed directly. If not, contrast medium may be introduced down the tube. It is desirable that all tubes to be used for aspiration purposes should be radio-opaque, for otherwise the aspirate may be contaminated with contrast materials. In rare circumstances the position of the tube may need checking by reinsertion of the endoscope. This method is obviously unsatisfactory, involving further discomfort to the patient and the possibility of dislodging an already accurately placed tube.

16.1.2 **Endoscopic guidance of previously inserted tube**

This method is suitable for all calibres of tubing. The tube is inserted prior to endoscopy and its distal tip is placed as closely as possible to the desired position. The endoscope is then inserted alongside the tube until the distal tip is visualized. (It is surprising how such a familiar object as a nasogastric tube can appear totally alien when viewed down an endoscope.) The tube may then be manoeuvred into position under direct vision and a variety of methods can be employed to achieve this. Small calibre tubing can be grasped with standard biopsy forceps but it is best to use 'alligator jaw' or 'rat tooth' forceps which give a much firmer grip and can be used for larger calibre tubes. If the gape of the forceps is still not sufficient to grasp the tubing firmly, then diathermy snare wires or 'basket' type graspers can be used.

When a twin-channel endoscope is used it is possible to use a combination of biopsy channel tube insertion with forceps manipulation. The lubricated tube is inserted down one biopsy channel of the endoscope and the forceps are inserted down the other. When the tube protrudes from the distal tip of the endoscope it is grasped by the forceps and manoeuvred into its required position. This technique allows larger calibre tubes to be passed down the biopsy channel because of the larger size of the channel in these endoscopes (3.6–3.7 mm) and the fact that the tubes may be pulled from the distal tip of the endoscope as well as being pushed proximally. It is also possible to repeat this last manoeuvre until the endoscope has been completely withdrawn over the tube.

16.1.3 **Insertion of large diameter tubes**

There are times when it may be necessary to pass large calibre tubes (e.g. pressure recording devices) into areas of the intestine where direct intubation and endoscopic manipulation are impossible. This usually means the colon but the technique may also be useful in the upper gastrointestinal tract. The tubes used are too wide to be inserted down the biopsy channel and therefore it is necessary to carry them with the endoscope during insertion and then release them at the desired position. One method of doing this is to use a 10–20 cm length of braided nylon. A terminal knot is made in the line so that it may be grasped firmly with the endoscopic forceps. The other end of the nylon line is firmly secured to the tip of the tubing. The forceps are passed down the endoscope until they protrude from the distal tip. The knot is grasped with the forceps which are then withdrawn a few centimetres into the intrument. The endoscope and tube are then ready for insertion into the patient. The presence of the forceps in the biopsy channel of the endoscope may attenuate the deflection of the distal tip making endoscopy more difficult. However, if the forceps are withdrawn too far down the biopsy channel, considerable difficulty can be encountered when the time comes for the forceps to be protruded from the distal tip and the knot released. This is because redundant line lying in the end of the biopsy channel may obstruct the passage of the forceps. A further problem with this method is that, when single channel instruments are used, aspiration and biopsy are impossible. Alternatively the tube may itself be gripped by the biopsy forceps which are then partially withdrawn into the endoscope biopsy channel. This has particularly been used for the passage of polyvinyl feeding tubes by Atkinson (see Chapter 3).

16.1.4 **Placing very large calibre tubes**

This method had only been used by the author on one occasion to relieve obstruction in a Koch's ileostomy pouch, but it may be helpful in other situations. The Koch's pouch was obstructed owing to a torsion of the distal ileum. It was possible to pass a GIF P2 endoscope into the pouch, but on withdrawal torsion recurred immediately. In order to maintain drainage a large calibre (1.2 cm internal diameter) well lubricated rubber tube was placed over the endoscope and moved proximally (in the way that a stiffening tube is used on a colonoscope). The rubber tube was made 30 cm in length so that an adequate amount of endoscope was available, beyond the tube, for insertion. The endoscope was inserted into the pouch and the rubber tube slid forwards into position until it was seen down the endoscope to be lying in the pouch. The endoscope could then be withdrawn and the tube secured.

16.2 USES FOR ENDOSCOPIC TUBE PLACEMENT

16.2.1 **Diagnosis**

(a) *Radiology*

Most radiological investigations using fibreoptic endoscopes can be carried out with catheters inserted through the biopsy channel of the instrument during endoscopy. On rare occasions the presence of the endoscope may obscure the necessary radiology, or films may have to be taken over a long period when the presence of the instrument would occasion discomfort to the patient. In these situations the endoscopic placement of catheters may be helpful. The author has used the technique for small bowel enemas through pyloric stenosis and for investigation of gastric emptying in the presence of oesophageal stricture.

(b) *Aspiration*

Endoscopic tube placement has been used successfully by the author for aspiration of pancreatic juice during secretin/pancreozymin tests and for the sampling of the upper small intestinal flora. Even under normal circumstances conventional intubation techniques may prove difficult for these investigations. However, the presence of stricture or postoperative alteration of the anatomy may render conventional intubation impossible. In these circumstances endoscopic tube insertion may be the only method of achieving success and our experience is that, even in normal patients, the time taken for intubation is considerably reduced.

(c) *Biopsy*

Endoscopes can be used to carry Crosby capsules to the duodenum by passing the tubing of the capsule and endoscope together. On reaching the duodenum the capsule can be advanced into the jejunum, fired and then withdrawn with the endoscope (see Chapter 14). We have found this method cumbersome and prefer to manoeuvre the capsule through the pylorus using a separately passed endoscope and 'alligator' forceps. Similarly the 'Quinton' multiple biopsy tube can be steered through the pylorus, when difficulty is encountered during conventional passage, by using a 'basket' type grasper through the endoscope. In addition, even when a degree of pyloric stenosis exists, the passage of a good size endoscope (GIF D3 or T X 8) through the pylorus, using persuasive pressure, may dilate the channel sufficiently to allow the Crosby or Quinton to proceed.

16.2.2 **Therapy**

Apart from some limited research procedures, the therapeutic uses of endoscopic tube placement are confined to feeding liquid diets into the upper small intestine. A major advance in patient comfort has been the ability to deliver high calorie fluid feeds through small calibre tubes (Table 16.1). These tubes can usually be passed satisfactorily using their respective introducers when the upper gastrointestinal anatomy is normal. However, where postoperative or malignant distortion is present or where stenosis exists, then endoscopic placement is essential. These small tubes can be passed easily through the biopsy channel of the endoscope and it is often useful to have their introducer wire present to assist passage. Alternatively they can be manoeuvred into position using forceps when the endoscope has been passed separately.

ACKNOWLEDGEMENTS

I would like to thank Dr. A. Ellis and Mead Johnson for help and technical advice.

EQUIPMENT SUPPLIERS

Aldon feeding tube – Aldington Labs Ltd., Mersham, Ashford, Kent. Tel. 023-372482.

East Grinstead feeding tube – Roussel Labs Ltd., Roussel House, Wembley Park, Middlesex. Tel. 01-903 1454.

Dobbhoff enteric feeding tube – Viomedex Ltd., The Old Post, South Chailey, East Sussex. Tel. 0273-400130.

Wallace feeding tube – H. G. Wallace Ltd., Chandlers Row, Port Lane, Colchester, Essex. Tel. 0206-45133.

17 Colonoscopic polypectomy

CHRISTOPHER B. WILLIAMS

17.1 THE POLYP PROBLEM

The precise incidence of colonic polyps is unknown and no single quotable figure will ever emerge since the numbers of polyps found will depend on the detection method used and the population studied. Series based on use of a hand-lens to identify minute lesions in postmortem material may show 40–60% of colons to contain polyps (Atwater and Bargen, 1945; Arminski and Mclean, 1964; Hughes, 1968) whereas some hospitals employing the single-contrast barium enema technique will rarely demonstrate them.

In older patients in Western societies, the incidence is high compared to that in younger patients or other ethnic groups such as Japanese eating a traditional diet (Wynder *et al.*, 1969).

A colon 'polyp', defined as a projection above the mucosal surface, is of interest because of the 80% likelihood that it will be an adenoma – a neoplastic and potentially cancerous lesion generally accepted as the benign stage of the 'polyp-cancer sequence' (Muto, Bussey and Morson, 1975).

Estimates of the incidence of colon adenomas suggests that about 10% of a Western population will form one or more adenomas during their lifetime (Arminski and McLean, 1964); 5–10% of snared adenomas prove already to contain invasive carcinoma (Gillespie *et al.*, 1979) and this finding alone justifies the aggressive policy of removal of all colonic polyps unless there is excessive risk in doing so. No diagnostic method except section of the whole polyp determines its benign nature with certainty. Prior to the availability of fibre-endoscopic snare polypectomy the low incidence of invasive malignancy in adenomas less than 1 cm in diameter was used to justify the policy of surgical removal only of large lesions inaccessible to the rigid sigmoidoscope (Enterline *et al.*, 1962), with radiological follow-up of small lesions at yearly intervals. These small polyps may grow so slowly between serial radiological examinations as not to reach significant size during the patient's life-time

(Welin, Youker and Spratt, 1963) and sigmoidoscopic studies of small rectal polyps have shown that some may disappear (just as occasional larger polyps may 'auto-amputate' themselves spontaneously after torsion of the stalk). Repeated barium enemas are a heavy sentence for the patient and there is inevitable danger that malignant transformation may occur before the radiologist sees any significant change in size or shape to suggest that trouble is brewing.

Colonoscopy has changed the picture radically (Williams and Riddell, 1976; Gabriellson *et al.*, 1978; Theuerkauf, 1978), since snare polypectomy or electrocoagulation of smaller lesions is normally a quick procedure little, if at all, more upsetting to the patient than a diagnostic barium enema. The relative ease and sophistication of the equipment for fibre-endoscopic polypectomy can make even rectal polypectomy sometimes preferable with a fibrescope rather than the rigid instrument, except for patients with lesions in the lower rectum (up to 7 cm above the anal margin) where the likelihood of pain and the physical problems of manoeuvring the flexible instrument make general anaesthesia and the rigid scope advisable. This is especially true for any *large* polyp accessible to the proctosigmoidoscope since in the event of haemorrhage the surgeon has infinitely better control with artery forceps and sutures than the endoscopist has without them.

Even if beyond the reach of the proctosigmoidoscope, almost any polyp is now within the grasp of the endoscopist and, since successful instrument insertion is usually possible, the position of the polyp in the colon makes little difference technically; 90% of all adenomas seen endoscopically are less than 2 cm in diameter (Gillespie *et al.*, 1979) and are easily dealt with. It follows that nearly every polyp, regardless of site or size can be dealt with. Logistical considerations, however, cannot be ignored, especially in view of the considerable cost of the instruments, and the expertise, time and possible trauma involved. If the object is to diagnose and treat malignancy, 95% of polypectomies are 'negative'. If to *prevent* colon cancer, it is doubtful that direct proof of prophylaxis will ever be possible; firstly it would be unethical to have a matched but untreated group of polyp patients and secondly, even after successful polyp 'clearance' and follow-up, adenoma-forming patients are likely to remain at high risk for colon cancer compared to the rest of the population (Sherlock and Winawer, 1977). Indirect evidence is available from the massive proctosigmoidoscopic screening surveys of Gilbertsen (1974) showing that the anticipated incidence of rectal cancer can be reduced by destruction of polyps, as Bussey and Morson (1978) have similarly described in the postoperative follow-up of the rectum of *polyposis coli* patients. Colonoscopic polypectomy patients are a particularly heterogeneous group, since colon polyps are usually symptomless and are either discovered by chance in patients presenting with functional bowel disorder (25% of our series), as a result of investigation of rectal bleeding (which sometimes appears to derive from coexisting haemorrhoids in 50%) or from follow-up examinations after previous polypectomy or cancer surgery.

The logistical implications and the need for a clear perspective about the polyp problem are intensified by the need for such follow-up regimens. Many authors such as Kirsner (1960) have described a 30–40% yield of adenomas over an average 8–10-year follow-up period after polypectomy using rigid proctosigmoidoscopy and barium enema. Fibreoptic endoscopy will make such follow-up more accurate but much more expensive; possible compromises will be considered later (see Section 17.8) but there is a clear need to decide among those requiring follow-up which factors constitute signs of 'high-risk', justifying extra expense and more frequent examination. Lovett (1976), for instance, has shown that a family history of colon cancer place first degree relatives at great risk; other predictive factors include previous cancer and numerous or malignant polyps. Gilbertsen (1974) wittily estimated the expense of his follow-up arrangements as being marginally cheaper than waiting to operate on eventual cancers. Bloom *et al.* (1973) could easily justify the expenditure on in-patient colonoscopic polypectomy compared with operative polypectomy, and the economics are actually more favourable than this, since most polypectomies can be performed on an out-patient basis. Taking both the initial polypectomy and life-long follow-up together, with increasing numbers of patients diagnosed by better endoscopic and radiological technique (towards a possible maximum 10% of the population) it is easy to understand Kern's (1976) nightmare vision of an endless chain of people colonoscoping people. His message is a good one: we have the means to attack and possibly prevent colon cancer (Wolff and Shinya, 1978) but our strategy must be as simple and as economic as possible. This chapter outlines some of the principles for the campaign.

17.2 SELECTION OF PATIENTS

Now that colonoscopy renders snare polypectomy or other methods of polyp fulguration so easily possible, nearly all colonic polyps should be dealt with, but there are exceptions. The commonest presentation is of one or more polyps seen, often by chance, on proctosigmoidoscopy or barium enema; colonoscopy is contraindicated only if the polyps are characteristic thread-like postinflammatory polyps in a patient with known ulcerative colitis or the hundreds occurring in classical (and histologically confirmed) adenomatous 'familial *polyposis coli*'. Even very large polyps often prove resectable and at least a diagnostic colonoscopy is indicated to check both the main lesion and for any smaller polyps missed on X-ray. A very elderly patient with a tiny 'ring shadow' on X-ray in the proximal part of a redundant colon or above severe diverticular disease might be spared vigorous colonoscopy. Dubious shadows on barium enema are sometimes better checked with repeat radiology if there is any reason against colonoscopy, since it can be tedious and difficult to be absolutely certain endoscopically that nothing has been missed. Paediatric colonoscopy and polypectomy presents no special difficulty (Burdelski, 1978; Deum *et al.*, 1977).

All available information is considered when planning the colonoscopy; some patients will need admission, blood-grouping, extra bowel preparation or special equipment and accessories. Any patient with a polyp of 2 cm or greater head-diameter may bleed and therefore needs overnight stay and blood available (Buhler *et al.*, 1979). Patients with a single small polyp demonstrated in the left colon on a high quality air contrast barium enema may need only limited preparation and no sedation, whereas others with poor X-rays, a tortuous colon or multiple polyps are likely to need both total colonoscopy and some sedation. Other complicating factors such as anticoagulant therapy, a cardiac pacemaker or cardiorespiratory disease may also modify arrangements, although with due precautions none of them contraindicate polypectomy.

17.3 SELECTION OF INSTRUMENTS

Colonoscopic polypectomy can be performed with any instrument, any snare wire and almost any electrosurgical unit; unnecessary mystique has grown up around what is usually a very rapid and easy procedure. Nonetheless polyps have a perverse habit of being situated around acute bends or behind prominent folds and it is desirable to have an up-to-date instrument in good condition so as to obtain the best possible view. Most endoscopists routinely use a single channel instrument for the purpose because it will angle and manoeuvre more easily, but in a few circumstances (e.g. during bleeding or for multiple polypectomies), a two-channel instrument does have advantages. The length of endoscope used is quite unimportant, but all accessories are bought long so that they will fit any instrument. The snare wires commercially produced by different companies are satisfactory; those with relatively thick braided-wire loops are safer than the thinner types which can cut through a stalk before enough coagulation has been produced. The handle of commercial snares has advantages for routine use (Cotton and Williams, 1980) over the handleless home-made snare (Sugarbaker and Vineyard, 1974; Bess and Spencer, 1979), because the position of the handle gives a good idea about the degree of snare-loop closure, which may be difficult to judge when managing awkwardly placed polyps. Modern small solid-state electrosurgical units also have a safety advantage over the older general-purpose operating theatre diathermy machines, mainly because they are less confusing to use and have a restricted power output, so that serious mistakes of power setting are unlikely; an apparently small adjustment on the dial of some older machines will result in a surprisingly large change in power output which can cause uncontrolled transection of the stalk. Some units have sophisticated inbuilt safety circuitry to warn of any failure including inadvertent touching of the instrument with a live snare-wire or loss of contact with the patient plate; these are theoretically attractive features but cannot prevent much more common and dangerous errors (such as forgetting to readjust the power dial before starting polypectomy) and may mean that the unit cannot easily be used with all endoscopes.

In equipping for polypectomy, apart from the colonoscope and electrosurgical unit, a single snare handle with several long teflon tubes and spare long wires are needed (check that the snare chosen will fit the particular instrument channel). Polyp retrieval is conveniently possible with the same snare loop, so 'grasper' or retrieval forceps are not really necessary, but insulated 'hot-biopsy' forceps (Williams, 1973) are invaluable for electrocoagulation of small polyps and telangiectases.

Some thought should also be given to the question of low-pressure carbon dioxide (CO_2) insufflation apparatus (Rogers, 1974); although this is not currently used by the majority of endoscopists there may be increasing medicolegal pressure to employ it in the future.

17.4 BOWEL PREPARATION

Polypectomy must take place in a clean field, both to see clearly what is going on and so that no fluid or residue is present to conduct 'leak currents' away from the polyp stalk, which will reduce heating efficiency very markedly. If CO_2 insufflation is not being used it is desirable that the proximal colon is also free of stool so as to remove the potential hazard of hydrogen or methane generation by colonic bacteria (Ragins, Shinya and Wolff, 1974; Bond and Levitt, 1975).

For total colonoscopy or total colon clearance relatively powerful measures are required, and the patient needs to understand the important role that he has in following the diet and purge regimes towards an eventually successful procedure. Most institutions and endoscopists (Teague and Manning, 1977) seem to have settled on much the same basic regime, starting with 24 hours of soft or low-residue diet, followed by a clear fluid regime (including alcoholic drinks if wanted) on the day before colonoscopy. The purgative dose (castor oil 30 ml, senna liquid 80 ml, magnesium sulphate or citrate) is taken either in the early afternoon, so as to get a diarrhoeal result before sleep, or last thing at night. Unfortunately the time-lag between dose and result will vary between 1–12 hours in different patients and adaptability is needed. The best final clearance is with one or more tap water enemas, sometimes with an added contact laxative (bisacodyl, oxyphenisatin) administered by the patient or a motivated nurse. The tube saline-lavage method (Hewitt, Reeve and Rigby, 1973) or drunk saline method (Levy *et al.*, 1976) have protagonists and can produce an impeccably clean bowel in a few hours, although a large quantity of clear fluid sometimes may require aspiration and some patients unpredictably dislike these regimes more than the purge-enema approach (Downing *et al.*, 1979). The drinking of 5–10% mannitol solution, a non-absorbed sugar with a sweet taste, is preferred by many patients but is theoretically unwise because of the danger of hydrogen production and explosion hazard during electrosurgery (Milito *et al.*, 1979; Bigard, 1979). Our experience is that *any* preparation regime gives poor results in 10% of patients, being more or less successful in the remaining 90%; the likelihood of good results will be improved by discussing with the patient what he is prepared to take, relating to the success or failure of previous preparations before X-ray.

Limited bowel preparation, using two disposable hypertonic phosphate (Fleet's, Fletcher's) enemas, given together 20 minutes before examination, and with no prior dietary regime or aperients, is highly successful in cleaning the left colon as far as the splenic flexure; provided that there is no diverticular disease or stricture to impede evacuation and no cause of diarrhoea (colitis, etc.) to make the distal colon refill at once, the view for limited examination or fibre-sigmoidoscopy is excellent. Polypectomy is justified with such limited preparation providing CO_2 is used, the right colon has been well seen on air-contrast barium radiography, and the polyp is not so big as to make a slow procedure likely – an avalanche is most unwelcome during polypectomy.

17.5 MEDICATIONS

17.5.1 **Sedatives**

The mucosal aspect of the colon has no pain sensation; the discomfort which occurs during insertion of the colonoscope is due to stretching of the serosa or the mesentery and no sensation of any kind should be felt during a normal polypectomy. If pain does occur, it may be due to overdistension with air (there is a subconscious tendency to be overactive with the air-button in the quest for a good view during polypectomy) or due to full thickness heating of the bowel wall by electrocoagulation; the first cause is rapidly reversed by aspiration so that if the pain does not disappear and heat damage is possible, further electrocoagulation is abandoned.

Diagnostic colonoscopy is frequently possible with little or no sedation but it is a mistake to have any dogmatic policy, either always to sedate or never to. Colonoscopy is an intrinsically unnatural act, sometimes exquisitely painful and often extremely uncomfortable for a short time; if the patient may need a follow-up examination it is unwise to risk alienating him on the first visit. After polypectomy repeated follow-up is likely so that if the initial examination was reasonably easy it is logical to try the *next* colonoscopy with little or no sedation so as to make subsequent visits possible without an escort.

Although very small doses of intravenous diazepam (3–7 mg) will often be sufficient to cause pain tolerance and a degree of amnesia it would be unsafe to allow car-driving afterwards. With the larger doses of intravenous diazepam (5–10 mg) and pethidine (25–50 mg) normally used it is essential that the patient is escorted so as not to fall downstairs or make other errors of judgement. The use of naloxone (0.4 mg i.m.), given towards the end of the procedure if the patient is obviously over-sedated, means that all patients are fit to walk out within half an hour, although a few may feel overdistended, sick or faint from residual air (if CO_2 has not been used) and the vasovagal stimulus of the procedure.

Acute over-sedation or respiratory depression are readily reversed with intravenous naloxone and the stimulant effect of inserting the colonoscope, but a ventilating bag (Ambu) is always available as well as an emergency box and well-rehearsed 'arrest' procedure. Even unsedated patients may become hypotensive and faint during either bowel preparation or colonoscopy and problems must be anticipated.

With the judicious use of kindness, talking and some sedation even the most apprehensive patient will tolerate colonoscopy and polypectomy well. Over-sedation or general anaesthesia is hazardous in concealing pain, which warns of errors of technique or impending bowel damage. On the other hand it may be unkind to subject even a very stoical patient to the hour or more of manipulation which may be required for several difficult polypectomies, without some sedation. The future trend should be towards rapid colonoscopy with little or no sedation, but never at the price of cruelty.

17.5.2 **Antispasmodics**

The other medication which is of great use during polypectomy is an intravenous antispasmodic such as hyoscine-*n*-butyl bromide (Buscopan) or glucagon. These agents greatly help the search for small polyps or the visualization of large ones, especially in the presence of an obviously 'spastic' colon or diverticular disease. Such spasticity is usually apparent during insertion, which is not helped by antispasmodics (Norfleet, 1978).

Since the effect of intravenous antispasmodics lasts only about five minutes it is logical to give them after full insertion, before inspection on withdrawal. Hyoscine (if available) is preferable, being cheaper than glucagon and without nauseating effect, but if the anticholinergic does not work well, glucagon will do so and is an excellent second-line agent.

17.6 COLONOSCOPIC TECHNIQUE

The details of colonoscopic technique (Cotton and Williams, 1980) are irrelevant to this chapter, but certain broad principles are, since they affect the timing and technique of polypectomy.

Every colon differs, so that there is never a single correct technique or strategy. Some apparently short colons on barium enema prove extremely difficult to intubate, whereas other redundant bowels or those with diverticular disease or previous pelvic surgery may be surprisingly easy. The view of the stretched colon during insertion may also be quite different to that of the straightened colon and convoluted mucosa on withdrawal. Therefore a luminal view and careful inspection should be sought as far as possible during insertion and any polyps which might be missed on withdrawal dealt with at once, especially any small ones suitable for 'hot-biopsy'.

By keeping loops to a minimum and straightening out the colonoscope where possible by 'pull back' after every major bend, manipulation of the instrument is made much easier, both for viewing and insertion. On the other hand if intravenous sedation has been used it will be maximally effective for only about five minutes and during this time the colonoscope should be inserted as far as possible without any avoidable delay. Once fully inserted, straightened out and withdrawn, reinsertion is usually (but not always) easy.

With modern very flexible and acutely angling colonoscopes it is often possible to ignore temporary formation of loops providing that the tip is progressing without pain, which indicates that the mesentery is sufficiently long and elastic. It is also unnecessary to resort to formal tricks such as the 'alpha-loop' manoeuvre which were previously required to coax the partially angling tip of a stiff instrument around the acute sigmoid-descending colon junction. Some colons however, have congenitally mobile mesenteries or 'mesocolons' causing normally retroperitoneal or fixed regions such as the descending or ascending colon to loop oddly, making normal straightening of the instrument impossible and persistent loops and some pain inevitable.

17.6.1 **Is total colonoscopy necessary?**

The goal for any screening examination of an organ must be to examine it completely; routine total colonoscopy is a desirable (Coller, Corman and Veidenheimer, 1975) but unfortunately unattainable ideal. Foregoing remarks on the logistics of polyp incidence and the unpredictable difficulties of colonoscopy mean that the potential patient load for colonoscopy and polypectomy is beyond the capability of the rather few individuals who can claim to be able to do total colonoscopy easily – then in only 95% of patients.

Even a high quality air-contrast barium enema can miss small polyps (Williams and Riddell, 1976; Thoeni and Menuck, 1977) but the miss rate for large polyps or cancers in the right colon on good films carefully reviewed is so low as to make total colonoscopy relatively unrewarding compared to the high yield in the left colon. If the right colon is poorly shown, or the patient has multiple polyps or malignancy in the left colon to increase the likelihood of synchronous cancer (Heald and Lockhart-Mummery, 1972), or polyps elsewhere in the colon, total colonoscopy *is* well justified. In high risk patients where the caecum cannot be reached during colonoscopy a barium enema can be performed immediately after colonoscopy; the radiologist will be helped if all air is aspirated and the examination finished using CO_2 insufflation, since this is rapidly absorbed and the colon deflates to make contrast coating easier.

In patients shown on a recent and convincing barium enema to have only one or two left colon polyps it is our practice to perform only limited colonoscopy to the splenic flexure, and after limited bowel preparation, which makes it a walk-in/walk-out procedure for the patient. By this means up to seven or eight patients can be examined, with any necessary polypectomies, in a half-day session, the decision having been taken during a previous X-ray review session as to which patients require full bowel preparation and total colonoscopy and which do not.

17.6.2 **Is fluoroscopy necessary?**

During the learning phase of colonoscopy, it is highly desirable to have access to fluoroscopy to understand the sequence of events during a 'difficult' colonoscopy, and also the logical remedies. With further practice it is not difficult to wean the procedure from dependence on X-ray, which often wastes more time than it saves. With a little thought it is obvious when a loop is forming during insertion, since the tip is seen to advance little when the instrument is pushed in a lot; the remedy is simply to pull back straight (at which time resistance is felt and the tip begins to slide back) and to try again. X-ray only proves that the loop exists and does not normally help in straightening it out or in steering in afterwards. X-ray does help to explain occasional complex loops and very rarely may give the endoscopist the courage and information with which to unravel them; it will also help to decide more quickly when pelvic adhesions are the cause of fixation of the colonoscope tip and the examination must be abandoned.

For localization of lesions found, the combination of endoscopic judgement, abdominal transillumination by the colonoscope, visualization of palpating fingers and distance (measured on the straightened colonoscope), combine to give a remarkably precise estimate of polyp site. The distance rules are surprising to anyone who has not seen them proved with fluoroscopy, because the caecum and ileocaecal valve are only 70–80 cm from the anus on withdrawal, the splenic flexure at 50 cm and descending colon at 40 cm (Fig. 17.1). During insertion or if a loop remains, the measurements will be much greater, so that the distance-rule presumes insertion beyond the splenic flexure and sufficient expertise to judge that the instrument is indeed straight. This does not mean that fluoroscopy is necessarily more accurate, because it can be equally difficult to interpret the site of the instrument tip from the limited view on the intensifier screen, and just as possible to make mistakes if the visual and distance rules are not also taken into account. Fluoroscopy is therefore a desirable luxury, invaluable for the beginner but dispensable thereafter.

A polyp is sometimes suspected of malignancy from its broad base, hardness or irregular configuration; although polypectomy is still indicated for histological confirmation it would obviously be useful for subsequent surgery to leave a site marker even if fluoroscopy has been used for localization. The use of submucosally injected Indian ink has been reported (Ponsky and King, 1975); others have passed the instrument to the site during operation, but failing this, the surgeon may

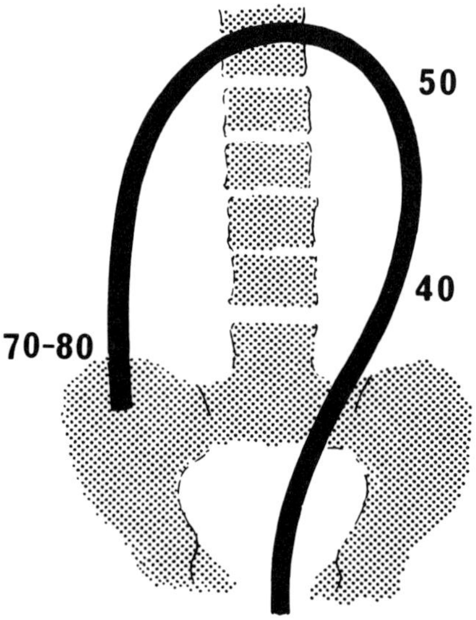

Fig. 17.1 Distances measured on the shortened colonoscope.

be forced (if he sees and feels no evidence of the polypectomy site) to make a suitably wide resection.

17.7 SNARE POLYPECTOMY TECHNIQUE

Once a polyp is seen, and the patient's position changed if necessary to make it hang down suitably, lassooing is usually not a problem. The use of rotatable snare is occasionally convenient but snare placement is normally by manipulation of the colonoscope tip. With the right combination of knob and shaft handling, using an assistant if necessary, the loop can be coaxed over almost any polyp. Since the loop emerges from the colonoscope tip and the tip steers it over the polyp, sometimes the view of the polyp must be lost completely before the loop is correctly placed, having then to be closed blindly.

The snare loop closes by pulling back into its teflon sheath, so that before closure the teflon should be pushed out onto the exact site on the stalk where snaring is intended. The correct sequence of events for polypectomy is shown step-wise in Fig. 17.2. The snare is ideally closed half-way down the stalk to avoid damage to the bowel wall while ensuring that all polyp tissue is removed together with any possible invasion into top of the stalk. If in doubt, especially if the stalk is thick or tapers to the top, the loop is placed *high*, which makes for easier and

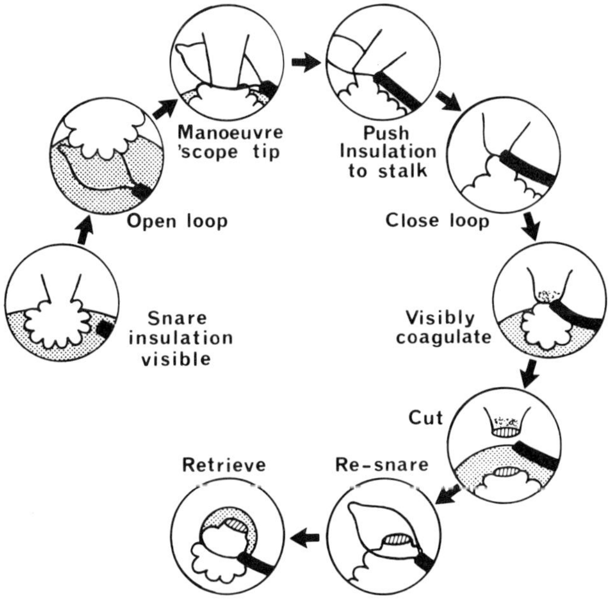

Fig. 17.2 The sequence of events during polypectomy.

safer electrocoagulation and also means that some stalk is left to resnare if there is any bleeding.

Once snared, the polyp is moved to and fro to check that the loop is correctly placed, and to find the best position which will hold the stalk and head as clear as possible from the bowel wall. The patient plate, connections and power setting are checked and electrocoagulation (Curtiss, 1973) starts on a low setting of 'blend' or 'coagulation' current. Current is applied in repeated short bursts, the setting being turned up if necessary so that gradual swelling and slow whitening of the stalk occur below the snare. Not until visible change (and often smoke) are apparent is it safe to tighten the loop further and start transection, still with very short current applications and turning down the power setting if too rapid cutting seems to be occurring.

If nothing happens after 15–20 seconds of action the circuit and snaring should be rechecked since either something is wrong or there is a larger than usual quantity of tissue within the snare loop (either a fat stalk or part of the polyp head also entrapped). Once closed the snare loop can often not be disengaged and replaced, having cut deeply into stalk tissue, which is why it is better to take time and care in placing the loop initially rather than regret it later. If any bad misassessment has been made it is possible either to cut the snare wire near the handle and to withdraw the colonoscope or to pass in a paediatric endoscope beside the colonoscope and use forceps to help disentangle the embedded loop.

Broad-based or sessile polyps with no stalk can often be removed piece-meal in multiple bites, if necessary in several sessions spread out over a few months so as to allow any heat-damaged tissue to separate; it is a well recognized phenomenon that on re-examination residual polyp tissue may have disappeared (Livstone, Greene and Troncale, 1973).

Very large polyps with head diameters over 4 cm are fortunately rare (Fig. 17.3) since they pose an awkwared dilemma for the endoscopist, tending to bleed (Buhler *et al.*, 1979) owing to the likelihood of a substantial leash of feeding vessels. For large polyps it is first necessary to decide whether the snare loop can be placed over the polyp head and then, if so, whether the stalk diameter will permit conventional snare electrocoagulation in one go. If in doubt the head is tackled piece-meal, taking only as much tissue at a time as can be seen; it is disastrous to end up with the snare embedded irrevocably and out of sight. Very large polyps in the low sigmoid colon can sometimes be intussuscepted and pulled out of the anus (Gillespie *et al.*, 1978). Others with a fat stalk (over 1.5 cm in diameter and at least 2 cm long) can be managed by a 'two-snare bipolar technique' (Williams and de Peyer, 1979; Williams, 1980), but this is technically difficult and only justified if there is judged to be a serious risk of bleeding. A loose home-made snare loop (Sugarbaker and Vineyard, 1974; Bess and Spencer, 1979) is first placed at

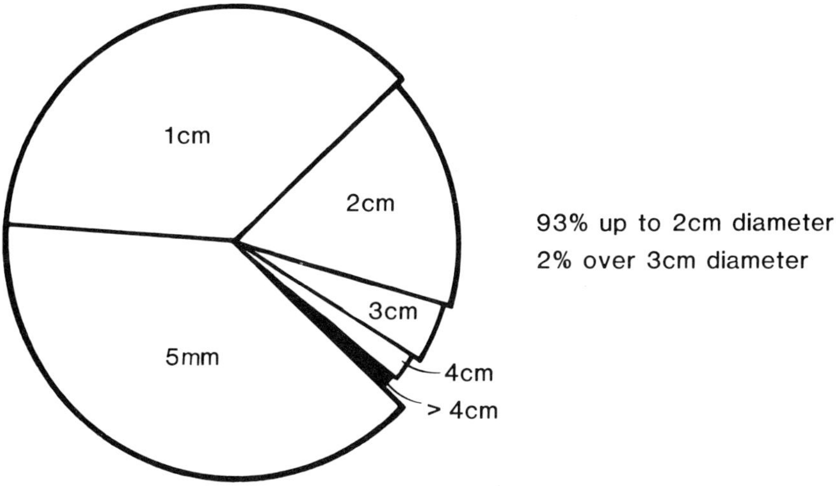

Fig. 17.3 Size and shape of polyps.

the base of the stalk and the colonoscope withdrawn leaving this loop in position and secured with an artery forceps. The colonoscope is then reinserted and the top of the stalk conventionally snared, electrocoagulation being normally managed between the tight apical snare and the loose basal one, *no patient plate being used* (Fig. 17.4). This technique avoids any leak currents, any danger of bowel wall damage and also means that the basal loop is available as an immediate tourniquet if there is bleeding.

Very large sessile polyps cannot usually be managed endoscopically (Buhler *et al.*, 1979), but it is justified to inspect them and attempt at least partial removal. When snaring a broad-based or sessile polyp the snared

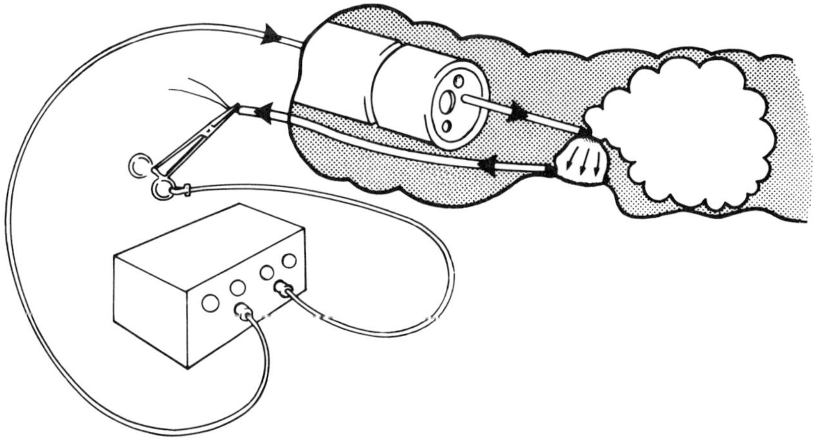

Fig. 17.4 Two-snare 'bipolar' polypectomy.

portion is moved to and fro with the teflon sheath; if the bowel wall moves too, the loop must be repositioned or there will be full-thickness damage. Although there are a few reports of success in removing large sessile lesions (Christie, 1978; Dagradi, 1976) such heroics should be left to experts and then only considered in patients where the endoscopic risk is justified but surgery is not.

17.7.1 **Management of small and multiple polyps**

Small (2–5 mm) polyps in the rectum are most commonly non-neoplastic 'hyperplastic' or 'metaplastic' polyps (Morson and Dawson, 1972); above the rectosigmoid junction biopsies of numerous similarly small polyps show that over 60% are adenomas and only 13% are metaplastic (Table 17.1). Snaring such small lesions is tedious and the specimen difficult to recover, although it can be aspirated into a 'mucus trap' placed in the suction line. A simpler, safer, and quicker technique is the use of the insulated 'hot-biopsy' forceps (Williams, 1973) to sieze, pull-up, electrocoagulate and biopsy the polyp in a sequence which takes only 5–10 seconds. The technique, conventionally used, will only biopsy and destroy polyps up to 7 mm diameter although a thin stalk of a larger polyp can be grasped and locally coagulated.

If 5–10 small polyps are seen it is prudent to check that there are not scores of even smaller ones present which may not be apparent to the naked eye. The 'dye-spray' technique, in which a non-absorbed blue dye (indigo-carmine 3% or dilute blue fountain pen ink) is washed onto the mucosal surface by a catheter, will sometimes reveal further otherwise transparent and invisible 1–3 mm polyps which can be biopsied for histological opinion. Although such tiny excrescences can also be seen projecting up in the reflected 'highlights' or 'light reflex' of the endoscope, only when outlined by the blue dye can they be acurately seen for biopsy taking. On histology some 'polyps' may prove to be normal mucosa or lymphoid follicles. Although conventionally the absolute diagnosis of familial adenomatous *polyposis coli* is said to rest on the presence (in the fixed colon specimen) of more than 100 adenomas as well as intramucosal microadenomas (Bussey, 1975), colonoscopy and

Table 17.1 Histology of 700 small colonic polyps (2–7 mm diameter) biopsied and destroyed by 'hot-biopsy'.

Adenoma	60%
Normal	19%
Metaplastic	13%
Heat-damaged	8%

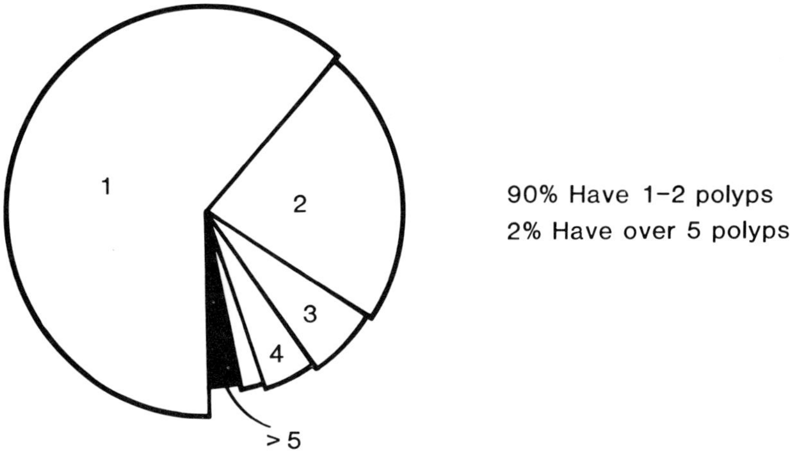

Fig. 17.5 Numbers of polyps snared per patient.

dye-spray reveals a 'multiple adenoma' subgroup of patients, often elderly, with 30–70 adenomas. These patients probably do not merit colectomy, but will need frequent check colonoscopy and destruction of polyps over some years.

Fortunately extremely few patients (Fig. 17.5) have five or more adenomas and of these several are usually tiny and rapidly managed by 'hot-biopsy' leaving only two or three for snaring and retrieval.

Multiple polypectomies present no problem, 30–60 or more hamartomas (Peutz-Jeghers, juvenile polyposis) being snareable in an hour or so because they need not be recovered; the problem is in individual retrieval of adenomas, which necessitates withdrawal and reinsertion of the colonoscope for each polyp. The overtube can be left *in situ* and the colonoscope withdrawn and reinserted through it for polyps in the proximal colon; several polyps can be caught in a single snare or basket but otherwise there is no obvious short-cut. The use of a wash-out enema has the obvious disadvantage that a malignant polyp may not be recovered. If the colonoscopy is difficult and multiple polyps are found the only solution is to retrieve the largest and most sinister-looking and to leave the others behind, washing out as many as possible thereafter.

17.7.2 **Management of malignant polyps**

Surprisingly often malignancy (carcinoma invading an adenoma) is only diagnosed by the histopathologist, and although a broad, firm stalk, a hard, ulcerated or irregular head or very pale colour all raise endoscopic suspicions, this can be in error. The pathology report thus often comes as a surprise after an apparently successful polypectomy and presents a difficult exercise in decision-making.

About 5% of colonoscopic polyps prove to be malignant (Wolff and Shinya, 1975; Gillespie *et al.*, 1979), 1% being polypoid carcinomas completely composed of cancerous tissue without any remnant of the adenoma from which they presumably arose (Muto, Bussey, and Morson, 1975).

In making his histological report, the pathologist will consider the grade of malignancy (well, average or poorly differentiated) the adequacy of resection and whether lymphatics or blood vessels in the head or stalk are invaded. A poorly differentiated (anaplastic) tumour, incomplete resection or involvement of lymphatics or blood vessels indicates survery, whereas a well-removed, well differentiated cancer has an excellent prognosis (Shatney *et al.*, 1974; Lock *et al.*, 1978; Wolff and Shinya, 1975), certainly better than that of colonic surgery with its well known risks, especially in elderly patients. Coutsofides *et al.* (1979) have suggested that malignancy in any villous adenoma or a sessile tubulovillous adenoma justifies surgery because of an increased tendency to early metastasis in such lesions.

Our own follow-up of more than 40 patients with malignant polyps over four years has resulted in only one known case of fatal metastases, a patient who had refused all forms of follow-up. Follow-up colonoscopy, other than a check examination at 2–3 months to ensure that the polypectomy site is healed, is unlikely in any case to affect prognosis, since the danger (if any) comes from spread to local lymph nodes – outside the endoscopist's territory. Such local spread is only rarely reported from pedunculated malignant adenomas (Jackson, 1970) and even more rarely if the above histological criteria are followed. In the individual case, especially a younger patient, full consultation is necessary between endoscopist, pathologist and surgeon to decide whether further resection is necessary; usually it is not.

17.7.3 **Complications of polypectomy**

Several large series have been published demonstrating a complication rate around 2% for polypectomy, haemorrhage being much the commonest problem, perforation unusual and mortality rare (Frühmorgen and Demling, 1979; Rogers *et al.*, 1975; Smith, 1976). The reasons for haemorrhage, largely occurring after snaring thick-stalked polyps, have been mentioned already and, except by the use of piecemeal removal (which is unpopular with the histolopathologist) or when two-snare techniques are possible, it seems likely that occasional bleeds will continue to happen.

(a) *Haemorrage*

Bleeding when it occurs, is usually visible immediately after transection. Any remaining stalk is quickly resnared and the snare handle taped shut for 10–20 minutes, after which the loop can usually be safely released. Local 'button' electro-coagulation is sometimes effective and the local infusion of 1–2000 ml of iced water and adrenalin solution is easy, although unlikely to influence an arterial bleed. The rule of thumb is that a 'spurter' *must* be actively controlled, but that an 'oozer' will stop of its own accord. Because bleeding can be expected to be self-limiting, albeit after several hours and 3–5 units blood transfusion, there is every reason to be slow in resorting to surgery. Blood loss can however be massive and careful patient assessment is essential. Arteriographic cannulation and infusion of pitressin is a more elegant alternative to surgery (Carlyle and Goldstein, 1975), but not often used, presumably because surgeons are more available than suitably skilled radiologists.

Secondary haemorrhage can occur 5–14 days after removal of large polyps, probably when local sepsis causes separation of the coagulum. This secondary bleeding can be substantial, but is normally self-limiting. It is rarely necessary either to transfuse or take any endoscopic measures, but after removing a large polyp the patient must be warned of the possibility and the potential need for observation in hospital. There is no evidence that a soft or low-residue diet is important in preventing trouble during the healing of postpolypectomy ulcer (Hambrick, 1976) but it seems sensible to avoid constipation or use of purgatives other than mild bulking agents or lubricants.

(b) *Perforations*

Perforations are rare, probably because most polyps are stalked, and this rarity suggests that thorough electrocoagulation is safe and desirable to avoid haemorrhage. Delayed perforation has however been reported (Dagradi, Norris and Weingarten, 1978) and coincidental operation after polypectomy not infrequently shows a full-thickness reaction with local adherence of small bowel loops or omentum to the polypectomy site. Sessile polyps should therefore be removed with caution in small bits, which can be fairly rapidly transected since the blood vessls are small compared to those in a stalk. The snared sessile polyp is moved around before starting coagulation to ensure that the bowel wall does not move too – a sign of 'tenting' of the full thickness of the wall into the snare loop.

(c) *Burns*

External burns to either patient or operator are unusual and of no consequence at the low power settings used. Pacemaker patients with modern units seem to be unaffected by high-frequency electrosurgical currents, but it is better to check with the manufacturers concerned before the procedure.

(d) *Carbon dioxide*

A single fatal explosion has occurred during colonoscopic polypectomy (Bigard, 1979) but with the increasing use of short instrument, rapid colonoscopy and limited bowel preparation the risks of residual hydrogen or methane must increase (Bond and Levitt, 1975; Ragins, Shinya and Wolff, 1974). The most effective reduction in explosive gas concentration should be achieved by several repeated aspirations with reinsufflation, and if bowel preparation is less than ideal aspiration/re-insufflation should not be forgotten even when CO_2 is used. CO_2, as a rapidly absorbed gas (Rogers, 1974), has advantages over air for routine colonoscopy, since, particularly in patients with diverticular disease, stricturing or functional bowel disorder, large quantities of gas can be trapped in the right colon and may cause worse symptoms after colonoscopy than the instrument does during it.

17.7.4 **Safety during polypectomy**

The patient, being conscious during the procedure, will warn of any local heating at the patient-plate contact, of any serosal pain or of over-distension. The electrosurgical unit is engineered to high standards and relatively unlikely to fail. By contrast, those parts of the system which are accessible to human manipulation and human failings are a source of accident – especially the leads, power-settings and the snare loop. The leads, especially to the patient-plate, are prone to fracture after repeated use, particularly if kinked or too tightly coiled. The resulting intermittent contact is potentially highly dangerous, since at one moment there is no effect, the power setting is increased and then at the next moment too-rapid cutting occurs. Faulty leads must be replaced and regular checks are recommended.

The basis of good electrosurgical practice is a regular routine, always checking connections and power-settings before starting, always ensuring that the snare insulation is kept in view so as to prevent contact between 'live' metal and endoscope. If obvious coagulation does not result in a reasonable time all factors are double-checked.

The use of 'safety-cord', 'by-pass wire' and other safety measures to avoid misuse of high frquency current is reassuring but of minor importance compared to the potential human errors in polypectomy.

17.8 FOLLOW-UP AFTER POLYPECTOMY – BARIUM ENEMA OR COLONOSCOPY?

With the passage of years all of us are more likely to form colonic adenomas, especially someone who has a previous history of adenoma or colon cancer. Follow-up studies with proctosigmoidoscopy or barium enema have shown up to 40% recurrence of adenomas over an 8–10 year period (Kirsner *et al.*, 1960; Brahme *et al.*, 1974), and the yield would presumably be even higher with the greater accuracy of colonoscopy. The intention of follow-up however is not simply to find small adenomas but to prevent cancer and the risk of this is small; Muto, Busse and Morson (1975) reported a 1.3% incidence of new cancers at an average interval of 12 years in patients with previous colon cancer. It is therefore necessary to keep a sense of proportion and to make arrangements for the individual patient which ensure that contact is not lost in the long-term and that the method and frequency of follow-up examinations are acceptable. It is certainly possible to miss polyps at colonoscopy (Laufer *et al.*, 1976; Miller and Lehman, 1978; Gelfand, Wu and Ott, 1979; Nivatvongs and Goldsberg, 1979); as well as on barium enema (Leinicke *et al.*, 1975; Wolff *et al.*, 1975; Williams, 1975; Thoeni and Menuck, 1977) so that a check examination is often advisable at six months to one year after polypectomy. What happens thereafter must depend on circumstances (Gabriellson *et al.*, 1978), depending on the degree of risk for the individual patient and on available facilities. The minimum reasonable follow-up would be an air-contrast barium enema every three years. An annual visit for procto-sigmoidoscopy is conventional, partly so as to give an opportunity to ask about rectal bleeding. Some patients, however, will have had inaccurate barium enemas in the past and may have no confidence in radiological surveillance; equally there are others who are impossible or exceedingly hard to colonoscope to the caecum. The choice must therefore relate to individual experience of the two techniques (Dodds, Stewart and Hogan, 1977), bearing in mind that it is possible to 'get the best of both worlds' by unsedated limited colonoscopy or fibre sigmoidoscopy (Lambert *et al.*, 1978, Marks *et al.*, 1979) (using CO_2) followed by immediate barium enema.

The frequency of examination is also a matter of judgement. A patient with multiple adenomas or one or more malignancies is presumably at 'high-risk' compared to another with only a single benign adenoma, although these risk-factors are not well-defined. It has been estimated that it takes 5–7 years for an adenoma to reach 'significant' size and longer still for it to become malignant (Muto, Bussey and Morson, 1975); exceptions seem to occur and we have experience of several patients developing a carcinoma within a year of an apparently normal total colonoscopy.

The frequency of examination must therefore be 'tailor-made' to the individual, maximum follow-up might involve annual alternating (or even combined) colonoscopy and barium enema lengthening the intervals between examinations if nothing is found. A few frail and elderly patients may not justify any follow-up at all. Most will need some modified regime coupled with a warning to report at once any rectal bleeding or change in bowel habit. The use of screening occult-blood tests (Haemoccult, Occultest) for follow-up is unproven, but although known to produce a significant yield of both false positive and negative results (Winawer *et al.*, 1976) may be a useful intermediate step, partly as a way of keeping in touch with the patient and focusing his attention on the need for prophylaxis.

REFERENCES

Arminski, T. C. and McLean, D. W. (1964). Incidence and distribution of adenomatous polyps of the colon and rectum based on 1000 autopsy examinations. *Dis. Colon Rect.*, **7**, 249–61.

Atwater, J. S. and Bargen, J. A. (1945). Pathogenesis of intestinal polyps. *Gastroenterology*, **4**, 395–408.

Bess, M. A. and Spencer, R. J. (1979). Colonoscopic polypectomies. *Mayo Clin. Proc.*, **54**, 32–34.

Bigard, M. A. (1979). Fatal colonoscopic explosion during colonoscopic polypectomy. *Gastroenterology* (in press).

Bloom, B. S. *et al.* (1973). Fiberoptics: morbidity and cost. *New Eng. J. Med.*, **288**, 368–9.

Bond, J. H. and Levitt, M. D. (1975). Factors influencing the concentration of combustible gases in the colon during colonoscopy. *Gastroenterology*, **68**, 1445–8.

Brahme, F. *et al.* (1974). Metachronous colorectal polyps. *Colon Rect.*, **17**, 166–71.

Buhler, H. *et al.* (1979). Large colonic polyp: endoscopic or surgical removal? *Schweiz. Med. Wschc.*, **109**, 619–20.

Burdelski, M. (1978). Endoscopy in paediatric gastroenterology. *Europ. J. Paediat.*, **128**, 33–39.

Bussey, H. J. R. (1975). *Familial Polyposis Coli*, John Hopkins University Press, Baltimore and London.

Bussey, H. J. R. and Morson, B. C. (1978). Familial polyposis coli. *Gastrointest. Tract Cancer*, Plenum Publishing Corporation, London, pp. 275–93.

Carlyle, D. R. and Goldstein, H. M. (1975). Angiographic management of bleeding following transcolonoscopic polypectomy. *Am. J. Dig. Dis.*, **20** (12), 1196–201.

Christie, J. P. (1978). Colonoscopic removal of sessile lesions. *Dis. Colon Rect.*, **21**, 11–14.

Coller, J. A., Corman, M. L. and Veidenheimer, M. C. (1975). Colonic polypoid disease: need for total colonoscopy. *Am. J. Surg.*, **131**, 490–4.

Cotton, P. B. and Williams, C. B. (1980). *Practical Gastrointestinal Endoscopy*, Blackwell Scientific Publications, Oxford.

Coutsotides, T. *et al.* Colonoscopy and management of polyps containing invasive carcinoma. *Ann. Surg.*, **188**, 638–41.

Curtiss, L. E. (1973). High frequency currents in endoscopy: a review of principles and precautions. *Gastrointest. Endosc.*, **20**, 9–12.

Dagradi, A. E. (1976). Colonoscopic polypectomy excision of a huge villous adenoma. *Am. J. Gastroent.*, **66**, 464–6.

Dagradi, A. E., Norris, M. E. and Weingarten, Z. G. (1978). Delayed ('blow-out') perforation of sigmoid following diagnostic colonoscopy. *Am. J. Gastroent.*, **70**, 317–20.

Deum, F. *et al.* (1977). Colonoscopic polypectomy in children. *Am. J. Dis. Child.*, **131**, 566–7.

Dodds, W. J., Stewart, E. T. and Hogan, W. J. (1977). Role of colonoscopy and roentgenology in the detection of polypoid colonic lesions. *Am. J. Dig. Dis.*, **22**, 646–9.

Downing, R. *et al.* (1979). Whole gut irrigation: a survey of patient opinion. *Brit. J. Surg.*, **66**, 201–2.

Enterline, H. T. *et al.* (1962). Malignant potential of adenomas of the colon and rectum. *J. Am. Med. Ass.*, **179**, 322–30.

Frühmorgen, P. and Demling, L. (1979). Complications of diagnostic and therapeutic colonoscopy in the Federal Republic of Germany. Results of an enquiry. *Endoscopy*, **11**, 146.

Gabriellson, N. *et al.* (1978). Malignancy of colonic polyps. Diagnosis and management. *Acta Radiol.*, **19**, 479–95.

Gelfand, D. W., Wu, W. C. and Ott, D. J. (1979). Extent of successful colonoscopy – its implication for the radiologist. *Gastroent. Radiol*, **4**, 75.

Gilbertsen, V. (1974). Rectosigmoidoscopy and polypectomy in reducing the incidence of rectal cancer. *Cancer*, **34**, 936–9.

Gillespie, P. E. *et al.* (1979). Colonic adenomas – a colonoscopic survey. *Gut*, **20**, 240–5.

Gillespie, P. E. *et al.* (1978). Snare polypectomy by sigmoid-rectal intussusception. *Br. Med. J.*, **1**, 1395.

Hambrick, E. (1976). The fate of colonoscopic polypectomy sites. *Dis. Colon Rect.*, **19**, 400–4.

Heald, R. J. and Lockhart-Mummery, H. E. (1972). The lesion of the second cancer of the large bowel. *Brit. J. Surg.*, **59**, 16–19.

Hewitt, J., Reeve, J. and Rigby, J. (1973). Whole-gut irrigation in preparation for large-bowel sugery. *Lancet*, **II**, 337–40.

Hughes, L. E. (1968). The incidence of benign and malignant neoplasms of the colon and rectum – a post mortem study. *Aust. N.Z. J. Surg.*, **38**, 30–35.

Jackson, B. R. *et al.* (1970). Adenomas of the colon the rationale for resection as the treatment of choice. *Dis. Colon Rect.*, **13**, 47–58.

Kern, F. Jr. (1976). Presidential address: good news and bad news. *Gastroenterology*, **71**, 537.

Kirsner, J. B. (1960). Polyps of the colon and rectum; statistical analysis of a long-term follow-up study. *Gastroenterology*, **39**, 178–82.

Lambert, R. *et al.* (1978). Fibrerectosigmoidoscopy: results of 47 cases. *Nouv. Presse Med.*, **7**, 4213–5.

Laufer, I., Smith, N. C. W. and Mullens, J. E. (1976). Correlation of endoscopy and double contrast radiography in the early stages of ulcerative and granulomatous colitis. *Gastroenterology*, **70**, 167–170.

Leinicke, J. A. *et al.* (1975). Comparison of roentgen and colonoscopic examination for demonstrating polypoid large bowel lesions. *Invest. Radiol.*, **10**, 448.

Levy, A. G. *et al.* (1976). Saline lavage: a rapid effective and acceptable method for cleansing the gastrointestinal tract. *Gastroenterol*, **70**, 157–66.
Livstone, E. M., Greene, F. L. and Troncale, F. J. (1973). Colonoscopic polypectomy: a caveat. *New Engl. J. Med.*, **288**, 1304–5.
Lock, M. R. *et al.* (1978). The treatment of early colorectal cancer by local excision. *Br. J. Surg.*, **65** (5), 346.
Lovett, E. (1976). Family studies in cancer of the colon and rectum. *Brit. J. Surg.*, **63**, 13–18.
Marks, G. *et al.* Sigmoidoscopic examinations with rigid and flexible fibreoptic sigmoidoscopes in the surgeon's office. *Dis. Colon Rect.*, **22** (3), 162.
Milito, G. *et al.* (1979). Is mannitol hazardous in bowel preparation? *Gut* (in press).
Miller, R. E. and Lehman, G. (1978). Polypoid colonic lesions undetected by endoscopy. *Radiology*, **129**, 295–7.
Morson, B. C. and Dawson, I. M. P. (1972). *Gastrointestinal Pathology*, Blackwells Scientific Publications, Oxford, p. 547
Muto, T., Bussey, H. J. R. and Morson, B. C. (1975). The evolution of cancer of the colon and rectum. *Cancer*, **36**, 2251–70.
Nivatvongs, S. and Goldberg, S. M. (1979). Management of patients who have had polyps containing invasive carcinoma removed via the colonoscope. *Minn. Med.*, **62**, 197–9.
Norfleet, R. G. (1978). Premedication for colonoscopy. Randomised double-blind study of glucagon vs placebo. *Gastrointest. Endosc.*, **24**, 164–5.
Ponsky, J. L. and King, J. F. (1975). Endoscopic marking of colonic lesions. *Gastrointest. Endosc.*, **22** (11), 42–43.
Ragins, H., Shinya, H. and Wolff, W. I. (1974). The explosive potential of colonic gas during colonoscopic electrosurgical polypectomy. *Surg. Gynec. Obstet.*, **138**, 554–6.
Rogers, B. H. G. (1974). The safety of carbon dioxide insufflation during colonoscopic electrosurgical polypectomy. *Gastrointest. Endosc.*, **20**, 115.
Rogers, B. H. G. *et al.* (1975). Complications of fibreoptic colonoscopy and polypectomy. *Gastointest. Endosc.*, **22** (2), 73–77.
Shatney, C. H. *et al.* (1974). The treatment of pedunculated adenomatous colorectal polyps with focal cancer. *Surg. Gynec. Obstet.*, **139**, 845.
Sherlock, P. and Winawer, S. J. (1977) The role of early diagnosis in controlling large bowel cancer *Cancer*, **40**, (suppl. 5), 2616–9.
Smith, L. E. (1976). Complications of colonoscopy and polypectomy. *Dis. Colon Rect.*, **19**, 407–12.
Sugarbaker, P. H. and Vineyard, G. C. (1974). Colonoscopy in the management of disease of the colon and rectum. *Surg. Gynec. Obstet.*, **138**, 581–3.
Teague, R. H. and Manning, A. P. (1977). Preparation of the large bowel for endoscopy. *J. Intern. Med. Res.*, **5**, 374–7.
Thoeni, R. F. and Menuck, L. (1977). Comparison of barium enema and colonoscopy in the detection of small colonic polyps. *Radiology*, **124**, 631–5.
Theuerkauf, F. J. (1978). Rectal and colonic polyp relationships via colonoscopy and fibresigmoisoscopy. *Dis Colon Rect*, **21**, 2–7.
Welin, S., Youker, J. and Spratt, J. S. (1963). The rates and patterns of growth of 375 tumours of the large intestine and rectum observed by double contrast enema study (Malmo technique). *Am. J. Roentg. Radiat. Ther. Nucl. Med.*, **90**, 673–87.
Williams, C. B. (1973). Diathermy-biopsy a technique for the endoscopic management of small polyps. *Endoscopy*, **5**, 215–8.

Williams, C. B. (1975). Evaluation of the colonoscopic examination. *Dis. Colon Rect.*, **18**, 365–8.

Williams, C. B. (1980). (In preparation).

Williams, C. B. and de Peyer, R. C. (1979). Bipolar snare polypectomy – a safer technique for electrocoagulation of barge polyp stalks. *Endoscopy*, **11**, 47–50.

Williams, C. B. and Riddell, R. H. (1976). Chapter: *Colonoscopic Polypectomy*, in: *Topics in Gastrointestinal Endoscopy*, Heinemann Medical, London.

Winawer, S. J. *et al.* (1976). Screening for colon cancer. *Gastroenterology*, **70**, 783–9.

Wolff, W. I. and Shinya H. (1975). Definitive treatment of malignant polyps of the colon. *Ann. Surg.*, **182**, 516–25.

Wolff, W. I. and Shinya, H. (1978). The impact of colonoscopy on the problem of colorectal cancer. *Prog. Clin. Cancer*, **7**, 51–69.

Wolff, W. I. *et al.* (1975). Comparison of colonoscopy and the contrast enema in 500 patients with colorectal disease. *Am. J. Surg.*, **129**, 181–6.

Wynder, E. L. *et al.* (1969). Environmental factors of cancer of colon and rectum. II: Japanese epidemiological data. *Cancer*, **23**, 1210–20.

Index